Supercharge Your Health with PEMF Therapy

The "Swiss Army Knife" Health Solution That Belongs in Your Home

Supercharge Your Health with PEMF Therapy

How Pulsed Electromagnetic Field (PEMF) Therapy Can Jumpstart Your Health, Banish Pain, Improve Sleep, and Help Prevent and Relieve Over 80 Common Health Conditions

By William Pawluk, MD, MSc

gatekeeper press™

Columbus, Ohio

Supercharge Your Health with PEMF Therapy: How Pulsed Electromagnetic Field (PEMF) Therapy Can Jumpstart Your Health, Banish Pain, Improve Sleep, and Help Prevent and Relieve Over 80 Common Health Conditions

Published by Gatekeeper Press
2167 Stringtown Rd, Suite 109
Columbus, OH 43123-2989
www.GatekeeperPress.com

The editorial work for this book is entirely the product of the author. Gatekeeper Press did not participate in and is not responsible for any aspect of this element.

Library of Congress Control Number: 2021944222

ISBN (paperback): 9781662916397
eISBN: 9781662916403

Disclaimer

The information in this book is not intended to replace the relationship between you and your doctor, nor as medical advice. You should regularly consult a healthcare professional in matters relating to your health, and particularly with any symptoms that may require a medical diagnosis or attention. Since this book focuses almost entirely on how pulsed electromagnetic fields (PEMFs) help the body, there is minimal discussion about other healthcare options. PEMFs may not be the only or best treatment available to you. Please carefully read Chapter 11 of this book and ensure you fully understand all the cautions and contraindications associated with PEMF therapy.

Table of Contents

Introduction

Learning all that you can do on your own to keep yourself and your loved ones healthy has never been more necessary than it is today. Why? Because the healthcare system is failing us, the costs are way too high, and conventional therapies are bound to industrial/regulatory controls, among many other issues, and, because of all these factors, innovation is very limited. One of the most important innovative, unconventional tools for helping us to be as healthy as possible is PEMF therapy.

PEMF stands for "pulsed electromagnetic fields." When these fields are applied to the human body using the PEMF devices, as this book will introduce you to, significant health improvements usually follow. As you will learn, PEMF therapy not only helps to improve and maintain your health, it is also effective for hastening recovery from numerous health conditions.

This is especially true when PEMF treatments are done on a regular basis. Frequent PEMF therapy sessions boost health right down to the cellular level, optimizing cell function by creating a dynamic cellular environment that improves cell function and enhances cellular resiliency. PEMF treatments also help to prevent cellular decline associated with the natural aging process. As we age, the body's replacement of aging cells with healthier new cells naturally slows down. Cell division happens more slowly and less efficiently until cells die faster than they are replaced. Cell communication and metabolism also slow down. As a result, energy production decreases and immune functions diminish. Regular PEMF treatments have been shown to protect against and counteract these consequences of aging.

Just as crucially, PEMF therapy can help protect you from the cumulative effects of stress, which physicians now recognize is the number one threat to good health and a primary cause of premature aging and disease. One of the most obvious reasons our bodies wear down over time is because of the cumulative effects of ongoing stress. Though your body's reactions to stress are immediate, recovery takes hours or even days. PEMF therapy offsets these effects before they make the body more susceptible to disease.

In addition to the above benefits, PEMF therapy offers many other vital health gains. Daily use of PEMF therapy restores neurotransmitters and brain function, increases blood oxygen levels, improves circulation, balances blood pressure, promotes energy production in the body by increasing levels of the energy molecule ATP (adenosine triphosphate), and helps to activate all of the body's antioxidant defenses to protect against free radical damage and chronic inflammation. Because of how versatile PEMF therapy is in its ability to provide such a wide range of health improvements, I have dubbed it the "Swiss Army knife" therapy. Just as a Swiss Army knife offers far more functions than a single knife alone, so too does PEMF therapy offer a much broader spectrum of health-enhancing benefits than other single therapies, both conventional and alternative/integrative.

As you will learn in more detail in Chapter 3, there are more than 25 mechanisms of healing action that PEMF therapy provides. These mechanisms address almost the entire range of factors that cause people to become ill, including pain, chronic inflammation, and circulatory problems. This means that there is virtually no disease condition that regular PEMF treatments cannot help prevent or improve. (**Note:** A full listing of the citations of the studies that support the information this book contains can be found in my previous book, *Power Tools for Health* and on my website www.DrPawluk.com.)

PEMF devices treat the body on all levels, regardless of whether the disease state is energetic, physiologic, pathophysiologic, or pathologic. PEMF therapy does not care what you perceive to be wrong with your body. It will provide stimulation to you whether you have a broken bone, failing heart, struggle with anxiety, or any other health ailments. It helps stabilize the body's systems while addressing the fundamental changes underlying almost all health conditions.

For all of these reasons, I recommend that every home have a PEMF device readily available for self-care health treatment and health maintenance. Compared to other modalities such as laser, ultrasound, TENS, and even acupuncture, PEMF systems provide the best value for the cost, because they penetrate all the way through the body, are very safe, and are easy to use.

Based on my experience as a holistic doctor and a medical doctor for over 50 years, I think having a PEMF system in your home is critical. It's rare that treatments in the doctor's office offer lasting relief, particularly with chronic health problems. Therefore, it's actually much better for patients and other individuals to own their own PEMF systems for daily use. Once you finish reading this book, I think you will agree with my recommendation.

How I Became a Recognized Medical Authority on PEMF Therapy

I began my medical career as a conventionally trained physician. In the 1980s, I was an academic family doctor, managing a multispecialty medical group of 30 other practitioners. We were the largest group of family physicians on the East Coast of the US at the time.

In 1985, within the same month, three of our group's patients were admitted to the hospital for gastric bleeding from the stomach. One of them died, and the other two almost died, all because they had been regularly taking lots of ibuprofen, a nonsteroidal anti-inflammatory (NSAID) drug, to manage their pain.

I was devastated and asked myself how this could this happen to my patients. The answer became obvious after a good medical workup. The patients' use of ibuprofen, aspirin, or both, had caused the gastric bleeding, along with kidney and liver damage. Why was I using these medications? Because that's what all doctors did at the time. It was the main solution that we had for helping people with their chronic pain problems.

Yet, even then physicians knew that stomach bleeding was a known side effect of these widely prescribed drugs. With no better options to help patients manage their pain, these complications were begrudgingly accepted. I remember thinking, *This is the actual definition of insanity!* Here we were, physicians sworn to protect our patients and, above all, do no harm, and we were doing the same thing over and over again, hoping for better or different results.

I asked myself what we doctors were doing by recommending ibuprofen and other NSAIDS to patients when it was clear these drugs were harming, even killing people. Every year in the U.S., over 16,000 people die from gastric bleeding caused by ibuprofen.

My colleagues accepted these side effects as a natural consequence of managing pain. I didn't. I thought there had to be a different, better solution and was determined to find it. I also realized that the solution I sought would probably have to come from outside the field of conventional medicine.

Stepping outside this "House of Medicine" was not a simple or easy decision for me. I knew I risked the ridicule, censure, and quizzical looks of my peers. How dare I say that conventionally-accepted medical practice was not good enough? After all, no self-respecting medical doctor would use any tools that did not require a medical license to use, prescribe, or recommend.

Even so, I was committed to finding a better and safer method for treating pain. And so I began my journey in search of better alternatives. I stepped well outside of my comfort zone, which until that point remained firmly within the confines of traditionally accepted medicine. I looked into tools my peers and I would have previously looked down upon. I made a decision to study several non-conventional disciplines, including acupuncture, hypnosis, and homeopathy. Along the way, I also explored energy medicine, spiritual healing and lifestyle, and nutrition. I was also impressed by reports out of the Roswell Park Medical Center of spontaneous recoveries of cancer that were not a result of conventional medical therapies for cancer. As a result, I decided to study acupuncture, because it was used in China for thousands of years.

At the time that I trained in the practice of acupuncture during the years 1989-1990, acupuncture was almost unknown in the U.S. When I approached people to do acupuncture, they refused, either because they didn't know what to think about it even after I explained it, or because they didn't want needles put in their bodies, thinking it would hurt them. Obviously, the needles didn't hurt, but they still had that fear.

Because the public was not yet ready for acupuncture, I started exploring other options of treating acupuncture points using alternative approaches. This included acupressure, heat, ice, friction, and magnets. I learned that in Asia, many acupuncture practitioners often used magnets to stimulate acupuncture points. I began experimenting with these and discovered that in fact, they did have a significant action on acupuncture points. I did a small experiment with an open-minded colleague using nerve-conduction testing to validate that a magnet did have an effect on an acupuncture meridian.

Since I could see no risk of harm, I began using magnet therapies on acupuncture points and meridians (the body's energy pathways) and then moved very quickly to treating many problematic tissues. I kept seeing major improvements in the problems I was treating using all kinds of static/permanent magnet devices. During this period of experimentation, a spider bit me on my leg, causing a huge welt to form. I placed a big magnet on the bite site. Within two hours, the welt was gone. Now I was really intrigued about what was happening with the magnets. There seemed to be actions happening beyond the principles of acupuncture. Wanting to know more, I studied the available scientific literature on magnet therapy but found a great deal of it to be in foreign languages and inaccessible to me.

Then I met Dr. Jiri Jerabek from the Czech Republic, who had translated and summarized a large body of work done in Eastern Europe. He shared my goal of getting this important work published in English. He gave me a copy of his manuscript and we agreed to edit it into an English-language book. The result was the publication of our book *Magnetic Therapy in Eastern Europe: A Review of 30 Years of Research*.

Most of the studies cited in that book were based on the use of PEMFs as opposed to static magnets. Around the time that it was published, nonmedical PEMF devices started becoming available in the US for the first time. Because of these studies, I had much more confidence in the huge range of benefits of PEMFs for helping all sorts of health conditions—a much greater variety of conditions than were possible with static magnets. So I decided to purchase some PEMF devices to further my research.

Since that time, I've purchased and evaluated a large number of different devices, spending hundreds of thousands of dollars. And I've used, treated, or supported the treatment of thousands of individuals—myself, family members, neighbors, patients and the curious, and even pets—using the PEMF systems my research and experimentation have shown me are most effective— more effective than anything I could do with most conventional medicine approaches. Still, I'm constantly looking at different systems to complement the ones I already trust.

Keep in mind that I'm not a physicist, engineer, research biologist, or mathematician. I am a practical, medically and holistically trained physician. My first priority is my patients, and my interest is in treating the whole person. While I continue to explore all the theories and science around PEMF and other energy medicine devices, ultimately the true test is whether or not they work.

I still routinely hear from people that they *BELIEVE* that PEMFs work. They need to be reminded that it's not a matter of belief. Based on my extensive exploration, I know that they *do* work. I have over 30,000 documents on the effects of magnetic fields in biology, and another 5,000 full-length articles of studies on different magnetic systems, that prove that fact. The therapeutic use of PEMF therapy is rooted in both science and history, with thousands of university-level controlled studies with PEMFs having been conducted on a large variety of health conditions and physical processes. Research continues to be done on the range of the ways that PEMF therapy affects the body.

Still, while PEMF therapy is great, like almost all other therapies, PEMFs are not a panacea. They do not raise the dead! But they have proven to be safe and amazingly successful, both as primary and complementary therapies.

Of course, proper instruction is an important part of individuals seeing success from doing their own home PEMF treatments. I wrote this book to provide you with that instruction.

What You Will Learn

This book is organized into two parts. The following chapters provide the information you need to understand PEMF therapy and, more importantly, teach you how to use it to improve your health and to help resolve over 80 of today's most common health complaints and diseases, starting with pain.

The chapters in Part One provide a deeper explanation of what PEMFs are, and how PEMF therapy works.

In Chapter 1, you will learn about the history of electromagnetic therapies in medicine dating back to their origins, millennia ago, and how they have continued throughout the centuries and have been promoted by notable scientists in modern times, including Nobel laureates. This chapter also discusses magnetics in relation to evolution, electromagnetic field science, and the natural electromagnetic fields (biofields) of humans and other living organisms.

You will also discover what conventional medical diagnostic tests, such as EKGs, have in common with PEMFs, and learn what PEMF therapy is, as well as the discoveries that led to the invention of today's PEMF devices and why they are increasingly being used by doctors and other health practitioners, as well as people at home, to maintain health and to help manage and reverse disease conditions.

In Chapter 2, you will learn the difference between health-enhancing pulsed electromagnetic fields versus the harmful electromagnetic fields (EMFs) that we are all now constantly exposed to. This chapter also explains frequency, modulation, wavelength, waveform, intensity, inverse square, "dose" of the magnetic field, coil configuration, and entrainment as they relate to PEMFs so that you will have a clear grasp of how PEMF therapy works.

In Chapter 3, you will learn the many ways that PEMF therapy can improve your health. This chapter builds on Chapter 2 and explains the many biological benefits and effects PEMF therapy provides. Just as importantly, it explains the levels (energetic, physiologic, pathophysiologic, pathologic) of the disease process or stage so that you have a better understanding of how disease unfolds, and how and why it is always best to address potential causes at the earliest disease stage, if possible.

You will also discover the fascinating parallels between your body's own electromagnetic system and its innate endocannabinoid (ECS) system, and learn what PEMF therapy and medicinal marijuana/CBD oil have in common.

Chapters 4 and 5 provide you with my recommended guidelines for using PEMF therapy and PEMF devices in order to obtain the most health benefits.

Chapter 6 explains how PEMF therapy can be used in combination with other therapies to enhance its effectiveness and vice versa. You will also learn what you need to know to create an overall healthy foundation for yourself via diet, nutrition, and other basic daily self-care measures so that you have enough "charge" in your body for PEMF therapy to work with.

In Chapter 7, you will learn about the different types of PEMF systems currently available and which systems I most recommend and why. Guidelines are also provided to help you choose the PEMF system that is best suited to your specific health needs and concerns. This chapter serves as a consumer guide that will educate you on what you need to know when selecting a PEMF system for home use. It includes a comparison of the PEMF devices and systems I have found to be most effective, criteria for choosing the system most appropriate for your needs, and precautions, safety, and contraindications you need to consider.

Chapter 8 concludes Part One. In it, you will learn why I recommend that you consider purchasing your own PEMF system. All of the reasons for doing so are covered here, including convenience, cost savings over time, and having a powerful self-care tool in your home "first-aid kit."

Part Two covers the numerous health conditions that can be prevented and reversed by regular use of PEMF therapy. Chapter 9 explains how to use PEMF therapy to prevent and resolve pain, one of the most widespread health complaints today. You will learn the mechanisms and factors that can cause and worsen pain, the types of pain (structural, neurological, inflammatory, etc.), what you must do to minimize your risk of developing pain, and what to do to gain effective relief should pain strike. You will be taught the specific ways PEMF therapy can prevent, reduce, and potentially reverse, numerous common pain conditions.

The primary focus of this chapter is to provide you with the how-to self-care information you need to use PEMF devices at home for pain management, including duration, wave forms, local versus whole-body systems, and the most beneficial applications to speed recovery. You will also learn more about the commonalities between PEMF therapy and the ECS.

Chapter 10 is the main section of this book. It addresses an extensive A-Z listing of the most common health conditions, covering their causes and risk factors, overall self-care preventive and recovery tips, and the information you need to achieve the best results for preventing and treating each condition at home using PEMF therapy.

Then, in Chapter 11, you will learn about the various factors that might prevent you from gaining benefit from PEMF therapy and what you can and must do to address those factors.

My aim in writing this book is to help you gain control over your health by adopting PEMF therapy as a primary self-care tool you can use to both prevent and reverse the widest range of health conditions. The information this book contains is supported by the most up-to-date research and science documenting the best systems of PEMF therapy, and the most effective PEMF methods of application.

My promise to you, if you take this information to heart and use PEMF therapy, is that you will soon notice measurable improvements in your health and overall well-being, just as I and the many thousands of patients I have treated with PEMF therapy have.

Now turn the page, and let's get started.

PART ONE

What PEMF Therapy Is and How It Works

A Brief History of Electromagnetic Therapies in Medicine

Although pulsed electromagnetic field therapy (PEMF) is relatively new to medicine, the use of magnetic fields for healing is not. In this chapter, I am going to take you on a journey through history, revealing the uses of the use of magnets as a health aid in many cultures around the world, starting thousands of years ago and continuing through to the present.

I will also explain why the principles of PEMF therapy are already known to you, though you may not realize it. These are the same principles that led to the development of a number of common conventional medical diagnostic screening tools and devices that you are likely familiar with.

Then I will explain what PEMF therapy is and share with you the discoveries that led to the invention of today's PEMF devices and how they are increasingly being used by doctors and other health practitioners, as well as people at home, to maintain health and help manage and reverse disease conditions.

Our journey begins more than 6,000 years ago.

Magnetic Field Therapy in the Ancient Past

The earliest recorded use of magnetic field therapy in rudimentary form dates back to approximately 4000 BC. At that time, healers in ancient India were known to use magnetized stones called *lodestones* to treat disease and ease symptoms.

A lodestone is one of the few naturally occurring magnets on Earth. It is derived from the mineral magnetite. Interestingly, magnetite itself does not typically become magnetized. Although scientists have yet to discover for certain how lodestones gain their magnetic properties, the most popular theory is that they do so as a result of lightning strikes to rocks containing magnetizable minerals, due to the strong electrical fields that make lightning bolts. Hence, the term *electromagnetic*. Supporting this theory is the fact that lodestones are mostly found on the Earth's surface, rather than beneath the ground. Humans first became aware of and began to find and use these lodestones many centuries ago, as evidenced in the earliest medical writings from India, China, and other countries.

As the oral traditions of healing in India were carried down the centuries, eventually they formed India's system of medicine, called *Ayurveda*, a Sanskrit term meaning "science of life." Ayurveda, along with traditional Chinese medicine (TCM), is one of the world's oldest, comprehensive, continually documented medical systems.

The earliest written Ayurvedic text dates back to approximately 3,000 years ago. It was written by the physician-sage Charaka. Known as the *Charaka Sambita*, this text guided the practice of healing for about one thousand years, until it was supplanted by the teachings of another physician-sage named Sushruta, author of *Sushruta Sambita*, a medical text that anticipated many aspects of today's modern surgery techniques, including procedures for mending broken bones and even techniques for plastic surgery. In the Sushruta Sambita and subsequent Ayurvedic texts, medical instruments called *ashmana* and *siktavati* are mentioned. Both of these instruments are thought to have been made of lodestone.

Around 2000 BC, while Sushruta was further expanding the teaching of Ayurveda, in China, the emperor Huang Ti and his court physician, Qi Bo, were establishing traditional Chinese medicine (TCM) as another complete system of medicine. In the process, they also developed the earliest written record of acupuncture theory. Their teachings were collected in the medical text known as the *Huang Ti Nei Jing*, more commonly known in the West as *The Yellow Emperor's Book of Internal Medicine*. This and other ancient Chinese medical texts describe protocols developed by Chinese physicians for using lodestones on acupuncture points.

Other medical texts from antiquity also provide evidence that lodestones and other "magnets" were commonly used for healing in ancient Egypt and Greece. In Egypt, for example, it was recorded that Cleopatra wore a small magnet in order to preserve her youth, while in Greece, Hippocrates, the "Father of Western Medicine," used magnets to treat pain and recommended that people lay down on lodestones or place them on their head to relieve headaches. Other texts and drawings from ancient Egypt and Greece indicate that magnets were also used to treat a variety of other health complaints.

What is fascinating about these ancient medical records is that healers of that time were incapable of understanding why magnet therapy worked in the same way that modern scientists are, due to modern research. Yet, nonetheless, the ancients obviously did recognize magnets' healing properties.

Magnet Therapy in the Middle Ages Through the 19th Century

A number of noteworthy European physicians and scientists promoted the use, and furthered our understanding, of magnet therapy through the centuries. Among them was the 16th century German-Swiss physician Philippus Aureolus Theophrastus Bombastus von Hohenheim, better known to us today as Paracelsus (1493-1541).

Paracelsus is credited with establishing the role of chemistry in modern medicine, and is considered to be the founder of toxicology. He also anticipated the field of homeopathy, declaring that, when given in small doses, "what makes a man ill also cures him," a statement that mirrors the basic homeopathic principle that "like cures like." In addition, his research and writings also contributed to the field of psychiatry—so much so, in fact, that Carl Jung wrote of him that "we see in Paracelsus not only a pioneer in the domains of chemical medicine, but also in those of an empirical psychological healing science."

Paracelsus theorized that the body and mind are connected by an invisible life force that he named *archaeus*. In TCM, this life energy is known as *Qi*, and in Ayurveda it is called *prana*. It is known by other names in various cultures around the world, and its existence has been validated by modern science, beginning with research conducted in the 20th century.

Believing that this life-giving energy could be strengthened by the use of magnets, and that magnets and lodestones were thus capable of promoting healing and treating disease, Paracelsus used magnets and lodestones to treat a wide range of conditions, including seizures and psychiatric disorders. He also employed the then-undiscovered or otherwise misunderstood, principles of magnetism to guide his practices in chemistry and symptom management.

Another noteworthy user of magnet therapy was William Gilbert (1544-1603). In addition to being the personal physician of Queen Elizabeth I, Gilbert was an accomplished physicist and natural philosopher. His most famous written work is *De Magnete, Magneticisque Corporibus, et de Magno Magnete Tellure* (On the Loadstone (sic) and Magnetic Bodies and on the Great Magnet the Earth), published in 1600. It provides a detailed account of his research on magnetic bodies and electrical attractions. As a result of that research, Gilbert correctly determined that compass needles point north-south and dip downward because the Earth acts as a giant magnet with magnetic north and south poles. In fact, Gilbert coined the term *magnetic pole, as well as the terms electric attraction and electric force. Due to his research, he is considered* the father of electrical studies, and a unit of magnetic potential was named the *Gilbert* in his honor. During his lifetime, he used and promoted magnet therapy as a means of improving health and treating illness.

By the mid-1700s, magnets composed of carbon and steel were common in many European countries. Interest in magnets' healing potential was also growing. During this time, the Jesuit priest, Maximilian Hell (1720-1792) of Hungary, an acclaimed astronomer and member of the Royal Danish Academy of Science and Letters, fashioned magnets in the shape of various body structures and used them to treat people, apparently with some degree of success.

Hell shared his work and ideas about magnetism with Franz Anton Mesmer (1734-1815), with whom he sometimes collaborated. Mesmer was a physician and a trained mathematician and lawyer. Hell's work with magnets influenced Mesmer's own explorations in this field.

Mesmer agreed with Paracelsus that there was a universal life force. He developed the theory of "animal magnetism" to describe what he saw as the natural energy transference between all things. Mesmer believed that this energy within the body's fluids possessed both positive and negative polarities that could be influenced by magnets, as well as by the animal magnetism emitted from his hands. (He termed the energy in minerals possessing magnetic properties "mineral magnetism.") His belief in a universal life force is similar to the concept of *Qi* in Traditional Chinese Medicine, while his theory of positive and negative polarities in the body is similar to TCM's theory of *Yin* and *Yang*.)

Throughout his controversial career, Mesmer used both external magnets and animal magnetism from the laying on of his hands to treat his clients, often succeeding in healing of their ailments, including, allegedly, deafness. Mesmer sometimes treated his patients with magnets alone, particularly in an effort to help psychiatric disorders. He also sometimes used magnets to increase the flow of universal life energy from his hands to those he worked on.

As word of his accomplishments spread, Mesmer's popularity with the general public grew. This led to an increasing number of people coming to him for treatments. Alarmed, the medical establishment criticized Mesmer's work. Eventually, they succeeded in convincing the public that both animal and mineral magnetism were hoaxes and that Mesmer's successes were actually due to the power of suggestion. This is how the term "mesmerized" came into being. Mesmer's work later influenced the Scottish physician James Braid (1795-1860) to develop hypnosis.

Another famous 18th century physician who explored magnet therapy was the German physician Samuel Hahnemann (1755-1843). Best known as the developer of homeopathy, Hahnemann was also reputed to use magnets in his treatment programs. In addition, he named one of the homeopathic remedies he developed *Magnetis Polus Arcticus* (Magnet of the North Pole), which today is prescribed by homeopathic physicians for people who appear to "lack an inner compass," such as in cases of vertigo and somnambulism (sleep walking).

In the 19th century, the scientific foundations about magnetic fields and electromagnetism began to come into focus. English scientist Michael Faraday (1791-1867) contributed a great deal to the study of electromagnetism, including the discovery of electromagnetic induction, diamagnetism, and electrolysis. Faraday went on to create the first electromagnetic rotary device, forming the basis of electric motors. His work in electromagnetism established for the first time that a changing magnetic field produces an electric field. This would later be named "Faraday's Law," one of the four Maxwell equations.

Shortly before his death, Faraday proposed the concept of electromagnetic fields, meaning forces extending into the space around a conductor. Unfortunately, he did not live to see the eventual acceptance of his theory.

In the late 19th century, the French-Russian engineer Georges Lakhovsky (1870-1942) became the first person to theorize that each cell had its own frequency oscillating at a specific amplitude. He proposed that cells also respond to oscillations imposed upon them from outside sources. Lakhovsky developed what is likely the first "energy medicine" device, called the Multiple Wave Oscillator or Radio-Cellulo-Oscillator. The device produced a wide range of therapeutic frequencies, from extremely low frequency (ELF) electromagnetic radiation all the way up to gigahertz radio waves. It was used in both US and European hospitals until the mid-20th century.

Magnetic and Pulsed Electromagnetic Field Therapies in the 20th and 21st Centuries

Perhaps the most important scientist in the late 19th and early 20th centuries whose work further laid the foundation for PEMF therapy was the Serbian-American inventor Nikola Tesla (July 10, 1856-January 6, 1943). Tesla was responsible for the development of the alternating current (AC) electrical system used all over the world today. Prior to his discoveries in this area, direct current (DC), pioneered by

Thomas Edison, was the only means of supplying electricity. But DC current came with many inherent limitations. Ironically, Tesla once worked as an employee of Edison and submitted his ideas for AC to him, but Edison rejected them. Thanks to Tesla, electricity became widely and inexpensively available, transforming the world even more than Edison's many inventions did.

Tesla also discovered the rotating magnetic field, which is now the basis of most AC machinery. Tesla had an intimate understanding of the relationship between electricity and magnetic fields, and developed ideas for a huge number of inventions that we use to this day, including dynamos, induction motors, radar, X-rays, and remote-control devices, to name just a few. While the classic electrical device named after him is the Tesla Coil (which produces streamers of electricity in a glass bulb – common attractions in children's museums), Tesla also invented a lesser-known electrical coil. This is the standard magnetic loop coil that is an essential element in all PEMF systems today.

In the 20th century, sophisticated static magnetic therapies were being developed in the Czech Republic, including checkerboard-designed magnetic foils. PEMF devices began there as well, and were introduced in Hungary in the early 1980s. Soon thereafter, PEMF therapy spread to other parts of Europe, with a wide variety of devices made available through a growing number of manufacturers. Simultaneously, Eastern European use and research into PEMF therapy began to blossom.

In 1954, scientists in Japan discovered the piezoelectric properties of bone. (Piezoelectricity is the electric charge that accumulates in various materials, including bone, in response to applied mechanical stress.) Following this discovery, further research demonstrated that damaged bone responds favorably to both electric fields and pulsed electromagnetic fields. Subsequent research showed that specific electromagnetic frequencies have a beneficial effect on all types of soft tissue in the body. The 1980s saw the introduction of the first FDA-approved PEMF system, which was intended for use as a bone stimulator to treat non-union fractures.

In 1986, the seminal book *Body Electric: Electromagnetism and the Foundation of Life* was published by Dr. Robert Becker and Gary Selden. This book provided one of the first scientifically-based descriptions of the human body as an electromagnetic apparatus that is very susceptible and amenable to magnetic field therapies. During this time, a wide variety of PEMF devices started to become available in Europe, and by the late 1990s, much of Europe was already familiar with PEMF therapy.

The 1990s also saw a discussion about the use of PEMF devices in space. It remains a common misconception that PEMFs were or are used in space. The international space station is in low Earth orbit, well within the Earth's magnetic field. As such, there really is little necessity for the application of external magnetic fields to maintain a functional biomagnetic field. In a discussion with the medical director of Russia's space program at a meeting in Germany, it was made very clear to me that PEMFs are not being used on astronauts, but that the study of what would happen to the body were it outside of the Earth's magnetic field is of great interest and importance as we consider venturing further out into space. The electromagnetic aspects, both from a treatment and prevention perspective, of humans outside the Earth's magnetic field (magnetosphere) are still being worked out.

Since the dawn of the 21st century, exciting new developments in the study of magnetic field stimulation of the body have continued. While debate continues about the value of low versus high magnetic field intensities, there is a rapidly growing body of scientific evidence to support the safe use of high-intensity PEMFs, especially for the brain. This technology was developed primarily to avoid the need for electroconvulsive therapy (ECT), which was effective but incredibly uncomfortable and widely considered barbaric. ECT had been used for decades to treat psychiatric disorders. High-intensity PEMF stimulation provides beneficial effects without the invasive or otherwise unbearable components of high electrical intensity ECT, such as convulsions.

This specific type of FDA-approved PEMF therapy is known as transcranial magnetic stimulation (TMS). A high-intensity coil is placed at the side of the head over the part of the motor cortex, the area of brain that controls movement of muscles. The intensity of the magnetic field produced by the coil placed on the head is increased until it is sufficient enough to cause a muscle contraction of the hand. Then the intensity is either maintained or lowered slightly, and the coil is moved to the part of the brain requiring the treatment, depending on the psychiatric indication of interest. Studies are also being done with these high-intensity magnetic fields to treat other parts of the body for a wide variety of medical conditions.

Other lower-intensity PEMF systems also continue to be developed, including for transcranial applications. Development of these new systems was made easier in the US by the recently updated FDA position, allowing PEMF systems to be marketed without FDA approval if their primary purpose is for health and wellness management.

Nobel Prize Science That Supports PEMF Therapy

Throughout the 20th and 21st centuries there have been a number of Nobel Prizes awarded in the field of Physiology or Medicine for discoveries that are relevant to and support the basis of PEMF therapy. Among the recipients and their discoveries are:

- Niels Ryberg Finsen in 1903 "in recognition of his contribution to the treatment of diseases, especially lupus vulgaris, with concentrated light radiation, whereby he has opened a new avenue for medical science." Ryberg Finsen's research serves as a basis for the use of electromagnetic "light" radiation and its use for healing. This is relevant since PEMFs are part of the electromagnetic spectrum.
- Jules Bordet in 1919 "for his discoveries relating to immunity." His work relates to the impact of PEMFs on immunity.
- Sir Charles Scott Sherrington and Edgar Douglas Adrians in 1932 "for their discoveries regarding the functions of neurons." Their work relates to the basic functioning of nerves and how PEMFs affect nerves and neurons, particularly in the brain.
- Joseph Erlanger and Herbert Spencer Gasser in 1944 "for their discoveries relating to the highly differentiated functions of single nerve fibres (sic)." This work relates to the basic functioning of nerves and how PEMFs affect nerves.
- Hans Adolph Krebs in 1953 "for his discovery of the citric acid cycle" (now also known as the Krebs cycle). Relates to the basic functioning of the body and PEMFs' effects on the Krebs cycle.
- Sir John Carew Eccles, Alan Lloyd Hodgkin, and Andrew Field Huxley in 1963 "for their discoveries concerning the ionic mechanisms involved in excitation and inhibition in the peripheral and central portions of the nerve cell membrane." This is relevant because of how magnetic fields interact with ions and their impact on nerve function, leading to improvement of neuropathy and pain.

- Albert Claude, Christian de Duve, and George E. Palade in 1974 " for their discoveries concerning the structural and functional organization of the cell." This is relevant because of the impact of PEMFs on cells, and in particular PEMF impacts on cell injury processes. Most of the actions of PEMFs relate to components of cell injury and their reversal or improvement with PEMFs.
- Paul C. Lauterbur and Sir Peter Mansfield in 2003 "for their discoveries concerning magnetic resonance imaging." This is hugely relevant because it demonstrates how high-strength magnetic fields interact with the body and can be used for assisting with diagnosis and assessment of physiological actions and anatomic conditions.

Two other Nobel Prize awards also relate to important actions of PEMFs in the body. The first is the Nobel Prize in Chemistry that was awarded in 1997(one-half jointly) to Paul D. Boyer and John E. Walker, "for their elucidation of the enzymatic mechanism underlying the synthesis of adenosine triphosphate (ATP)," and to Jens C. Skou, "for the first discovery of an ion-transporting enzyme, NA+K+-ATPase." This is relevant because of the effect PEMFs have on stimulating ATP production, the body's "energy currency."

The second is the Nobel Prize in Physiology or Medicine awarded in 1988 to Robert F. Furchgott, Louis J. Ignarro and Ferid Murad for their discoveries concerning "nitric oxide as a signaling molecule in the cardiovascular system." This is relevant because it relates to PEMFs' stimulation of the production of nitric oxide, which leads to the widening of blood vessels (vasodilatation), helping them to maintain healthy blood flow, and various immune functions.

What Is Magnetic Field Therapy?

Now that you have learned the history of magnetic field therapy, let's examine what it actually is before we get into the specifics of PEMF therapy and how and why it works in the body.

The first basic principle of electromagnetism to understand is that all life, including plants, animals, and human beings, evolved on a planet that is a giant magnet of its own. In addition to the Earth's own static magnetic field, the planet's magnetic rock formations, Schumann resonances, geomagnetic storms, and natural electric currents that flow on and beneath the surface of the planet, called telluric currents, all contribute in significant ways to the overall magnetic environment in which we humans have arisen, evolved, and thrived.

Our dependence on these magnetic fields has been demonstrated in research by shielding the body, depriving it of Earth's magnetic fields. Of particular significance to our well-being are the Schumann Resonances. These are atmospheric PEMFs crucial to human functioning and are an important background within which the human brain maintains homeostasis. Research confirms that the range of Schumann Resonance frequencies are an important factor in how the body heals itself. The seven peak resonances are 7.8 Hz, 14 Hz, 20 Hz, 26 Hz, 33 Hz, 39 Hz and 45 Hz. The "average" or major peak Schumann Resonance is 7.8 Hz. Schumann Resonance frequencies (often separated into the brainwave state bands) are found in many PEMF devices.

In addition to naturally occurring magnetic fields, the Earth is now also bathed in artificial electromagnetic fields (EMFs) created by humans. Such EMFs are emitted by televisions, computers, Wi-Fi, power lines, microwaves, cell phones, and smart meters, among many other sources. Especially in densely populated areas, this global aura of manmade magnetic fields easily overpowers the life-giving and life-sustaining value and importance of the Earth's natural magnetic field sources. The difference between healthy PEMFs and harmful EMFs are discussed in Chapter 2.

We can't escape our basic nature and the forces of nature surrounding us. All the processes that make us functional as human bodies are part of, interact with, and are dependent upon the magnetic fields around us. When we are deficient in electromagnetic energy, or when there is insufficient electromagnetic energy around us to help us with the health conditions we are dealing with, aging accelerates, illness is more likely, and our body's ability to recover and repair is decreased. Since the Earth does not always provide us with the energy we need, external local and controllable sources of comparable energy, such as those provided by PEMFs, can be helpful.

On the simplest level, magnetic field therapy refers to using magnet fields to treat illness and maintain health. This includes the minimally helpful static or permanent magnets and the much wider potential and value of pulsed electromagnetic fields. Both the Earth and the human body naturally produce electromagnetic fields. However, we can also produce more dynamic electromagnetic fields using specifically designed technology. Practitioners of magnetic field therapy recognize that interactions between the human body, the

Earth, and other electromagnetic fields can cause both physical and emotional changes in humans. They also understand that the body's electrical and electromagnetic fields frequently, and perhaps continuously, need to be balanced to maintain optimal health. To this end, they apply magnetic field therapy from outside the body using electromagnetic fields that can be:

- Electrically charged, which deliver magnetic pulses to the treatment area.
- Stationary and static (not electrically charged), which deliver continuous treatment to local areas of the body for longer periods.
- Combined with acupuncture needles for treating energy pathways within the body.

Electromagnetic Field Science: As you will discover in Part Two of this book, magnetic field therapy, and especially PEMF therapy, can be an effective treatment for a wide range of health conditions. But before it is used for healing, it is important to have a basic understanding of some of the physical characteristics of magnetic science, including electric and magnetic fields and their actions on the body. This knowledge will allow you to choose the best solutions for your health needs. Unfortunately, too often, people make their choices based on cost alone. This results in false starts and inadequate benefits. There are so many choices and so much conflicting information available today that you need to educate yourself adequately to make the best value decisions.

All matter is made up of moving particles. Forces exist in the space around these moving (electrical) particles. Those forces are magnetic fields. By definition, force is an interaction that changes the motion of an object.

An electric field is the force field created by the flow of electricity (caused by the attraction and repulsion of electric charges). A magnetic field is the force field created as a consequence of the flow of electricity or electrical charges. Electric fields and magnetic fields always exist in tandem – one cannot exist without the other. An electromagnetic field, then, is the combination of an electric field and a magnetic field.

Let's back up briefly and talk about charge. Electric charges can either be positive or negative. Positively charged substances repel other positively charged substances, but attract negatively charged substances. Conversely, negatively charged substances repel other negatively charged substances, and attract positively charged substances.

Our bodies are fundamentally electric. When a person goes into cardiac arrest, for example, a defibrillator is used to apply electrical energy to the heart so that it can reestablish a normal rhythm.

The electricity that flows through our body creates electromagnetic fields. External magnetic fields and the body's native magnetic fields interact regularly. Because of these interactions, a magnetic field passing through the body will have an electromagnetic effect on a cellular level and expand to function at an organ level.

Electric and magnetic fields control our chemistry by changing and influencing the motion of charged particles. This movement stimulates a vast array of chemical and electric actions in tissues, helping them rebalance or heal themselves where necessary. Additionally, this increased motion of ions and electrolytes helps cells increase their available energy by as much as 500 percent.

Electromagnetic fields affect the charge of the cell membrane, rebalancing it so that membrane channels can open up. These channels are like the doors and windows of a house – by opening them, oxygen and nutrients are better able to enter the cell, and carbon dioxide and waste are more easily eliminated from the cell. This helps to rebalance and restore optimum cell function.

If you restore and rebalance enough cells, they will all work more efficiently. Cells of the same type come together to make tissues, which come together to make organs. By restoring or maintaining cellular function, you will in turn restore or maintain organ function, allowing the entire body to function better. This is the basis for magnetic field therapy – affecting and improving basic cellular function in order to combat a variety of health conditions and, when possible, to prevent cellular damage from happening in the first place.

At the start of this chapter, I mentioned that the principles of magnetic field therapy led to the development of a number of common conventional medical diagnostic screening tools that you are likely familiar with. One example is how unshielded electric fields or current can be designed to contact the body and are used therapeutically that way (as with electro-stimulation from a transcutaneous electric-nerve stimulator—or TENS—unit).

A cardiac defibrillator is another example of electric charge being used directly to electrically reset an organ (in this case, the heart). Another example includes magnetic resonance imaging (MRI) scans that take advantage of multiple electromagnetic fields within the body (each tissue and organ in your body has a unique electromagnetic signature) to create a map of the body's tissues using pulsed electromagnetic fields. Electric charges are also applied in medicine to burn off warts or other skin lesions, or to cauterize blood vessels.

Bioelectromagnetic Fields and Healing

To understand how the body interacts with and responds to magnetic fields, we must appreciate how much our bodies themselves are electromagnetic. This brings us to the final example of magnetic fields that are present on this Earth: the body's own internal magnetic fields.

To exist in an electromagnetic world, our bodies have to be an intimate part of it. The extraordinary amount of internal electrical activity that keeps our bodies alive naturally generates its own magnetic fields. Most people assume that this electrical activity is confined to the nervous system, but the vast majority of chemical reactions in the body are accompanied by the movement of charge. When you consider that most of the fluids in the body are actually electrolytes, it is easy to see that the body is like a large battery, constantly active, producing current and occasionally needing recharging.

Once the connection is made between the magnetic aspects of the human body and its biophysical chemistry, it becomes easier to see the body as a dynamic, ever-changing bioelectric and biomagnetic organism, subject to all the physical laws of electromagnetism. That means that the body not only has a vascular system and a nervous system, but also a less obvious, complex electromagnetic system, in, among, and in between its cells and tissues. The biomagnetic fields of the body, though extremely tiny in intensity, have been measured with techniques including magneto-encephalography (MEG)and magneto-cardiography (MCG). These devices measure the magnetic fields produced by the electrical activity in organs of the body and are used diagnostically today in medicine.

The body's electrical activity (and therefore its electromagnetic activity) happens primarily in the cell membrane—the shell of molecules surrounding each individual cell in the body. This membrane is critical to maintaining the cell's structure and to protecting its contents. It also acts as a sort of gatekeeper, opening and closing channels (sometimes called "membrane pumps") through which ions can flow.

The cell membrane itself has a voltage called a "potential" (or membrane potential, or transmembrane potential). Membrane potential refers to the difference in electrical charge between the inside and outside of the cell. The channels in the membrane are opened or closed based on the polarity of the membrane. When the channels are closed, a cell membrane is at its "resting potential" and when it is open, it is at its "action potential."

Action potential occurs in excitable tissues, such as nerve or muscle fibers, when a changing resting potential reaches a firing threshold. The process of a nerve or muscle cell moving from resting potential to action potential is all or none—it either happens or does not, like a light switch. Membranes cannot be half open or half closed; there is no in-between state. A nerve stimulus will show several phases, beginning with a rising potential (depolarization), causing a nerve impulse to occur. Then it proceeds to rebuild the charge (repolarization), even sometimes to the extent of hyperpolarization.

Besides action potentials, membranes require charge to open their channels. During this process, the electrical potential of the membrane rapidly rises, allowing the channels to open. As they do, ions flow into the cell, causing a further rise in the membrane potential, prompting even more channels to open. This process produces an exchange or movement of charge, another non-nerve form of electric current (and therefore resulting magnetic field) across the cell membrane, and the cycle continues. Once all channels are open, the membrane potential is so great that the polarity of the membrane reverses, and then the channels begin to close. As they do, exit channels are activated. Once the process is complete, all channels close and the membrane returns to its resting potential. This is an ebb and flow cycle of cell energy activity, and is the basis for all organisms being alive.

Charge potentials play different roles depending on cell type, but are generally responsible for cellular communication or to activate cellular processes. Muscle cells, for example, use charge potentials as the first step to achieving action potentials and therefore muscle contraction. Since all potentials are controlled by charge, they can be influenced by magnetic fields.

To sum up, the term "magnetic therapy" refers to various health and wellness practices that make use of electromagnetic fields, ranging from wearing a magnetized bracelet to sleeping on magnetized mattresses to therapy involving pulsed electromagnetic field (PEMF) devices, small and large.

When it comes to the effects that magnetic fields have on the body, there are multiple theories, all correct to some degree, yet none of which completely explain the magnetic phenomena. However, the general consensus is that magnetic fields act upon the body at the molecular level by enhancing or affecting the natural electrical charges in the tissues that correct disruptions or imbalances. According to laboratory studies, magnetic fields can modulate the transport of ions and related neuronal and cell activity. Through these actions, magnetic field therapies have been found in hundreds of research studies to have benefits in numerous health conditions.

Scientific evidence is constantly accumulating to support positive results of magnetic therapy. You could even say that magnets and other electromagnetic devices are approaching mainstream medical acceptance for both diagnostics and treatment. They are certainly in common use in complementary or alternative health practices, not the least of which includes acupuncture. My hope is that the medical community will soon begin to understand and that this type of therapy provides effective and predictable results. Furthermore, I hope that more physicians will understand the safety of magnetic therapy, since it doesn't introduce foreign substances into the body as long-term medications do.

And now that you understand how and why electromagnetic fields can play such positive roles in human health, I hope that you will consider PEMF therapy to improve and maintain your own well-being. Read on to learn how and why.

Health-Enhancing PEMFs vs. Harmful EMFs

One of the most common concerns people have about the value of PEMF therapy is its association with the negative effects of other man-made EMFs in the environment and the so-called "electro-smog" they create. In this chapter, I will share with you the difference between the beneficial electromagnetic fields (EMFs) that are used in PEMF devices, and the harmful EMFs that are becoming increasingly prevalent in our world today. Then I will explain the many ways that you are being exposed to harmful EMFs, and, most importantly, provide you with action steps you can take to protect yourself from them.

To begin, let me emphasize that it is a scientifically proven fact that PEMF therapy can improve and maintain your health.

Moreover, the PEMF devices that you will learn about in this book are perfectly safe to use.

You learn about the many ways that PEMF therapy can benefit you in Chapter 3. For now, let's examine the differences between harmful EMFs and the therapeutic EMFs generated by PEMF devices.

The first point to understand is that all EMFs interact with living systems, affecting enzymes related to cell division and multiplication, growth regulation, and regulation of the sleep hormone melatonin (controlled by pineal gland metabolism), among many other effects. Depending on their nature, electromagnetic fields, frequencies, and waveforms will either amplify or diminish your body's own signals. Harmful EMFs negatively affect the body's natural functions, while therapeutic EMFs act in positive, supportive ways, enhancing cellular communication and overall health. The balance of the human organism can easily be negatively affected by electromagnetic changes in the environment, and an unbalanced body is more susceptible to disease.

To further clarify terminology, health-enhancing PEMFs are really extremely low-frequency (ELF) PEMFs. Harmful EMFs are very high-frequency. For simplicity, I will frequently use the term "EMFs" to signify the environmental, high-frequency EMFs. PEMFs which are ELFs can be considered beneficial and safe, whereas EMFs from a health perspective would be considered mostly undesirable.

The exception to being considered undesirable is when high-frequency magnetic fields are used for directed medical applications. Directed medical applications are used in radiofrequency ablation for intended tissue destruction, such as burning nerves, skin lesions, or warts. Directed medical application extremely high frequency (EHF) EMFs also include therapeutic lasers (more than one trillion (10^{12}) Hz), infrared light, and LED (400-600 terahertz which equals 400-600 trillion Hz) light therapies. Here is a chart showing frequencies in the electromagnetic spectrum, including infrared, visible light, ultraviolet, and X-rays:

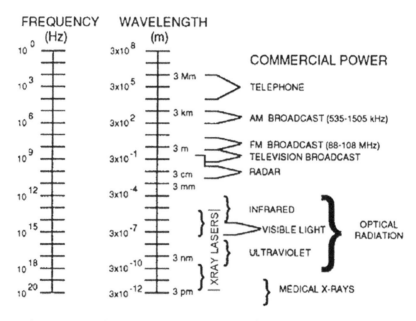

Figure 1. Electromagnetic Spectrum. From *https://fas.org/man/dod-101/navy/docs/laser/fundamentals.htm*

It can be seen that lasers range in frequency, depending on color, from $10^{13} - 10^{17}$ hertz. So, from here on out, I will use the term EMFs for environmental magnetic fields. Therapeutic extremely high frequency electromagnetic fields will be referred to as EHF EMFs.

The primary differences between harmful and therapeutic EMFs are exposure time, wavelength, and frequency. Confusion often stems from the fact that our electric power grids generate 50-60 Hz frequencies, which fall within the same frequency range as many therapeutic PEMFs. There are a few important distinctions to keep in mind when comparing these EMF sources. By far, the strongest manmade magnetic fields are emitted from high voltage transmission lines (which are the big metal towers, not the single wires that tend to run through neighborhoods on wooden poles).

It is generally accepted that a "safe distance" from large power lines is about 700 feet (or 0.1mile), and a "safe distance" from the neighborhood lines is as little as ten feet. The intended 50-60 Hz frequency of power lines is becoming increasingly contaminated with transient surges of high frequency wave radiation, often referred to as "dirty electricity." Modern electrical devices tend to induce high levels of these surges or spikes back into the electrical system. Therefore, our power grids and home wiring are contaminated with frequencies much higher than the intended 50-60 Hz, and ongoing research indicates that these high-frequency, very short-wavelength surges can pose potentially serious health risks. But power grids are hardly the only source of EMFs you need to be concerned about.

Sources of Harmful EMFs

Unless you are living completely "off the grid," you are exposed to EMFs on a constant basis via your cell phone, laptop, or computer tablet, Wi-Fi, smart meters used by water and utility companies, and the many wireless devices, including home appliances, baby monitors, and fitness bands and watches, that are found in many homes today. Even new cars expose you to EMFs due to the now-standard features of satellite tracking and Bluetooth they include.

Further compounding this problem is "dirty" electricity that is all too commonly found in houses, apartment complexes, and other buildings. Living in close proximity to power lines and/or cell phone towers is another danger, as are the blue light emissions from cell phone, computer, and TV screens, as well as compact fluorescent light (CFL) and older-model LED light bulbs. Since electromagnetic fields are able to penetrate through walls, EMFs from outside sources can enter your home and workplace.

Another type of EMF that poses a threat to your heath is radio-frequency/microwave electromagnetic radiation (RF). Sources of RF exposure include mobile and cordless phones, microwave ovens, wireless networks, portable radios, radio and radar transceivers, Wi-Fi, Bluetooth, GPS devices, and smart TVs and TV antennas.

To make matters worse, with the advent of 5G, or the "fifth generation" of cell phone technology and global satellite 5G that is rolling out, and now the earliest stages of the roll-out of 6G, your EMF exposures and their associated health risks may increase, especially if you live in a large urban area. These new electromagnetic frequencies have never been tested for long-term safety on humans.

The bottom line is that we now live in a world that is inundated with health-sapping "electrosmog," and knowing how to protect yourself and your loved ones from it is an important and necessary step you must take to safeguard your health.

Health Risks of Harmful EMFs

Martin L. Pall PhD, Professor Emeritus of Biochemistry and Basic Medical Sciences, Washington State University, has been studying the biological effects that man-made EMF exposures have on humans and other living organisms for years. Based on his extensive review of the scientific literature, along with his own research and published studies, he points out that there are eight distinct and primary ways that man-made EMFS can cause harm, which he outlined in *5G Risk: The Scientific Perspective—Compelling Evidence for Eight Distinct Types of Great Harm Caused by Electromagnetic Field (EMF) Exposures and the Mechanism that Causes Them*. Specifically, these EMFs:

1. Attack the nervous system, including the brain, resulting in a wide range of neurological and neuropsychiatric effects.
2. Negatively impact the body's endocrine (hormonal) system.
3. Cause oxidative stress and free radical damage, both of which are causative risk factors for virtually all chronic diseases.
4. Attack and damage DNA, including causing both single strand and double strand breaks in cellular DNA, as well as oxidation of DNA. This increases the risk of cancer and other harmful cellular mutations.
5. Cause higher than normal levels of apoptosis (programmed cell death), increasing the risk for both neurodegenerative diseases and infertility.
6. Lower male and female fertility and libido, reduce sex hormones, attack DNA in sperm cells, and increase the risk of miscarriage.
7. Produce excessive intracellular calcium and excessive calcium signaling.

8. And directly attack the cells of the body to cause cancer. According to Dr. Pall, "Such attacks are thought to act via 15 different mechanisms during cancer causation."

The first six of the health risks listed above were originally verified by research conducted by the United States Navy's Medical Research Institute that was published in June, 1971.

There is also a substantial body of scientific literature demonstrating that such EMFs can cause life-threatening heart attacks, cardiac arrhythmias, hypertension (high blood pressure), and other cardiac events; Alzheimer's, dementia, anxiety, depression, concentration problems, and other neurological conditions; and early childhood autism and ADHD.

Environmental EMFs can also make anxiety worse. One important aspect in managing anxiety successfully is the need to consider outside electromagnetic influences that may contribute to the anxiety. Some individuals, regardless of how much they try to reduce their anxiety with any particular therapeutic approach, just do not respond. Many times, this can actually be due to the background EMFs in their environment. EMFs that enter the bedroom in particular can be incredibly potent irritants to the nervous system. Unless these EMFs are dealt with and reduced or eliminated, it becomes challenging for any treatment to work.

If PEMFs are being used for anxiety and they don't appear to be working, a key element to consider is the possibility of extraneous high frequency EMFs contributing to the situation. These EMFs include living near power lines, routers and cell phones near the bed, smart meters, and contaminated home wiring as potential contributing factors for their anxiety.

External EMFs above the range of 50-Hz and EMF intensities encountered in homes of >1-100 milligauss (mG), with daily magnetic-field exposure, may be associated with poorer health and more "chronic anxiety" symptoms. This is consistent with a direct effect of continuous long-term 50-Hz or 60-Hz magnetic field exposure on the nervous system.

Cumulative exposure—hour after hour, day after day—to EMFs is of the greatest concern. Ordinary household appliances tend to generate larger cumulative EMF exposures than power lines, as most people do not live close enough to power lines to be dramatically affected by them. The same cannot be said of kitchen appliances, computers, televisions, cell phones, and even electric outlets (especially if it's directly behind the headboard of a bed). Though EMFs from appliances drop off to negligible levels at a distance of about sixteen feet, people are regularly much nearer than that to the source of the electromagnetic field—typically no more than eighteen inches from computers, a few feet from televisions, and practically no distance from cell phones.

The Problem of "Dirty" Electricity

Dirty electricity is a term that used to describe spikes and surges of electromagnetic energy that travel along power lines and into buildings. It is also referred to as dirty power, electrical noise, and electromagnetic interference (EMI).

Under normal conditions, electricity traveling through wiring and power lines should be between 50 to 60 Hertz AC (alternating current). Spikes and surges above these levels create a type of EMF pollution caused by electrical devices that change or manipulate standard electrical current in order to operate. Many home and other building electronic devices today operate in this fashion. Rather than running on standard AC electricity, the devices must convert it into other forms of electricity—often either low voltage direct current (DC) or higher Hertz level AC— in order to function. In addition, many electronic devices today draw power in short bursts instead of continuously, fluctuating the flow of electricity to the devices in much the same way that one turns a power switch on and off repeatedly. It is not uncommon for this process to occur as often as thousands of times per second. This interrupts the flow of standard electrical current to cause erratic surges and spikes of electrical energy known as high frequency voltage transients (HFVTs).

Once created, this unusable dirty electricity spreads throughout a building and even to other buildings via wiring and power lines. As it travels, it radiates potentially harmful electromagnetic fields into home and work environments. Not only does dirty electricity interfere with the proper functioning of appliances and electronic equipment, it has also been shown to disrupt the human body's own bioelectric processes to cause or exacerbate a wide variety of health problems, including ADD/ADHD, allergies, asthma, blood sugar imbalances, brain fog and memory loss, cancer, depression, diabetes, fatigue, headaches, hearing problems, muscle and joint pain, rashes, uncomfortable tingling sensations, sleep disturbances, and suicide. Dirty electricity has also been shown to be a potential cause of amyotrophic lateral sclerosis (ALS, or Lou Gehrig disease).

Common sources of dirty electricity in homes and other buildings include battery charging devices for cell phones, tablets, etc., blenders, cordless phone systems, computers and laptops, fluorescent light bulbs and tubes, hair dryers, home entertainment and video game systems, light dimmer switches, multispeed fans, smart meters, new model appliances and televisions, and Wi-Fi routers and modems.

Ungrounded or improperly grounded wiring in the home is another major cause of dirty electricity, as are power lines near homes and other buildings.

Dirty electricity can be detected using an oscilloscope or spectrum analyzer, although such devices can be expensive and usually require the assistance of an electrician or other professional trained in their use. Fortunately, a less expensive, do-it-yourself option is also available, called an EMI meter. These devices plug into electrical outlets and measure the level of electrical "noise" that may be present on nearby wiring.

Note: EMI meters are not the same as meters designed to measure wireless, radio frequency, and microwave radiation. These latter types of meters do not provide an accurate measurement of dirty electricity.

The Differences Between Harmful EMFs and PEMFs

The types of EMFs associated with the harmful effects noted above have significantly shorter wavelengths and higher frequencies than therapeutic PEMFs. The electromagnetic spectrum is huge, encompassing all possible wavelengths and frequencies, including X-rays, microwaves, radio waves, visible light, and infrared. (See Figure 1.)

Practically speaking, for therapeutic magnetic field applications, the spectrum is very narrow. The goal of a PEMF system is to produce a magnetic field that will not only be supportive to the body's natural functions, but also to use magnetic field strengths that will go all the way through the body with sufficient intensity, called magnetic flux density, to create the desired actions in the body.

An EMF frequency broadcast into air of 1 Hz has a wavelength of 100 million meters (more than 62,000miles). At the upper range of what would be produced by an ELF EMF, the frequency can be about 10,000 Hz or so. The wavelength there would be 10,000 meters (about 6.2 miles). For comparison, a low-end microwave-range frequency would be about100,000,000 Hz (1×10^9 Hz). This would correspond to a wavelength of about 1 meter (0.00062 miles). So, ELF EMFs have long electromagnetic wavelengths that go completely through the body.

However, ELF PEMFs in applicator coils don't broadcast into the air in the same way that radio and microwave antennas do. The magnetic field produced around a PEMF treatment coil is a closed, not open, loop. It does not broadcast out into open space. A closed loop means that the magnetic field is effectively going around in a circle, repeatedly expanding and collapsing on itself based on the frequency it "pulses." The size of the generated magnetic field loop depends mostly on its intensity and its frequency, the diameter of the coil loop, and the number of turns of the coil's wire. A slower frequency pulsing magnetic field will mean that for a given control unit power output producing the magnetic field intensity, the size of the magnetic field loop can reach its full potential, being larger. For a faster pulsing rate, for the same control unit power output, the magnetic coil intensity, because it is pulsing at a higher rate (frequency), the magnetic field cannot reach its full potential intensity, so the actual magnetic field intensity will be weaker and the magnetic field will have a smaller loop.

Electromagnetic radiation is classified into two types (ionizing and non-ionizing) based on the radiation's capability of ionizing atoms and disrupting chemical bonds. Ultraviolet and high frequencies, like X-rays or gamma rays, are ionizing. They pose their own health hazards, the most common of which is tissue burning, like sunburn, but may also include the induction of cell transformation, leading to possible cancers.

Non-ionizing radiation doesn't carry enough energy to disrupt chemical bonds. It only has enough energy to excite electrons into a higher energy state, increasing charge in the tissues, through the process of inductively coupled electrical stimulation (ICES). Almost all therapeutic ELF PEMF systems are non-ionizing and use the principle of ICES.

Most therapeutic PEMF systems have pulse rates or frequencies in the Extremely Low Frequency (ELF) to Very Low Frequency (VLF) range on the electromagnetic spectrum. These pulse rates/frequencies (below 10,000 Hz or 10 kHz) do not induce damaging heating actions in cells or tissues. PEMF devices also contain various levels of filtering inside the control unit or frequency generator portion of the system, which clean up the surges/spikes, mentioned above, that often come out of the household outlets we use to power the device itself.

Protecting Yourself From Harmful EMFs

One of the biggest obstacles people face when it comes to minimizing their exposures to harmful EMFs is their reluctance to forsake the many conveniences that Wi-Fi, cell phones, computers, and other wireless-enabled devices provide.

A leading researcher into the potential health risks of EMF is Magda Havas, PhD, of Trent University in Canada (https://magdahavas.com). Dr. Havas has been researching the biological effects of electromagnetic pollution since the 1990s.

A video presentation Dr. Havas posted on YouTube, entitled *Wi-Fi in Schools is Safe. True or False?* offers compelling evidence that Wi-Fi and other sources of EMFs damage human health. But as she states in this video, "(W)henever I talk to health-conscious people about the importance of eating organic food, avoiding chemical contaminants, and drinking clean water, most will agree with me. Yet when I talk to these same people about the importance of detoxifying the home of excessive electromagnetic radiation, they will look at me sideways or debate about how we need Wi-Fi and smart phones to survive in today's world."

Perhaps you feel the same way. If so, keep in mind that I and other doctors who warn about the health risks EMF pose are not against these modern technological advances. Rather, we simply want people to know the risks and to take sensible precautions by doing all they can to reduce those risks. The following action steps can help you to do so.

Know the Sources of EMFs in Your Home: It is important to recognize the devices that emit the vast majority of the EMFs that you are exposed to in your home are. The most common devices include:

Cell phones, laptops, and tablets.
Wi-Fi routers.
Cordless DECT phones (digital enhanced cordless technology).
Microwave ovens.
Bluetooth devices, such as headphones, AirPods, fitness trackers, keyboards, wireless mice, printers, baby monitors, hearing aids, speakers, gaming consoles and controllers, Amazon Echo and Alexa-enabled devices, and any "smart" device, including virtually any new TV.
Smart electric, gas, and water meters.

Make the Invisible Visible: If you're concerned or have electromagnetic sensitivity or health problems that are not responding to treatments, you may want to determine your level of EMF exposure in your home. This can be done using devices that can accurately locate and measure hidden sources of EMFs.

To detect and measure sources of EMFs, you can either hire a professional building biologist to measure EMF levels for you, or you can do it yourself. The most affordable option is to purchase your own EMF meter and do the measuring yourself.

There are different types of meters designed for consumers. Among them are multifield (also called trifield) meters, which measure wireless (radio frequency, or RF), electric, and magnetic field strength, and EMI meters that measure dirty electricity. Both types of meters can easily be found on online, such as at the website RadMeters.com. High-frequency EMFs can be measured with the EMFields Solutions Acousticom-2.

In addition, you can use a gauss meter to measure the levels of AC (alternating current) magnetic fields in your home, such as those given off by home appliances, as well as outside power lines below or above your homes. The maximum safety threshold for this type of field inside homes is 1.0 mG (milligauss), and the ideal reading over beds should be no higher than 0.2 mG. You can purchase a gauss meter from LessEMF.com.

Alternatively, you could hire a professional building biologist who is trained and certified to analyze indoor environments and systemically reduce EMF exposures. Such professionals can also teach you how to use your own meters. Another advantage of working with a building biologist if you can afford and locate one in your area is that he or she can also help you work with your utility company to find and repair power line connections if they are found to produce AC magnetic fields above 1.0 mG. The Building Biology Institute (www.buildingbiologyinstitute.org) offers a nationwide directory of certified building biologists. You can also Google "EMF building biologist."

Reducing EMF Exposures From Computers, Laptops, Tablets, and Wi-Fi: Wi-Fi and the computing devices that operate on them are one of the largest contributors to EMF exposure in your home. The general principles of reducing EMF exposure are:

- Switch off or reduce the source
- Increase your distance from the source

- Reduce the time of exposure
- Use shielding.

Especially for people with significant sensitivities or more severe autoimmune diseases, you could consider grounding the device and/or your own body, too. There is more information about electrically grounding the body at https://www. ultimatelongevity.com/earthing-grounding/clint-ober.shtml. Grounding advocates sometimes make claims for "curing" all sorts of problems. Grounding can be useful to offset environmental challenges but does not create enough healing charge in the body to do the healing work that PEMFs can do. However, they can be used together to produce even better results than just PEMFs alone, especially, as I said above, when there are significant environmental stressors, especially EMFs.

You can reduce your exposure to EMFs by doing the following. If possible, use a hard-wired Ethernet cable (local area network, or LAN) to connect your home computer and printer to the Internet instead of wirelessly through a Wi-Fi-enabled router. Be aware, however, that many newer laptops do not have an Ethernet port. If you own one, you will need to purchase an inexpensive adaptor that fits into the USB A, USB C, or Thunderbolt port.

The more you use computers, laptops, and tablets, the more EMF you will be exposed to. If possible, reduce the amount of time you use them. In addition, do not place laptops and tablets on your body, especially the lower abdomen or lap, as doing so directly affects your reproductive organs. Ideally, you should place your computer, laptop, or tablet at least 12 inches away from you when you use it. This can reduce your exposure to the EMF the devices, especially laptops, emit by as much as 80 percent.

To further reduce EMF, choose a mouse and keyboard that plug into your computer or laptop, rather than wireless versions. Then, if your computer has a Bluetooth feature, disable it. Otherwise, it will continue to transmit even when your mouse and keyboard are plugged in.

When using laptop computers, avoid using them when they are plugged in and charging. The radiation emitted by laptops when they are plugged in can be up to 100 times higher than the EMF you are exposed to from them when they are operating on battery power. The same is true for tablets and Kindle devices, as well as cell phones.

Also consider using a shielding computer or laptop pad to further block radiation. Shielding pads cover the bottom surface of these devices, which are the prime source of the emitted EMF associated with them. You can find such pads online. However, their effectiveness varies, depending on the brand, so research them before purchasing them.

Finally, when you are not using your computer, laptop, or tablet, turn it off. In addition, if you have a Wi-Fi-enabled printer, connect it to your computer using either an Ethernet or USB printer cable and then turn off the Wi-Fi feature on the printer.

Reducing Cell Phone Risks: Despite the many advantages your cell phone provides, protecting yourself from the EMF radiation it emits is another important step you need to take.

Whenever you don't need to use your cell phone, switch it to airplane mode in order to avoid the continuous radiation it emits, especially when you carry it on your body.

Avoid using your cell phone when the signal is weak. In these moments, as the phone works harder to establish a connection to the cell tower, it emits higher levels of radiation. A 2019 study found that phones emit up to 10,000-fold more EMF radiation when the connectivity is low. It is much better to wait until you're in an area with full bars, and even then, to use speakerphone so that the phone is farther away from your body.

Don't sleep with your cell phone in your bedroom. If you can't do this, make sure it is in airplane mode, with Wi-Fi, NFC, and Bluetooth switched off. Also don't use your cell phone as an alarm clock.

Never use wireless chargers for your cell phone, especially anywhere near your bed, as they also will increase EMFs throughout your home. Instead, use a standard plug-in charger and keep that charger and its cord well away from your bedroom.

Pregnant women should also limit their cell phone use and be sure to keep cell phones away from their bodies by using the speakerphone mode. Research has established that cell phone radiation can damage the brains of the developing fetus as well as damaging the mother's reproductive system during pregnancy. (To learn more about the dangers of cell phone use during pregnancy, visit www. babysafeproject.org.)

Protecting Yourself from EMFs From Other Household Appliances: Various home appliances can also be sources of EMF. These range from new model "smart" TVs and refrigerators, front-load washing machines, microwave ovens, fluorescent light bulbs, compact fluorescent lamps, and certain LED and halogen fixtures, to any other wireless-enabled home device.

Microwave ovens are particularly dangerous because of the high levels of EMF they emit when in use. Over time, the seal on the door of microwave ovens can also wear down, causing radiation to leak out even when they are not in use. Your best option is to avoid using a microwave oven altogether, and cooking your food on a stove. If you do choose to use a microwave, leave the kitchen while it is turned on to reduce your EMF exposure, and have it serviced once a year to ensure the door seal is fully intact.

Also, stop using fluorescent light bulbs. Besides emitting EMFs, these bulbs contain mercury, a dangerous toxin which is released into the environment when the bulbs break. Old-fashioned, incandescent bulbs and new-model LED or incandescent halogen bulbs are much safer lighting choices.

If you have a smart TV, limit how often you use it, and when it is on, sit as far away from it as possible.

Smart Meters: Many utility companies across the United States and other countries have installed or are in the process of installing smart meters on their customers' homes without informing the public about the inherent health dangers these meters can cause.

Unlike analog meters, smart meters contain electronic components that are energy intensive and can emit extreme levels of EMF radiation. This toxic exposure has been shown to cause a variety of serious health problems, including heart palpitations, insomnia, ringing in the ears, anxiety, nausea, dizziness, tingling in extremities, and memory loss, as well as increasing the risk for cancer. Smart meters are also privacy-invading and have been known to spontaneously cause electrical fires. Thousands of home fires caused by smart meters have been documented, as have cases of smart meter explosions near gas lines.

A number of states across the U.S. have passed laws that allow consumers to refuse smart meters being installed on their homes. To learn more about this and the steps you can take to refuse a smart meter or have one removed, visit StopSmartMeters.org and TakeBackYourPower.net. The latter website features a free, full-length documentary that explores the dangers of smart meters in greater detail.

If you live in a state that has not passed such laws and still have an analog meter on your home, you have the right to secure it behind a lock and key so that your utility company cannot remove and replace it. You can also write and send a certified letter to your utility company stating on the record that you refuse to consent to have a smart meter installed.

If you already have a smart meter on your property, you can revoke your consent by sending a certified letter to your utility company, demanding that they remove the meter by a specified deadline. Your home is your property, and your utility company has no right to harm your health.

If you cannot get your utility company to comply with your demand, you can shield your meters by placing EMF-shielding material (such as High-Performance Silver Mesh Fabric) on the inside wall where the smart meter is located on the other side of the wall. It is most effective to use an alligator clip attached to an insulated copper wire that can then be attached to the ground hole in an electrical plug or to a copper rod driven in the earth outside the window in that room. You can find shielding material at www.lessemf.com.

Dirty Electricity (DE): Following the precautions outlined in this chapter thus far can help reduce the health risks of dirty electricity in your home. To fully address the problem of DE, there are additional steps you might also consider. The first is to purchase and install DE plug-in filters in your home. Doing so can greatly reduce DE and the amount of EMFs generated by the appliances and wiring in your home. Two of the best sources of DE plug-in filters are StetzerElectric.com and GreenWaveFilters.com.

As an alternative to DE plug-in filters, you can also consider purchasing Memon transformers. Based in Germany, Memon manufactures a variety of EMF-protection products, including transformers. For more information, visit www.memon.eu/en. In the U.S., Memon products are also available at www. totalharmonywithnature.com.

Another option is to install a whole-house DE protection device. Such products connect directly to your home power panel. Not only do these devices significantly reduce DE, they may also result in utility bill savings. One such device is the SineTamer. To purchase or find out more about it, visit www.poweremt.com.

Stay Informed: The above recommendations can go a long way to helping you to minimize your exposure to harmful EMFs. However, our understanding of the risks these EMFs pose continues to grow as further research is conducted. Therefore, it is best to stay informed about this issue. The following organizations can help you do so:

Americans For Responsible Technology (americansforresponsibletech.org)
BioInitiative 2012 (bioinitiative.org)
Electromagnetic Health (electromagnetichealth.org)
EMF Consultancy (emfacts.com)
Environmental Health Trust (ehtrust.org)
Lloyd Burrell/Electric Sense (electricsense.com)
Dr. Magda Havas (magdahavas.com)
Dr. Joseph Mercola (mercola.com)
Physicians For Safe Technology (mdsafetech.org)
Take Back Your Power (takebackyourpower.net)

To learn more about EMF's, I also recommend the book *EMF'd*, written by my colleague and friend, Dr. Joseph Mercola. You can also listen to an interview I conducted with Dr. Mercola here: www.DrPawluk.com/podcast/emfs-and-the-pain-connection-dr-joseph-mercola/

It's important to know that EMF protection and mitigation is still in evolution and there are no perfect solutions. There are many opinions and positions taken on this highly emotional topic. Numerous products are being promoted with the claims of neutralizing the detrimental effects of EMFs or electrosmog. It is possible that there may be some benefit but there have been almost no science or credible independent studies to back these claims.

The problem with these claims has to do with the tremendous number of variables involved in both the EMFs and the circumstances in which they are encountered—for example, being near or far from a microwave mast, length of exposure, dose of exposure, as well as the condition of the body at the time and the biological processes being affected. So it's hard to conceive of a single piece of equipment being able to provide perfect protection and mitigation.

Sadly, this may lead to a sense of complacency and unrealistic expectations regarding EMF exposures, such that appropriate avoidance and control steps are not taken. While this book is about PEMFs and the benefits PEMFs provide, PEMFs are also not adequate to completely protect against all the possible effects of EMFs. And, as with PEMFs, lifestyle factors are very important for protection, including adequate nutrition, stress reduction, appropriate supplements, appropriate rest, adequate activity, etc.

My goal in presenting this EMF and electrosmog discussion is to increase awareness both of the issues and also of possible solutions. Once someone has significant health issues, particularly significant autoimmune problems, multiple chemical and environmental sensitivities, nervous system hyper-excitability and EHS, it will be very challenging to remove or reverse the conditions. A reasonable and important strategy is to decrease aggravating factors to decrease symptoms as much as possible and reduce progression.

Regular PEMF treatments can also mitigate many of the risks harmful EMFs pose, helping to keep your body more resilient in the face of EMFs and other health threats. The many ways that PEMF therapy can benefit you is the topic of Chapter 3.

The Many Ways That PEMF Therapy Can Improve Your Health

In this chapter, we are going to explore the multiple ways that PEMF therapy can improve and maintain your health.

Ongoing research into PEMFs has identified more than 25 ways that PEMF therapy supports both physical and psychological health. My own investigations, as well as my work as a physician who treats patients with PEMF therapy, has confirmed these research findings. PEMF therapy is one of the most effective health treatments available to us today, as well as one of the most versatile. The fact that it also readily lends itself to home treatment as a significant self-care tool significantly adds to its overall value.

Most of the beneficial effects of PEMFs occur through the basic actions of magnetic fields and electrical charge on cellular biology. All cellular communication in our bodies requires an electrical signal which triggers the release of chemicals. In turn, these chemical reactions cause a change in the neighboring cells. This chain of electrical signal actions continues rapidly until the cell's function has been completed. PEMFs enhance and support this charge activity when it is out of balance, causing cells to function more efficiently, but only when they need extra help. Research studies have confirmed that the appropriate therapeutic use of PEMFs only affects or improves body systems that are compromised, while not affecting normal or healthy systems or tissues, unlike even properly prescribed medications and other medical interventions.

The benefits of this type of electrical charge support are both big and small. From the tiniest molecule or enzyme up to the largest organ system (skin), you can find a process PEMFs either streamline, correct, improve, or don't affect. Therefore, PEMFs have the potential to positively affect an extremely broad range of physiological and biological actions. Any negative or non-reaction effects PEMFs have on these processes are usually self-limited and do not result in any significant problems. In general, when used appropriately PEMF therapy is extraordinarily safe.

The Top 10 Benefits of PEMF Therapy

As you will learn in Part 2 of this book, PEMF therapy has been shown by research to be an effective treatment for both preventing and helping to reverse over 80 serious health conditions. What follows are ten of the most powerful benefits that explain why.

Pain Relief: Pain management is one of the most common applications for PEMFs. Whether the pain is acute or chronic, inflammatory, or vascular, musculoskeletal, or in the nervous system, PEMFs help address both pain perception (pain blocking) and the cause of the pain itself (pain reduction). I have fairly often seen people get miraculous, sudden, and complete relief of pain after only one treatment of even low-intensity PEMFs.

Pain mechanisms are extremely complex, but on the most basic level they involve a signal being transferred to a receptor and causing a change in cellular behavior. My goal is always to help my patients prevent cellular injury in the first place, which is why, in many cases, daily treatment with PEMF therapy is essential. Cellular injury means cellular damage from any cause. The term injury is usually quantitatively used to mean trauma, but injury in this context means anything that damages the cell, including sun exposure, freezing, poisoning, burns, and hypoxia, as well as various other factors besides, of course, trauma. In cases of acute injuries, or for those people who have found PEMF therapy after an injury or disease condition has already taken hold of the body, the goal changes from prevention to injury resolution and pain management.

The body normally does its own pain blocking in response to pain signals through an increase in levels of serotonin, dopamine, endorphin, and encephalins, along with a decrease in cortisol and noradrenaline.

The primary mechanisms for pain in response to cell injury are edema, apoptosis or necrosis, diminished circulation, decreased cellular metabolism, and impaired cellular repair processes. PEMF therapy addresses each of these mechanisms in very basic and measurable ways.

In addition, PEMFs help to manage and relieve pain because of their positive effects on adenosine, a molecule that plays a vital role in controlling inflammation that triggers pain. Adenosine acts through its receptor, the *adenosine receptor (AR), and is a* building block for RNA/DNA. It is also a part of the energy molecule ATP and regulates the function of every cell, tissue, and organ in the body. Because of this regulatory role, adenosine has been called the "guardian angel" protecting against human disease.

Through various metabolic processes, adenosine is released by the breakdown of ATP to create energy and then is re-used to create more ATP in a perpetual cellular cycle. The concentrations of adenosine are naturally at low levels in body fluids between the cells of unstressed tissues. These concentrations increase rapidly in response to cell injury-causing stress conditions such as low oxygen (hypoxia), lack of blood supply (ischemia), inflammation, or trauma. Adenosine has a short half-life in the blood (a few seconds) and in spinal cerebrospinal fluid (10 to 20 minutes). Once released into the extracellular space, adenosine functions as an alarm or danger signal, and then activates specific adenosine receptors, causing numerous cellular responses that aim to restore tissue homeostasis. When adenosine production drops off or is low, inflammation persists and produces chronic inflammation.

Adenosine acts through four subtypes of adenosine receptors: A1, A2A, A2B and A3. PEMFs appear to primarily influence the A2A and A3 receptors, stimulating their activation, increasing their functionality, and augmenting chemical agents that also stimulate them. Stimulation of A2A and A3 receptors by PEMFs in cells throughout the body reduces inflammation by lowering many pro-inflammatory tissue cytokines, including tumor necrosis factor-α (TNF-α), interleukins (IL-1β, IL-6, and IL-8 in microglial cells; IL-6 and IL-8 in cartilage and bone cells; IL-8 and NF-kappa B in skin cells); and synovial fibroblasts.

Most research to date has been done on PEMF stimulation of A2A receptors, which has been shown to be especially helpful for chronic inflammation. That's because the A2A receptor, under normal conditions, is naturally stimulated by acute inflammation-producing molecules to inhibit or control the inflammation. Most notably, PEMFs, by increasing adenosine receptors, enhance adenosine's functional efficiency, resulting in a stronger physiological action than the use of pain-relief drugs. A PEMF intensity of about 15 gauss (1.5 mT) has been found to be optimal to affect the adenosine receptors. The anti-inflammatory effect of adenosine enhanced by PEMF is less likely to have the side effects, desensitization, and receptor resistance than drugs designed to be used to act on adenosine receptors. Prolonged stimulation of adenosine receptors with a drug can dampen the ability of the receptor to function. Prolonged use of drugs decreases the quantity of receptors, thereby reducing the effectiveness of the drug over time.

A more complete explanation of how and why PEMF therapy is so effective for pain prevention and relief is presented in Chapter 9.

Healthy Heart Function: Heart attacks continue to be the leading cause of death in the United States, and this toll is even larger when deaths from other heart diseases, such as stroke, congestive heart failure, coronary heart disease, etc., are taken into account. Helping to maintain healthy heart function is one of the most significant benefits PEMF therapy provides.

Because the heart is an electrically dynamic organ, it is most susceptible to PEMFs. The heart muscle itself, because of its dynamic electrical activity, also creates its own internal PEMFs that have their own healthful effects on cardiac tissue. The heart contributes between five and ten percent of the total electromagnetic field brought about in the human body by externally applied electric and magnetic fields.

The reaction of the cardiovascular system to external PEMFs is complex and includes direct responses of many tissues including, cardiac muscle, the autonomic nervous system, blood vessels, and reflex responses processed by the central nervous system among others. Studies have shown that the natural PEMFs of the heart become much larger when exposed to external PEMFs.

Studies show that PEMFs can affect the function of the centers of the autonomic nervous system that control heart rhythm. A temporary increase in blood pressure is seen with clinical exposure to industrial EMFs, but extended exposure causes the systemic pressure to decrease. The heart has both macro (large) and micro (tiny) blood vessels. PEMFs dilate the macro blood vessels, acting just like nitroglycerin used for angina chest pain.

Microcirculation is often compromised by diabetes. Microcirculation dilatation also occurs, with increased blood flow and an increased permeability of the vascular wall. Even lymphatic vessel flow increases. These changes decrease the workload of the heart, which is especially important when the heart is already damaged or in danger of failing.

The heart has its own "nervous" system, the conductive pathways of the heart. This system controls the natural rhythmic and coordinated beating of the heart. PEMFs help to make this system function better and decrease its sensitivity to the external, body-wide autonomic nervous system.

Another reason why PEMF therapy can support heart function is because of its beneficial effects on the functional state of the body-wide nervous and endocrine systems, as well as on heart tissue metabolism. PEMF stimulation activates the parasympathetic nervous system, the part of the autonomic nervous system responsible for the body's rest and repair mechanisms. This activation, in turn, causes heart rate and blood pressure to decrease and the cardiovascular system to become less reactive to adrenaline and acetylcholine, while also reducing the stress hormones cortisol and aldosterone. This likely explains why it is so common for people to report significant relaxation and feelings of stress reduction following treatments with whole-body PEMF systems.

PEMFs have also been shown to improve microcirculation in people with ischemic heart disease and vascular diseases in their extremities, and to improve both lipoproteins and cholesterol levels. In people with low blood pressure, PEMFs improve heart contractions and help normalize bioelectrical function. In most people, PEMFs lower blood pressure by lowering vascular resistance with vasodilatation. Hypertension is improved, depending on the function of the heart before treatment. PEMFs normalize heart function and circulation in people with high blood pressure, and at the same time improve circulation. People with normally functioning hearts have improved blood flow, as well. The improvements in blood pressure, as well as lipid metabolism and coronary circulation, make PEMFs a useful treatment for people with the combination of hypertension and ischemic heart disease.

Improved Circulation and Blood Flow: The majority of the body's functions are handled by blood cells moving freely throughout the various systems such as the neurological, cardiovascular, nervous, digestive, and many others. These cells need to be able to travel unimpeded by blockages and other issues which cause restrictions in flow. This can only occur when blood vessels are healthy and wide enough to allow blood cells to easily circulate.

A class of drugs known as vasodilators widen (dilate) blood vessels, preventing the muscles in your arteries and veins from tightening and their walls from narrowing. As a result, blood flows more easily through your vessels. Your heart doesn't have to pump as hard, reducing your blood pressure.

Abnormal or diminished production of nitric oxide (which occurs in various disorders) can cause blood vessels to become constricted, adversely affecting blood flow and other vascular functions. In a healthy cellular environment, blood vessels continually produce nitric oxide. The inner lining of the blood vessel (endothelium) produces and uses nitric oxide to signal the adjacent smooth muscles in the blood vessel wall to relax, causing blood vessels to widen.

The subsequent increase in blood flow leads to an immediate decrease in both blood pressure and heart rate.

Improving circulation is considered one of the most essential mechanisms of the healing effects of PEMF therapy. Research shows that therapeutic PEMFs enhance delivery of nutrients as they pass through the bloodstream, repairing molecules, stimulating growth factors, increasing oxygen, eliminating waste, and achieving many other actions that support healthy circulation.

Improved Sleep and Better and Fuller Sleep Cycles: Studies show that nearly two-thirds of all adults experience some level of sleep deprivation. Of those two-thirds, nearly one-third of them experience chronic sleep deprivation. PEMF therapy can not only help people struggling with issues falling asleep, but also *staying* asleep. This nocturnal cycle is when all of the body's regenerative and restorative processes take place. Keeping it in balance is critical to overall health.

Research studies support the value of PEMF therapy to enhance sleep and show that using it before going to sleep or during bedtime can enhance and balance circadian rhythms. Sleep disturbances can affect daytime functioning, psychologically and cognitively. Since PEMFs at desired, low brainwave frequencies (below 7 Hz) and higher intensities can improve sleep, PEMFs can also improve psychological and cognitive daytime function through better sleep.

I have found that presenting the brain with one PEMF frequency of 3 Hz throughout the night anchors the brain into delta levels and lower theta levels. Not only does this result in better and deeper delta, you also get longer periods of delta, and you also then begin to have a deeper theta level of sleep. What wakes people up during the night the most is the fact that when you're aware of your dreaming you are in high levels of theta. When you anchor or tether more of the brain in delta throughout the entire night using PEMF, people get a much longer night's sleep.

Improved Mental Focus, Concentration, and Cognitive Function: PEMF therapy around 10 Hz promotes the alpha state in neurological function, which is when the mind is relaxed and at its most aware and its senses are the most heightened. The alpha state is one of the peak times for learning and retaining information. Unfortunately, one of the many issues that go along with blood cells that are not properly charged is the inability to create and maintain this state.

PEMFs between 14 to 30 Hz can also increase the brain's beta waves. By doing so, PEMFs improve the brain's ability to process information analytically, problem-solve, and multitask much more efficiently.

PEMF stimulation impacts psychological and cognitive function both directly and indirectly. Indirect benefits are especially significant when other symptoms are present. For example, if you're experiencing chronic pain, you're more likely to also experience some depression or anxiety. As PEMF therapy addresses your pain, it will also improve your psychological function. Another indirect benefit is from improved sleep, as mentioned above.

Direct benefits result from PEMFs' actions on the brain and nervous system. Whether these actions are because of changes to the brainwave levels or actions on the brain cells themselves, either way, the effects are measurable. Through entrainment, PEMFs can quickly shift dominant brainwaves from beta to alpha or theta, and even down into delta (deep sleep).

Since different parts of the brain function at different frequencies, stimulation at a given frequency will either stimulate or depress brainwave frequencies to match the stimulation frequency. PEMF exposure in the alpha and beta rhythms will likely have a positive effect on long-term memory, making us better able to see relationships between ideas and memories, and enhancing other cognitive processes. Even a single session of theta frequency (5-8 Hz) stimulation to the brain affects numerous measures of cognitive function.

Even weak PEMFs appear to help cognitive function, including short and long-term memory, word-finding, attention, and concentration. Recollection seems to improve more dramatically with higher-intensity stimulation. Studies show this to be true even in cases of people with mild to moderate Alzheimer's disease. In fact, PEMFs alone worked better than PEMFs and medications together.

Other people that benefit from lower frequency (alpha, theta, delta) PEMFs include those with stress-induced anxiety (in which patients have been shown to respond significantly even from a single session), day surgery patients, healthy individuals, ADHD children with behavior problems (up to 70 percent benefit), and women suffering with premenstrual symptoms.

I routinely hear from people using PEMFs for the first time that they feel more relaxed and pleasant. A sensation of congeniality is especially common with PEMF treatment directly to the head with frequencies at 10 Hz or below.

While PEMFs are not the same as counseling or resolving personal and interpersonal issues by working through them, they can help to change the state of the brain, making it more receptive to finding new solutions. Some psychologists use PEMF stimulation prior to doing their counseling sessions and report that their patients/clients have much better working sessions and are better able to resolve emotional and cognitive blocks.

In addition to beta, alpha, theta and delta brainwave patterns, neuroscientists have more recently been doing extensive evaluations of gamma brainwaves, often called gamma brain oscillations (GBOs). These, too, are important for optimal brain function. How PEMFs enhance GBOs is discussed later in this chapter.

Improved Muscle Performance: When all of the positive and negative electromagnetic charges are working properly in healthy cells, muscle performance improves. This includes everything from mobility and flexibility to increased stamina and strength. This is critical as you age and lose this type of function and ability, or after injuries requiring rehabilitation. PEMF therapy applied regularly can help prevent such losses and keep your muscles strong and healthy.

Reduction in Stress and Anxiety: PEMFs not only offer incredible benefits for physical well-being, but also for stress, anxiety, and other mental/emotional issues. This is especially necessary in a time of unprecedented anxiety over the state of the world. In addition to worries over the global pandemic and keeping themselves and their loved ones safe and healthy, the economic impact of various shutdowns has also increased the stress levels of many people.

PEMFs change the stress responses in the body, resulting in a more efficient function of the nervous and endocrine systems. In addition, in 2011, the FDA-approved high-intensity transcranial PEMF therapy to treat severe depression.

PEMFs help with stress in three basic ways. First, they reduce the brain's reaction to it. Second, they help the body eliminate the neurotransmitters and hormones produced by stressful fight-flight reactions. Third, they help defend the cells and tissues of the body from the physical changes induced by stress chemicals and hormones.

In addition, PEMF stimulation of the kidneys accelerates the excretion of stress hormones. The same thing happens with the hypothalamus in the brain, which has a central role in controlling the brain's responses to stress. In many individuals, the brain is in a heightened state of expectancy for stress.

In people prone to anxiety, alpha brainwaves appear to be lacking. PEMF therapy has been shown to help entrain alpha brainwaves, thereby alleviating anxiety.

Stress clearly causes significant disruptions in normal brain rhythms. Research in Germany found that 10 Hz PEMF stabilized circadian rhythms. Use of this frequency can treat jet lag and other sleep disturbances. Circadian rhythms control the hormone balance of the body. When they are out of alignment or not in their proper phase, many problems begin to show up in the body. Stress is a clear example of how circadian rhythms and brainwave frequency patterns can become disrupted. A 7 or 10 Hz PEMF can be useful for reducing many of the physical effects of stress, circadian disruption, and tissue regeneration.

Enhanced Healing, Repair, and Recovery: This is one of the most common uses of PEMFs. In addition to the fact that PEMF therapy can improve muscle strength and endurance, as noted above, energy production in the muscles themselves can increase by as much as 500 percent with regular treatment sessions.

By triggering the production of heat stress proteins (natural tissue- protective proteins) before exercise, PEMF therapy assists in not only preventing the wear and tear and breakdown of cells, it also promotes accelerated restoration and recovery. For people struggling with chronic injuries or continual pain, it means finally having the relief they so desperately seek. For fitness enthusiasts and athletes, it means performing at a higher level with less recovery time.

One of the most important research findings is that PEMF signals appear to have therapeutic effects on damaged tissue, but do not seem to affect normal tissue. Under normal conditions, PEMFs interfere only moderately with enzyme activity but greatly enhance activity when enzymes function under less-than-optimal conditions due to tissue damage. When tissue is damaged and ion leakage results in altered ionic concentrations at cell sites, data show that PEMFs markedly increase the enzymes' activity.

Reduction of Inflammation and Swelling: When the body's repair and recovery process are not working properly, inflammation and its associated swelling are often the main culprits. It is very hard for the body to heal inflammation and reduce swelling when there are issues with blood flow, as well as with the health of the blood cells themselves. As discussed above, PEMFs can improve blood flow and also improve of the health of blood cells, most notably red blood cells (discussed later in this chapter).

Athletes and others who regularly engage in physical activities are particularly prone to inflammation and swelling. Recognizing this, physical trainers and practitioners at pain clinics are increasingly using PEMF therapies and systems for their clients, a growing number of whom, including many professional athletes, also have their own PEMF devices and systems in their homes. Regular home therapy produces more consistent and enduring results.

Cellular Restoration: Every function in the body relies on its cell membranes and their electromagnetic charges. When these charges are out of balance, any or all of the issues mentioned above can occur. When these cells are working properly, they are able to do everything from processing nutrition better to carrying much-needed chemicals to the various parts of the body. This one improvement alone, which PEMFs can and do provide, can lead to better oxygenation, better circulation, and more efficient productivity in every aspect.

Other Health Benefits of PEMFs

In addition to the above benefits, PEMFs support health in other significant ways, as well, including:

Acupuncture Stimulation: Tens of thousands of scientific articles confirm the clinical benefits of acupuncture. Many people, however, are uncomfortable with the idea of needles, making PEMF stimulation an excellent alternative to traditional acupuncture.

Acupuncture points have electrical characteristics, which means they are susceptible to both electrical and magnetic stimulation. Acupuncture points lie along energy pathways in the body known as meridians, and have shown corresponding electrical conductivity. Stimulating these acupuncture points with PEMFs can improve the flow of charge, clearing out any blockages.

Using appropriate applicators, PEMFs can be targeted directly at specific acupuncture points, stimulating both the acupuncture points and all the tissues in the area of the magnetic field, providing a dual benefit. If PEMFs are used for other tissue or organ stimulation purposes, all acupuncture points or meridians in the magnetic field will also be stimulated. This is true whether the stimulation is local or whole-body. When whole-body PEMF therapy is used, all the acupuncture points and meridians in the body are stimulated at the same time, creating a simultaneous rebalancing of the meridian system. This creates a major secondary benefit of PEMFs over acupuncture alone. In fact, I know of acupuncturists who combine PEMFs with acupuncture and claim that their results are even better than usual.

Since there are so many acupuncture points in the body, almost any PEMF stimulation will include acupuncture points and meridians in the magnetic field. Therefore, PEMFs provide the advantage of both acupuncture-type stimulation simultaneously with direct cellular stimulation.

Antibacterial, Antifungal, Antiviral, and Anti-Parasitic Benefits: Research has shown that PEMFs can help the body resist harmful bacteria, fungi, viruses, and parasites. A wide range of PEMF frequencies and intensities has been studied in this regard. Growth inhibition occurred in each bacterial culture exposed to PEMFs, but was much more dramatic with higher-intensity magnetic fields, with effects becoming evident within six to ten hours after the initial exposure. Although the studied microorganisms were not killed outright by the PEMFs, there was some killing action. The same is true for many antibiotics and antivirals, many of which only inhibit growth but don't actually kill the organisms. In this sense, PEMFs can act like some antibiotics.

In addition to hindering bacterial growth, research also shows that PEMF exposure improves the function of cells that kill bacteria (phagocytes). One type of phagocyte, the monocyte, had higher levels of stress proteins, leading it to become a better bacterial hunter. PEMF stimulation has also been shown to improve the function of the specific type of white blood cells that trap bacteria (neutrophils). These neutrophils create neutrophil extracellular traps (NETs), which act like spider webs to bind pathogens. Studies confirm that the formation of NETs is enhanced by PEMFs and that PEMFs improve the innate immune system .This is yet another example of how PEMFs deal with infections in a number of different ways, even if they don't kill bacteria, viruses, or fungal infections directly.

Blood cell investigations were done to evaluate the effect PEMFs have on the body's ability to engulf yeast cells (phagocytosis). Even the first treatment with PEMF enhanced phagocytic activity. Another study of PEMF applied to herpes virus-infected cells showed that, though PEMF did not affect the growth and viability of the cells, the viruses developing under PEMF exposure had mainly defective viral particles. This indicates that PEMF therapy can heal the tissue, while at the same time potentially rendering the virus less active. Antibiotics and antivirals do not have this dual action.

Numerous stimuli may cause bacteria to mutate and become resistant to drug treatments. Research shows that PEMF exposure inhibits mutagenic transformation in these bacteria. PEMFs do not appear to increase the risk of bacterial resistance that happens with antibiotics and, in fact, at least experimentally, do the opposite.

Other research showed that combining PEMFs with antifungal agents increases their effectiveness for killing the fungi. The combination treatment killed almost 90 percent of the fungi rapidly, versus only 43 percent with the medication alone, even after a much longer exposure. Since antifungal therapies can be toxic, PEMF therapies combined with them could allow for much lower dosing with less risk of toxicity. In addition, while systemic therapies are often used for local tissue problems, PEMFs may allow for local tissue treatments, further reducing the risk of toxicity while improving benefit.

Early in my work with magnetic fields, I read a research study that found that magnetic fields caused parasites to be eliminated in children, somewhat better than medication alone. The researchers did not study the combination of magnetic fields and medication but it can be reasonably assumed that the combination would work even better.

Anticoagulant Effects: PEMF therapy addresses many of the mechanisms that lead to increased blood viscosity (thickness) and clotting, including the reduction of platelet adhesiveness, reduction of fibrinogen and improvement of fibrinolysis, improving the pliability of red blood cells (allowing them to move through capillaries more easily), and increasing the saline content of the blood, decreasing viscosity. PEMF therapy reduces the stickiness of platelets, thus decreasing the risk of clotting by an amount almost equivalent to taking aspirin. It works through a different action so, if aspirin is added, the benefit about doubles. In addition, PEMF therapy does not have the risks associated with aspirin use, particularly gastric bleeding. These anticoagulant effects appear to be universal to virtually all types of PEMFs.

Anti-Edema Activity: Edema is swelling caused by excess fluid trapped in tissue. Tissues with edema are deprived of oxygen, nutrients, and circulation. PEMF therapy has a positive effect on swelling and edema by improving cellular metabolism through direct actions on the sodium-potassium pump in the cell membrane. Any kind of cell or tissue damage causes edema due to leakage of fluids from the cells and blood vessels. Improving circulation helps to remove this excess fluid and prevent further fluid accumulation. Anti-edema effects happen rapidly after starting the use of PEMFs.

In addition to improving blood circulation, PEMFs also have a positive effect on lymphatic vessels, stimulating lymph drainage and reducing production of lymph edema, and therefore simulating the immune system and correcting the edema.

Anti-Spasm Activity: Muscle spasms can occur in either smooth muscles or skeletal muscles. Smooth muscle spasms include those in the GI and urinary tract, muscles controlled by the nervous system, and the muscles in arteries. Skeletal muscle spasms (cramps) are generally associated with overworked muscles, as commonly happens with athletes or those working in extreme heat. Spasms tend to happen when muscle cells are depleted of energy or electrolytes, causing them to become hyper-excitable. Another major cause of muscle spasticity is brain lesions, such as seen in spinal cord injuries, multiple sclerosis, or cerebral palsy.

Because PEMF stimulation has a direct effect on cellular charge, it improves calcium flow in and out of the cell and therefore impacts cell depolarization and action potentials. When nitric oxide is formed in the blood vessel, it diffuses into muscle cells, where it binds to and activates cellular enzymes. This chain of events leads to the cell signaling for muscle relaxation, preventing or relieving muscle spasms.

Autophagy: Autophagy is the natural, regulated process in the body that disassembles and eliminates unnecessary or dysfunctional cellular components, resulting in the orderly breakdown and recycling of these components. Autophagy may also be responsible for clearing out dysfunctional cells in the body that, when they accumulate and clog up tissues, can lead to the development of cancer. Japanese scientist Yoshinori Ohsumi received the 2016 Nobel Prize in Physiology or Medicine for his pioneering work on autophagy.

There is not much research at this point on the effects of PEMFs on autophagy, given how new the science is, but some experimental studies provide support for its use in helping to maintain healthy cells.

To assess the impact of PEMFs on autophagy, one study looked at their effects on human neuroblastoma cells. Neuroblastoma cells are often used in research into Alzheimer's disease (AD). In these cells, a specific PEMF induced a pro-survival autophagy process that was cell-protective by removing damaged proteins and cell organelles and removing beta-amyloid cells. The same PEMF had previously been found to improve resistance to induced cellular oxidative stress, which is damaging to cells. This study not only demonstrated the potential benefit for PEMFs in protecting against and possibly slowing the progression of AD, but also that it does this through the improvement of autophagy.

In another study, authors investigated the effects of a PEMF on mouse embryo fibroblast autophagy. Fibroblast cells, a major structural component of skin and soft tissue, exposed to a PEMF were found to cause a significant increase in autophagy markers starting at six hours after exposure.

If PEMFs can improve autophagy at a basic level, as they did in these studies, then they are likely to help with many of the conditions of aging and cell breakdown and injury. This is another basic mechanism through which PEMFs help to maintain health, improve poor health conditions, and have an anti-aging benefit.

ATP and Mitochondria: Mitochondria are often called the powerhouses of the cell because they are the major generators of adenosine triphosphate (ATP), a key molecule in energy storage and energy transfer in the tissues of the body. Mitochondria are tiny and the number inside a cell vary significantly from cell to cell, depending on the level of activity of the cells. The liver cells, for example, have about 2000 mitochondria. The organs with cells that have constant activity, such as the brain, heart, arteries, lungs, and kidneys, have the most mitochondria. The only cells of the body that do not have mitochondria are the red blood cells. Mitochondria are constantly regenerating themselves using their own DNA. Mitochondria have been associated with a number of human diseases and conditions, such as mitochondrial disorders, cardiac dysfunction, heart failure, and autism. PEMFs have been found to increase of the number and size of mitochondria that then promoted cellular and intracellular regeneration.

Aside from blood cells, all other cells in the body need ATP to function properly, especially brain, heart, and muscle cells, which have the greatest need for ATP. One of the most important functions of PEMFs is enhancing the production and use of ATP, and therefore the body's energy supply. Research has shown that PEMFs can induce between 100 to 600 percent more ATP production within a short time after stimulation.

We make approximately our body weight in ATP per day. Each ATP molecule recycles about 200 to 500 times per day. Inflammation places a huge demand on the need for ATP and the fatigue often seen with inflammation can be at least partially attributed to the lack of ATP needed by the body. People using PEMFs frequently report significant increases in energy, most likely due to the significant increases in ATP production.

ATP needs to be broken down into adenosine diphosphate (ADP) to release the stored energy. This process is called ATP hydrolysis and the enzyme that performs this task is F1Fo-ATPase. When F1Fo-ATPase is exposed to PEMF stimulation greater than one gauss, ATP hydrolysis activity is enhanced. Even when researchers deliberately inhibited the enzyme chemically, its hydrolysis activity was still enhanced with the PEMF stimulation. So, in addition to helping with ATP synthesis, PEMFs increase the production of energy from the ATP itself, when the stimulation is above a specific intensity threshold.

Mitochondrial energy production also depends on an enzyme called cytochrome oxidase.

Measurement of the levels of cytochrome oxidase in cells is an indicator of the level of energy production in the cell. PEMF exposure significantly increases the level of cytochrome oxidase energy production above the average level.

Research has also demonstrated that sperm motility is improved with PEMF exposure because of increased mitochondrial membrane charge. Overall, research into the effects of PEMFs on ATP and mitochondria show that PEMF stimulation elevates energy metabolism-related molecules in all treatments.

Circadian Rhythms: Some of the effects of PEMF treatments on cellular processes impact the natural daily cyclical rhythms of the cells, called circadian rhythms. Circadian rhythms have a length of around 24 hours. The body responds to both external stimuli, like light, and natural internal stimuli. The external stimuli affect the master clocks of the body and the pituitary and pineal glands. Many of the body's naturally produced rhythms exist without any external stimuli and happen because of natural clocks in the cells and tissues throughout the body. These cellular clocks are controlled by genes that coordinate and regulate themselves through feedback loops.

PEMF treatment stimulates biological clock genes. This has been shown experimentally where a PEMF signal entrained clock genes. Since an important aspect of PEMF's ability to entrain is by acting on the circadian rhythms of the body, we expect that PEMFs used regularly, particularly to the whole body, will help maintain and optimize the natural health of the body. One study showed that 10 Hz was the most likely frequency to restore circadian rhythm. In addition, by affecting and restoring impaired or dysfunctional clock genes, PEMF stimulation may help prevent and reverse obesity, hypertension, type II diabetes, coronary heart disease, and possibly even cancer.

Collagen, Hyaluronic Acid, and GAGs: Collagen, hyaluronic acid (HA), and glycaminoglycans (GAGs) are molecules that play many important roles in the body. These molecules are found widely throughout the body in the connective, skin, and neural tissues. Collagen tissues may be rigid (bone), compliant (tendon), or range from rigid to compliant (cartilage). Collagen is mostly in fibrous tissues such as tendons, ligaments, skin, corneas, cartilage, bones, blood vessels, the gut, intervertebral discs, and in teeth. The fibroblast is the most common cell that creates collagen. Fibroblasts are an important constituent of skin that help to form it and maintain it.

Collagen, and its related molecules and structures, actin and microtubules, are considered as bionanowires. These bionanowires are formed into a matrix throughout all the tissues of the body, potentially capable of high-speed electrical, protonic, and ionic signaling. This bioelectrical signaling system is critical to the regeneration and ordering of the cells, tissues and organs. The messaging systems of the body that rely on chemical signals have limited speeds. Bionanowires have much faster message passing speeds. Bionanowires have significant electrical activity and therefore their activity is dramatically impacted by PEMFs. In fact, these tissue bionanowire structures create their own internal electromagnetic fields, because of their electrical activity, even to the point of impacting or generating brainwave patterns. Therefore, PEMFs have a strong effect on improving the vitality of the body by acting on the bioelectromagnetic nature of these bionanowires, present throughout the whole body.

Hyaluronic acid (HA) is found widely throughout connective, skin, and neural tissues. One-third of HA is turned over (degraded and synthesized) every day. The size of HA molecules in cartilage decreases with age, but the amount increases. HA is a major part of the synovial fluid in our joints. HA along with other associated molecules absorb water and are responsible for the ability of cartilage to compress. The loss of HA with aging is a major contributing factor to arthritis. HA is also a major component of skin, where it is involved in tissue repair. The skin damage seen with aging is often related to the loss or breakdown of HA. When a tissue is wounded the amount of HA increases as part of the acute inflammatory repair process. HA forms the granulation tissue in a wound allowing it to heal itself by filling in the space in the wound.

Glycaminoglycans (GAGs) are important in providing support and adhesiveness in bone, skin, and cartilage. GAGs have widespread functions within the body. GAGs also decrease with age. GAGs attract water, used in the body as a lubricant or shock absorber. They play a huge role in communication among cells, regulation of cell growth, proliferation, promotion of cell adhesion, anticoagulation, and wound repair. Chondroitin sulfate, HA and heparin/ heparan are GAGs. Heparin and heparan is found in mast cells that release histamine. Heparan has numerous biological activities and functions, including cell adhesion, regulation of cell growth and proliferation, cell development, new blood vessel growth, viral invasion, and tumor metastasis. Clinically, heparin is used as an anticoagulant.

PEMFs have been shown in humans to increase collagen, HA, and GAGs, along with elastic fibers and soluble matrix. One benefit of this is plumping of skin and a decrease in wrinkles.

Animals with burns and patients with spinal cord injuries and pressure sores have been shown to heal faster when HA is used along with PEMFs. The use of HA and PEMFs resulted in a 90 percent reduction in wound area by the 30th day of treatment. This is a rapid recovery since pressure sores usually require months to heal. Early on in the course of treatment most of the PEMF effects relate to the increased production of HA, while in the latter stages, when HA production has plateaued, the PEMFs trigger increased growth of new tissue, demonstrating that PEMFs have a multilevel role in wound healing.

Detoxification: Detoxification is what your body constantly does to neutralize, transform, or get rid of unwanted materials or toxins, in order to maintain optimal health. A large percentage of the molecules made by our bodies every day are used for getting rid of waste products. We need hundreds of enzymes, vitamins, and other molecules to help rid the body of unwanted waste products and chemicals. The bulk of the detoxification work is done by the liver and the intestinal tract.

The kidneys, lungs, lymphatic system, and skin are all also involved in this complex detoxification process.

Our liver is the main detoxification organ. Apart from synthesizing and secreting bile, its primary waste product, the liver acts as a filter for toxins and bacteria in the blood and chemically neutralizes toxins, converting them into soluble substances that go back into the bloodstream so that they can then be eliminated by the kidneys. The liver has a large variety of chemical-transforming enzymes that change these molecules through oxidation, reduction, and hydrolysis (Phase I) and then through conjugation (Phase II). This two-phase process handles the vast array of different chemicals in the environment to which we are exposed daily.

Because PEMFs improve inefficient or suboptimal liver and kidney function, they clearly help the body to detoxify. PEMFs also improve cellular detoxification because they improve the ability of cell membranes to open and rebalance themselves. In addition, because they optimize the function of all cells in the body, PEMFs further enhance detoxification by improving blood and lymph circulation, decreasing inflammation, rebalancing cell energy, helping to restore cell function, improving skin respiration, and repairing damaged cells of tissues involved in detoxification.

Gamma Waves: Gamma waves are specific patterns of electrical activity in the brain that occur at frequencies between 30-100 Hz. The term "gamma frequency" is most often assumed to be 40 Hz, when not otherwise specified. More recently, a "high-gamma" label has been applied to frequencies between 80 Hz and 200 Hz. Gamma and high-gamma activity can occur simultaneously in the brain.

Gamma brainwaves are required to process information in different areas of the brain, particularly in the higher-level tasks needed for cognitive functioning, learning, memory, and the processing of information by the brain. Gamma waves are also involved with sensory perception, memory formation, and voluntary movement.

There is an optimal range for gamma activity, which leads to better focus, attention, sensory processing, cognition, information processing, learning, perception, and REM sleep. With too little gamma activity, problems such as ADHD, depression, and learning disabilities result, while too much gamma activity can lead to anxiety, stress, and hyperarousal. Cognitive function is complex and effective cognitive function leads to proper attention and memory and the necessary grouping of constantly changing thoughts and processes. Awareness requires this integration to make sense of the inputs into the brain. This integration is facilitated by gamma activity, which aids the processing of the barrage of sensory information that the brain constantly receives from the external world.

PEMF therapy, using an appropriate frequency, can help synchronize neuron firing throughout the brain. The amount of gamma production, as well as synchronization of signals, impact attention. With more gamma production and better synchronization, attention becomes stronger. The basal forebrain, which is located at the bottom part of the front of the brain, provides vital input for both attention and gamma activity. Stimulation with PEMF therapy over the temples can increase gamma activity in this area, which may benefit those with attention, memory, and focus issues.

Applying adequate specific stimulation to the brain can create entrainment, the natural synchronization of brainwaves. Research has shown that entrainment is more noticeable in the thalamus during gamma stimulation than with other frequency brainwave patterns. Entrainment with gamma frequencies also seems to be easier to achieve than entrainment with other brainwave frequencies.

There have been many types of stimuli used for entrainment, most commonly audiovisual, pulsing lights, sound, and transcranial electrical stimulation. PEMFs have many advantages over some of these other forms of stimulation for inducing gamma brainwaves. In addition to being extremely safe, PEMFs can either target specific areas of the brain or penetrate and pass through the entire brain, a major difference from other approaches. Other entrainment approaches are absorbed by the brain, which can produce harmful heating effects. They also produce indirect effects through interactions with the nervous system, probably accounting for a large part of their actions. PEMFs, on the other hand, can be more directly controlled and targeted to act on the brain, while simultaneously being available to treat other parts of the body. This adds great value to the use of PEMF therapy for gamma brainwave entrainment.

Gamma waves also reduce the level of a sequence of amino acids that are the main component of the amyloid plaques found in brains of those with Alzheimer's disease (AD). In a study of healthy individuals (Barr 2009). A 20 Hz high-intensity PEMF repetitive transcranial magnetic stimulation (rTMS) significantly increased gamma oscillations produced during a working memory test. This means rTMS could be a strategy useful for enhancing cognition.

40 Hz oscillations in the brain have been found to be abnormal in patients with Alzheimer's disease. This 40 Hz response is a major mechanism in brain functioning. In the early stages of neurodegeneration, daily gamma entrainment maintains the number of neurons and synapses in multiple areas of the brain and modifies cognitive performance. Regular gamma entrainment produces many benefits including improved synapse function, greater neuroprotective factors, and decreased DNA damage in neurons. This suggests that daily gamma entrainment could be very helpful in reducing the progression of Alzheimer's for those in the early stages of cognitive decline. Based on research around the benefits of gamma stimulation, it can be expected that routine daily PEMF stimulation at 40 Hz could produce positive results that would safeguard against Alzheimer's disease, such as preventing the development of new plaque, reducing existing plaque progression, and preventing mild cognitive impairment from becoming AD.

Growth Factors and Nitric Oxide: Growth factors are substances (primarily hormones and proteins) that regulate and stimulate various cellular processes. They are essential for the regeneration and healing of tissues after injury. Typically, growth factors act as signaling molecules between cells, binding to receptors embedded in the cell membranes of their target cells. PEMF stimulation fine-tunes growth factors in many ways, but one of the best-understood is by increasing nitric oxide production.

Calmodulin (CaM) is a messenger protein in the cell that binds calcium. It mediates various biologic processes. Once CaM binds to calcium (a process PEMF therapy increases by supporting the necessary electrical charge activity), the resulting cascade catalyzes the release of nitric oxide, and therefore improves growth factors.

A NASA PEMF neural stem cell stimulation study using a 10 Hz square wave PEMF signal found that this PEMF application increased production of over 160 different growth factors that may facilitate nerve regeneration. Evidence to date also shows that PEMFs can significantly increase growth factors throughout the body, whether in the brain, nerves, bones, etc., all contributing to tissue regeneration and healing.

Healing and Regeneration of Tissue: Basic regeneration (that which does not happen because of injury) is part of normal cell function. Cells are always dividing, growing, and eating up their older or injured neighbors (see autophagy above). This does not require any outside stimulation, although it can enhance and ease the process. Injury-induced regeneration and wound healing require significantly more energy and adaptation and, therefore, time.

The body is constantly regenerating itself even without injury; we become completely new bodies about every seven years. This concept is based on the bones recycling completely in seven-year cycles. All organ tissues have their own unique organ repair and regeneration cycles. The cornea of the eye, for example, regenerates every twenty-four hours. Intestinal cells can repair within seventy-two hours. Skin and muscle cells may repair in two to three weeks. Cell turnover slows as we age, but never stops completely, continuing until death.

Injury-induced regeneration and wound healing require a significant amount of energy. To regenerate, a cell's contents must be copied. DNA synthesis or replication requires existing proteins to split and reassemble. RNA messengers help with the transfer of genetic information from the existing cell to the nucleus of the newly formed cell. Regeneration and wound healing also require a great deal of cellular communication and adaptation to take place and rely significantly on the stimulation and production of stem cells and growth factors.

Healing of tissue and regeneration take time and energy. Patience is required. Often, though, this healing process can happen faster, and in some cases in about half the time it would normally take. The FDA–approved PEMF devices for healing nonunion fractures had to be used for between 4 to 12 hours per day to the fracture site. It could take up to 12 months for these nonunion fractures to heal, which may be understandable given the severity of the problem. The time it takes to heal tissue completely depends on the severity of the problem and the health status and age of the person. Youngsters heal much faster than the elderly. We have seen the same healing timeline principles applied above for many of these actions of magnetic fields.

When it comes to healing and tissue regeneration, addressing and resolving the cause of the problem is the goal all physicians aspire to achieve. PEMFs go a long way in helping us to do that, whereas typical conventional treatments infrequently cannot or do not. In fact, physicians rely almost solely on the body's natural capacity to heal, regardless of the age or health status of the person. This is basically like rolling the dice, hoping for the best to happen naturally. PEMFs dramatically improve on leaving healing to chance.

Many of the problems PEMFs are used to address involve musculoskeletal and neurologic tissues, which can be stubborn to treat. We cannot push the tissue to regenerate beyond its optimal capacity. However, PEMFs can stimulate damaged tissue to heal faster, become healthier, and be less likely to have complications beyond what is considered the norm without stimulation. In other words, PEMFs can set new tissue-healing norms. Since magnetic fields interact with and increase natural electrical charges, PEMF therapy can amplify this information transfer. These benefits of PEMF therapy are frequently and, often dramatically, seen with wound healing and tissue regeneration.

PEMF therapy has been used to heal bones, ligaments, and tissues in almost every imaginable situation. Therapeutic magnetic fields accelerate healing through their effects on reduced inflammation, improved circulation, streamlined cellular communication, and growth factors. Magnetic stimulation increases stem cell production, differentiation and maturation, and growth factors.

As mentioned above, PEMF signals have therapeutic effects on damaged tissue but do not seem to affect healthy tissue. This activity of PEMFs primarily on abnormal tissue or functions is another aspect of the appeal of PEMFs for healing.

Immune Function: The body's immune response to disease, especially infection, requires nitric oxide for a variety of reasons. PEMFs assist with this on a basic level by increasing nitric oxide production. This helps lay the foundation for a healthy immune system and is part of why PEMF therapy is so important for prevention.

PEMFs also positively affect white blood cells (WBCs), which play important roles in the body's immune response. In addition, PEMF stimulation can assist with "rolling adhesion." Part of the body's immune response involves a natural inflammatory response characterized by vascular permeability, which, in turn, allows white blood cells (leukocytes) to move through tissues and collect at the site of injury or disease. During rolling adhesion, the WBCs bind to the inner wall of the blood vessel and slowly roll along its surface, inducing chemical changes in the surface of the vessel. These changes result in the WBC migrating through the vessel wall and into the target tissue. The basic actions PEMFs have on transmembrane potentials and ion flow improve this process by increasing the adhesion properties of WBCs and by improving the overall permeability of the vessel walls themselves.

Free radicals are known to interfere with cellular communication and mitochondrial function, damaging the immune system. PEMFs support cellular metabolism, making the body better able to adapt to the presence of free radicals.

Cytokines are chemical messengers in the body that are part of the inflammatory process. Wherever there is significant inflammation, whether it's from obesity, trauma, infections, cancer, toxins, autoimmune disease, etc., cytokine levels are elevated. PEMFs have been found to reduce cytokine levels in areas of inflammation.

Autoimmune disease is indicative of an overactive immune system. So, while we want to enhance immune function in other situations, in the presence of autoimmune disease, the goal is to suppress or reduce overactive immune reactions. PEMFs do not appear to increase autoimmune reactions. On the other hand, PEMFs are unlikely to turn off autoimmune reactions that have already started. The goal in this situation is to help the body to deal with the damage caused by the immune reactions, by reducing inflammation and initiating tissue repair and regeneration. Resolving the autoimmune damage and decreasing inflammation will reduce the related physical and psychological stress in the body and as a result help to tone down the autoimmune activity.

Nerves and Nerve Conductivity: Studies conducted on bone and soft tissue healing using PEMFs in the 1970s found that nerve function improved as a byproduct. After this, researchers began to study PEMF therapy on nerve regeneration directly. Much of the early research was done on animals or in a laboratory.

Damaged nerves repair at extremely slow rates—on average, about 1 mm per month. The body will work to regenerate all nerve injury, even nerves that have been cut through completely. This happens through a process called nerve sprouting.

In the laboratory, research on damaged nerves found that even low-intensity PEMF stimulation produced a 50 percent enhancement in the growth of new nerves. In animals, a slightly higher-intensity PEMF signal produced a 22 percent increase in the rate of nerve regeneration. Other research found that nerve growth factor (NGF), which is lost after major nerve injury, increased in the first 72 hours after the injury using a PEMF signal.

The conduction of currents through nerves follows the same principles as any electrical

current. That means that nerves not only produce charge that creates actions in tissues such as affecting muscles that open or close blood vessels, generate muscle actions, or carrying sensations, but also produce their own tiny but dynamic magnetic fields that affect all the surrounding tissues. This is especially important in the brain, where the different regions constantly talk to each other through nerve conduction and the magnetic field effects produced by neural activity.

Charge movement through nerves involves both action potentials and activity involving synapses. These are called action potential currents and post-synaptic currents. Synaptic currents follow a much slower recharging process and usually involve several thousand adjacent nerve processes. PEMFs affect both of these types of currents or nerve activity.

Damage or injury to nerve fibers causes nerve pain (neuropathy). The damage to nerves can be due to trauma, infection, metabolic changes, burns, radiation, autoimmune reactions, or toxicity. So, any treatment that improves the cause of, or reaction to, the nerve damage will improve nerve function. Inflamed or irritated sensory nerves tend to be hyperactive. PEMFs often help to resolve the underlying cause of the nerve problem and quiet the overactive nerves.

Slowing down nerve firing was shown in research on myelinated nerves. Nerve traffic decreased to zero after five minutes in a relatively high-intensity magnetic field and after ten minutes in a lower-intensity field. It is thought this is caused by the displacement of calcium ions across the nerve cell membrane. This is another example of how stronger PEMFs produce faster results.

High-intensity PEMFs rely heavily on activation of neurons by the high-intensity magnetic fields. The number of neurons stimulated depends on the intensity of the stimulus. These high-intensity stimuli have a net result of disruption of any abnormal pattern of neuronal activity occurring in the brain at the time of the stimulus. Simultaneously, there is activation of current in many nerve cells that release multiple neurotransmitters. The release of the neurotransmitters then causes their own beneficial actions in the brain.

Oxygenation: Low oxygen levels in the body cause cell injury, with the degrees and lengths of time tissues are oxygen-deficient determining the degree of damage. The vast majority of cellular functions depend on an adequate supply of oxygen.

PEMFs can significantly increase oxygen levels in tissues by improving circulation, helping the body transfer oxygen from the air into the lungs and blood, affecting the ability of hemoglobin to carry oxygen, and helping the oxygen in hemoglobin to transfer into the tissues. One study focused on the effect magnetic fields have on the gas-transport function of blood during oxygen deprivation. They found that magnetic field therapy changed the shape of the hemoglobin molecule from a form that was less reactive to oxygen to a form that was more reactive, positively influencing the gas-transport function.

In bronchitis and emphysema or pulmonary edema with heart failure, there is poor oxygen exchange from the air into the air sacs in the lung and then into the blood. This is called oxygen exchange. PEMFs reduce the inflammation in these conditions, allowing better oxygen exchange and improving the saturation of oxygen in the blood, that is, as measured by pulse oximetry.

A study was done on patients with terminal emphysema. These patients received PEMF therapy (just thirty minutes per day for seven days) in addition to their standard medical care. The addition of the magnetic therapy improved blood oxygen levels by as much as 21 percent, and all patients reported greater stamina. It's likely that these results would have been even more dramatic if the treatments were done earlier in the disease state and for longer times since the oxygen exchange mechanisms in the body would be better overall.

One of the earlier demonstrations of the benefit of PEMFs in improving oxygenation was done in Germany in the early 1990s using a large PEMF plate. They found that PEMF effects could be increased during periods of high muscle activity, after drinking alcohol, while sleeping, or after inhaling CO_2. Hyperventilation and large meals would reduce the magnitude of the effects. In their studies, they found that blood volume increased, oxygen levels increased, and pH became more alkaline.

PEMFs can help with oxygenation during exercise with oxygen therapy (EWOT) and hyperbaric oxygen therapy (HBOT). Unfortunately, PEMFs, unless they are battery-operated, cannot be used inside HBOT chambers because of the electrical risk. PEMF therapy may be used before and/or after HBOT. It may be best to do PEMF therapy before HBOT to increase the oxygen in the blood and tissues first, followed by the pressure therapy to drive the oxygen better into the tissues. Most of the conditions benefiting from HBOT are also benefited by PEMFs, even without HBOT. The combination of the two would be expected to produce even better results.

Ozone therapy is used to increase the delivery of oxygen into the body. There are other benefits from ozone therapy, as well. Since both ozone therapy and PEMFs increase delivery of oxygen into the body, it makes sense to combine these therapies. There is research to show that PEMF therapy combined with ozone therapy produces better results than either one alone.

Red Blood Cells: Red blood cells (RBCs) are the primary transporters of oxygen to tissues. They make up 70 percent of all the cells in the body. The sheer number of red blood cells we carry and produce is astounding: upwards of two million per second. Through all the basic mechanisms it affects, PEMF therapy helps facilitate the formation, function, and reabsorption of RBCs.

The majority of oxygen transfer happens as red blood cells travel through the microcirculatory system, made up primarily of capillaries. Capillaries are so incredibly small that red blood cells often must contort themselves, almost folding in half, to squeeze their way through. A phenomenon known as the "rouleaux effect" makes this process difficult or impossible.

A rouleaux formation is a stack of red blood cells stuck together. It closely resembles a stack of coins and is therefore commonly referred to as "coining." Capillaries can only accept a single RBC at a time, so healthy circulation requires that coining or rouleaux be prevented from happening as much as possible.

Because PEMF therapy facilitates a balanced cellular membrane charge, it has a direct effect on RBC activity. Properly charged red blood cells will repel from one another. There are many examples of this on the internet shown by practitioners using dark field microscope samples. Aside from preventing rouleaux, PEMFs' separation of RBCs allows for a greater available surface area for oxygen and nutrients to be absorbed and exchanged. PEMFs can enhance the release of oxygen from hemoglobin, with only ten to thirty minutes of exposure increasing the rate of oxygen release for several minutes to several hours.

Skin: The skin is the largest organ in the body in surface area. It consists of three layers: the epidermis, the outermost layer that provides a barrier between us and the outside world; the dermis, the middle layer, made up of connective tissue; and the hypodermis, the deepest layer, made up of connective tissue and fat. Skin also contains a variety of structures including nerves, blood vessels, hair follicles, sweat glands, oil glands, and lymph vessels. In addition to protecting our bodies from the environment, skin regulates body temperature through sweating and blood vessel dilation to allow for evaporation and radiation of the body's own heat. Plus, it allows for the release of toxins in perspiration.

In humans, only the cells in the outermost 0.25–0.40 mm of the skin are exclusively supplied by external oxygen, although this amount relative to total body respiration is negligible. Therefore, any stimulation that increases blood supply to the skin, such as PEMFs, also improves respiration. PEMF therapy can increase the respiratory rate of regenerating skin by as much as 70 percent, preventing skin breakdown.

PEMFs also inhibit a process called lipid peroxide oxidation, which destabilizes cellular membrane charge and inhibits respiratory enzymes. Lipid peroxide oxidation, which is the process of breaking down fats in the tissues, generates damaging free radicals in the tissues. This is considered one of the key processes for aging of the skin.

PEMFs have been used successfully in the treatment of eczema and psoriasis by reducing the number of mast cells (a type of white blood cell that causes allergic symptoms) in the skin. PEMFs decrease the number of mast cells in skin by as much as 200 percent.

As part of the healing process, skin cells migrate in response to the level and direction of charge in the tissue. Since electrical charges interact so dynamically and directly with magnetic fields, PEMFs have a direct effect on skin wound healing rates. Healing rates vary depending on the location of the skin wound. Wounds in the hands and feet will heal faster than the skin in other parts of the body.

The general actions of PEMFs also provide a variety of other benefits to skin, including improving circulation, reducing edema and inflammation, resolving infections and the impact of insect bites, stimulating tissue regeneration and healing of cuts and wounds by increasing collagen production, improving cellular nutritional status, and much more.

Whenever you're treating any part of the body with PEMFs, the skin in the area is, of course, also getting treatment. Regular use of PEMFs will keep the skin younger-looking by slowing down the natural aging breakdown of repair processes. Although a study has not been performed on this directly, clinical experience and feedback from people using PEMF therapy suggests their skin feels and looks younger. This is an exciting area to explore in future studies.

Stem Cell Stimulation: Stem cells are able to become (differentiate into) specialized cells and can divide to produce more stem cells. In humans, the two main types of stem cells are embryonic (found in the developing fetus) and adult (found in various tissues). Adult stem cells act as the body's repair system, replenishing damaged tissues. They are found in bone marrow, adipose tissue, and blood and in the umbilical cord immediately after birth. All undifferentiated stem cells in the blood have to be turned into differentiated stem cells in the tissues or organs needing repair or regeneration.

Adult stem cells have less differentiation capacity than embryonic stem cells, so stem cell therapies don't always work well without additional external stimulation, such as with PEMFs. PEMF therapies help stem cells differentiate themselves into specific tissues to help with regeneration and healing. This can be used as a therapeutic modality to address an injury or disease state, and also as a health maintenance modality.

Every tissue has its own supply of stem cells available and ready to regenerate and repair tissues as they are injured or die off naturally. The goal with PEMF therapy is to stimulate stem cells that are already present in tissues to keep those tissues healthy. It takes less energy to maintain health constantly than to repair or regenerate tissues after injury. Either way, health maintenance or repair/ regeneration using PEMFs has been shown to be possible and effective.

PEMFs also increase RNA building blocks of neuronal progenitor embryonic stem cells. Human bone marrow stem cells (hB-MSCs) can differentiate into nerve cells and PEMFs induce this differentiation. Proteins turned on through PEMF stimulation may help as a therapeutic option for treating neurodegenerative diseases. PEMF stimulation increases the amount of viable stem cells by 40 – 59 percent and results in up to 60 percent higher cell densities. The PEMF exposed hB-MSCs have the ability to differentiate into multiple types of cells. PEMFs also differentiated neural stem cells and neurons.

NASA studied the use of 10 Hz PEMF stimulation on the growth of nerve stem cells. With their particular 10 Hz signal, NASA discovered about a 400 percent increase in neural stem cells and this signal turned on about 160 growth and regeneration genes.

In line with the NASA research, PEMF stimulation of Schwann cells was studied. Schwann cells are a variety of nerve-associated cells that keep peripheral nerve fibers alive. PEMF stimulation produced high regeneration ability. A PEMF has an additive effect on human dental pulp stem cells. The stimulated Schwann-like cell improved nerve regeneration after transplantation into a body. Therefore, PEMFs improved peripheral nerve regeneration.

Ongoing research on PEMF stimulation of stem cells demonstrates that PEMFs not only helps for health maintenance by enhancing stem cell function and production, but also helps with tissue healing. In the future, we will see a lot more use of stem cells to heal various parts of the body. It appears that PEMFs can help with increased stem cell harvest, increased differentiation, and better preservation of the tissues into which the stem cells are being implanted, and likely will increase the ability of those stem cells to be successful.

It is said that "you can't grow a garden in the swamp." Anybody planning on getting stem cell therapies should consider using PEMFs beforehand to prepare the "garden" before planting stem cells. Then after stem cell therapy, when PEMF therapy is continued, the cells are more likely to differentiate, growing in number, surviving better, and maintaining healthier tissue.

PEMFs and Water

Another noteworthy way in which PEMFs can improve and help maintain your health has to do with their beneficial effects on water, both the internal water of our bodies and through drinking magnetically treated water. Up to 60 percent of the human adult body is water. The brain and heart are composed of 73 percent water, and the lungs are about 83 percent water. The skin contains 64 percent water, muscles and kidneys are 79 percent, and even the bones are watery, at 31 percent.

Since water is the medium through which all electrochemical activity in the body takes place, its ability to respond to an electromagnetic field is a major aspect of the actions of PEMFs in the body and critical in the body's health maintenance and healing process. Research shows that all magnetic fields, including PEMFs, are capable of changing the properties of any solution with charge, and thus will have a direct effect on the water in our bodies.

When cells are studied under an MRI (which replicates a powerful PEMF treatment), water is observed to act differently from when it is not exposed to a magnetic field. Molecules are re-formed in smaller clusters in a linear arrangement. The molecules are lined up and move in and out of the cells easily.

In contrast, when water is photographed after being removed from MRI exposure, molecules are randomly ordered and cluster with neighboring water molecules to form large molecular clusters. Interestingly, when cancer cells are studied under MRI influence, its water molecules are also organized and calm, in contrast to their aggressive, violent movement without MRI exposure.

I have read unpublished reports that Eastern Europeans and Chinese have, since the 1980s, found that magnetically-treated water may help to dissolve kidney stones and gallstones. Since calcified stones in the body are often associated with nano-bacteria, water may help to gradually degrade the stones through a process of erosion, similar to the wearing action of water on rocks in nature. In addition, the ability of oxygen to dissolve in water has been demonstrated by the use of magnetic fields.

Since the 1980s, it has been well-documented that magnetic fields can change various physical, chemical, and obvious properties of liquid solutions, including surface tension, electrical properties, and the ability of substances to dissolve in magnetic field-exposed solutions. Calcium compounds demonstrate long-lasting changes in conductivity on exposure to magnetic fields. Subsequently, when these magnetically exposed solutions are applied to nerve cells, they have been shown to cause both physiological and biochemical changes. Even when water is studied outside the body, research shows that a brief magnetic field exposure can create changes in fluid conductivity for at least two and half hours after the exposure. Water-salt interactions may well underlie biological magnetic field sensitivity. The solutions altered by PEMFs can produce changes in cell membranes and metabolism. These findings explain why PEMFs can positively affect the water in our bodies' cells, tissues, and organs.

Then there are the effects that PEMFs and other magnetic fields have on external water supplies, beginning with the way these fields are capable of restructuring water. For example, research demonstrates that magnetically restructured water produces a synergistic effect on the insecticidal activity in solutions. These results imply that magnetically restructured water could play a significant role in managing different crop pests, as well as human and animal diseases, allowing less than the recommended concentrations of insecticides, antibiotics, fungicides, and other pesticides to be used.

Growth of algae, a form of bacteria, in solution has also been shown to significantly affected by direct and indirect magnetic field exposure. Indirect exposure was done by exposing the solution the algae were to be grown in first and then after the algae were introduced into the treated solution. The results showed that the magnetic field influenced "structural chemistry" of the water to produce "live water" structures. This is significant because different water structures can influence bacterial nutrient uptake, enzyme activities, and the orientation of precursor biomolecules in the liquid crystalline phase during growth. This means that biochemical processes in organisms are affected both directly and indirectly.

The degree of these effects increased with increasing duration of magnetic field exposure.

Water treated with magnetic fields will first affect whatever grows or lives in that water, including cellular molecules, making the water "live." Even the growth of fungal spores is decreased by up to 83 percent if the water is pretreated with magnetic fields. Research also suggests treating drinking water with PEMFs will positively alter its molecular composition, making it more readily absorbed by the body and having positive therapeutic effects.

In one experiment, water exposed to 0.1 T and 0.25 T magnetic fields increased activation of chick pancreas digestive and salivary enzymes, enhancing the breakdown of the substances these enzymes work on, and at a faster than normal rate. Similarly, pretreatment of drinking water before eating can improve digestion.

Magnetically treated water (MTW) has been used for therapeutic purposes at a health resort for several years. Drinking magnetized water and taking magnetized water baths produced favorable results in patients with hypertension, gastrointestinal, and skin diseases. Their overall health improved, and they also experienced decreased fatigue and improved sleep.

Researchers also studied whether there might be a direct bactericidal effect of MTW. This was confirmed by experiments with mineral water. The maximum gross concentration of bacteria decreased from 60/ml in untreated samples to 40/ml, 8/ml, and 2/ml at field intensities of 50, 115, and 140 mT, respectively.

At the same health resort, detailed analysis was done of the health of patients treated with and without MTW. Those receiving MTW had a decrease in heart rate, improved cerebral blood vessel tone, and a decrease in systolic blood pressure.

In addition, water in an oral irrigator treated with magnetic fields was shown to significantly decrease formation of supragingival calculus and its accompanying plaque. This is important, since plaque and gum disease are major contributors to heart disease and other health conditions.

The probable mechanism for this effect of magnetically treated water involves calcium ions. The magnetically affected ions reduce the attachment of plaque and calculus to the gingiva. This effect may be similar to that seen in the use of magnetic fields in industrial water storage tanks to reduce slaking, or clogging of the storage tanks with calcium deposits.

PEMFs and Marijuana (Cannabis)

Marijuana (cannabis), both for medical and recreational use, has become legal in many states in the US and throughout Canada. Though the debate continues about the potential risks and benefits of recreational marijuana, the medical uses of marijuana are increasingly recognized and accepted by researchers. Marijuana acts throughout the body on tissue and cell receptors in what is known as the human endocannabinoid system (ECS). Research is now revealing that PEMFs, in addition to their health-enhancing actions described above, also act on the ECS, and that some of the common actions of marijuana/cannabis are also seen with PEMFs.

Why the Endocannabinoid System (ECS) Is Important to Your Health: Substances called cannabinoids (CBDs) were first discovered in marijuana/cannabis plants in the 1940s. Since then, we have known that cannabinoids help the plants ward off predatory insects, while attracting pollinators, and help them survive harsh environmental conditions, including frost, heat, and dehydration. In 1988, researchers discovered cannabinoid receptors in animals. They also found that these receptors outnumbered all other receptors in animal brains. Since these receptors were inside the body, they came to be called endocannabinoids. Endocannabinoids are found in all animals except insects, as well as in human beings, with their locations being unique to each species' endocannabinoid system.

Research indicates is that the ECS can be activated or enhanced both by acting internally on endocannabinoid receptors already active in the body, and through the intake or application of external cannabinoids, including cannabis and hemp-derived CBD. Cannabis/marijuana contains both THC (tetrahydrocannabinol) and CBD, the most active components, among many other compounds.

Hemp plants contain more CBD, and cannabis plants contain more THC, the compound that causes the "high" that people associate with cannabis use. Hemp-derived CBD products with less than 0.3 percent THC are legal under federal law. The benefits of CBD do not depend on whether it is cannabis-derived CBD or hemp-derived CBD. Common side effects, such as an upset stomach, feeling tired, or feeling on edge, remain the same. This is because the chemical make-up of CBD does not depend on which plant it comes from. It is generally thought that THC acts mostly on the nervous system, whereas the CBD also acts more commonly on the rest of the body.

Types of Cannabinoid Receptors: A receptor is like a lock that has to be opened or activated, usually by a molecule, to create its actions. There are two basic types of endocannabinoid receptors, CB1 and CB2. CB1 receptors are found mostly in the brain and spinal cord, while CB2 receptors are found everywhere else throughout the body.

The first receptor-activating molecule was discovered in 1992 and called anandamide (AEA), *ananda* being the Sanskrit root word for "bliss." Years later another important activating molecule called 2-AG was found that activated both CB1 and CB2 receptors. There are many other endocannabinoids with lower levels of activity, primarily acting to boost the activity of the main endocannabinoids. Lipid molecules normally in the cell membrane are converted into the endocannabinoid receptors, and the body produces endocannabinoids as needed.

Endocannabinoid Functions: The ECS helps maintain functional balance in the body (homeostasis), and plays vital health-enhancing roles via it actions on sleep, mood, memory, appetite, physical activity, pain perception, and immunity, among many other functions. An adequately functioning ECS also helps us to be energetic, focused, and healthy. When the ECS function is impaired, whether due to problems with producing ECS receptors or their proper functioning, many problems can occur.

People with various conditions have deficient cannabinoid numbers or function. Common conditions include irritable bowel syndrome (IBS), fibromyalgia, and migraines. Inflammatory nervous system conditions, such as Parkinson's, Alzheimer's, multiple sclerosis (MS), and Huntington's disease, are being studied to see if cannabinoids can help slow or stop them. Even depression and PTSD are thought to have an endocannabinoid deficiency aspect. In addition, certain cancers have higher levels of cannabinoid receptors, meaning that they are seeking more of the activating molecules, AEA and 2-AG. Research shows that supplying the body with cannabinoids or stimulating their production not only helps with symptom management in individuals with cancer, such as pain, sleep, anxiety and nausea, but can also help ease the side effects of chemotherapy and directly attack cancer cells.

The ECS also plays important roles in brain function, including memory. The development of plaque in the brains of Alzheimer's patients may be caused by endocannabinoids blocked in the brain. In addition, one of the best-known effects of cannabis is to help with fear, anxiety, and depression.

The ECS also helps energy production, storage, and expenditure, and may be useful for dealing with metabolic disorders, such as obesity, diabetes, and cardiovascular disease. However, the low-grade inflammation and insulin resistance associated with these conditions can be aggravated by overactivity of the ECS. In obese patients with type-2 diabetes, for example, a CB1-blocking drug has been found to help decrease blood glucose levels and lower inflammation beyond what weight loss alone could do. On the other hand, the CB1 blockade can cause significant psychiatric problems.

PEMFs and ECS Activation: Although there is very little research yet on the impact of PEMFs on the endocannabinoid system, since the ECS is so important and extensive in the human body, it is hard to imagine that PEMFs don't have some effect on these ECS receptors. I was encouraged when I saw the paper *"Repetitive high-frequency transcranial magnetic stimulation reverses depressive-like behaviors and protein expression at hippocampal synapses in chronic unpredictable stress-treated rats by enhancing endocannabinoid signaling"*(Xue). This research article tells us that PEMFs have an effect on the ECS receptors in the brain If that's true for humans, PEMFs will almost certainly also have a positive impact on ECS receptors and actions throughout the body. This makes a lot of biologic sense and may be one of the important reasons for the vast range of actions of PEMFs on human function and physiology. It's known that PEMFs have actions on many different types of receptors, not just in the ECS, and with a lot of overlap of action among them.

A specific form of PEMFs, called repetitive transcranial magnetic stimulation (rTMS), is FDA-approved for the management of treatment resistant depression. In addition, TMS is being studied for a large range of different types of neurological and other health conditions. A study was done to evaluate the impact of rTMS on the ECS of the brain related to the management of depression. Previous research has definitely shown the involvement of the ECS in depression. Chronic stress in both humans and in animals increases the risk of depression. Much of the effects of chronic stress impacts the hippocampus of the brain. The hippocampus regulates emotion and susceptibility to chronic stress through its connections with the amygdala and limbic hypothalamic-pituitary-adrenal axis.

The major findings of this study were as follows: (1) rTMS improved depression-like behaviors induced by chronic stress; (2) the expression of various ECS-enhancing receptors increased in the hippocampus following rTMS treatment; on the other hand, the amount of enzymes that break down endocannabinoids decreased after rTMS treatment, thus showing a dual action of rTMS; (3) rTMS elevated the amount of CB1 in hippocampal astrocytes and neurons. These data together indicate that the activation of the ECS in the hippocampus is involved in the antidepressant effects of rTMS treatment.

In addition to rTMS affecting the ECS, another study found that longer-term use of lower-intensity PEMFs also affects the ECS, especially neural brain cells. Glutamate is an excitatory neurotransmitter in the brain. Glutamate-induced neural overstimulation (excitotoxicity) is a common cause of many neurological diseases. The role of PEMF in glutamate-induced excitotoxicity was evaluated in relation to the ECS. (Li) PEMF exposure of mouse hippocampus neural cells (HT22 cells) in cultures was studied, with a 15 Hz, 9.6 gauss peak magnetic field for four hours in two protocols, plus 20 and 24 hours of glutamate treatment. In another protocol, PEMF was for four hours, followed ten hours later by another four hours plus 24 hours of glutamate treatment. The most significant effects were seen in the extended PEMF exposure of a total of 8 hours.

The PEMF stimulation improved the life span of mouse hippocampus neural cells (HT22 cells) and reduced cell death after induction of excitotoxicity. A CB1 receptor-specific inhibitor suppressed the protective effects of PEMF exposure. AEA and 2-AG were elevated following PEMF exposure, showing that the neuroprotective effects of the PEMF were related to modulation of the ECS. These results suggest that PEMF exposure leads to neuroprotective effects against excitotoxicity by acting on the ECS. The ECS can regulate glutamatergic synaptic transmission and neural plasticity. Activation of ECS signaling inhibits excitotoxicity and therefore plays an important role in neuroprotection against ischemic stroke or traumatic brain injury.

The most encouraging aspect of these studies using different intensities of PEMFs is the strong probability that PEMFs applied anywhere in the body are likely to have impacts on ECS receptors anywhere in the body. There is also a strong probability that PEMFs can work synergistically with the intake of cannabinoids, whether marijuana- or hemp-derived CBD. This could also mean that dosing with marijuana and/or hemp CBD may be able to be reduced when combined with PEMFs. It could also mean that PEMFs may be able to reduce the side effects of marijuana /CBD when used in combination.

To summarize the health and wellness benefits that PEMF therapy can offer, the main thing to point out is that addressing even one of the above issues can have a tremendous impact on the rest of your life. Oftentimes, these issues can be intertwined with one another. This means that treating one concern effectively can lead to solutions for others, with the same general treatment able to be used on a number of problems. And in terms of prevention and health maintenance, because of the subtlety and widespread effects of PEMFs, you may never know what you prevented.

With so many possible benefits of using PEMF therapy, there is little reason not to at least consider it. The difference it can make for you could be life-changing. Because of the many benefits it provides, I am confident that appropriate PEMF therapy will supplant many traditional therapies and health maintenance approaches in the next few years.

How to Apply PEMF Therapy to Obtain the Most Benefit

In the previous chapter, you learned about the many ways that PEMF therapy supports and enhances health. In this chapter, you will learn how to best apply PEMFs in order to get the most benefit from each of those mechanisms of action, using local, regional, or whole-body applications.

Every time PEMF therapy is performed anywhere on the body, many or most of these actions are activated. The body decides which ones are given priority and will occur before others. For example, while you may desire improvement in your circulation as a priority when PEMF is applied, your body may prioritize pain reduction. Even so, you will still receive both benefits, as well as the benefits from all the other mechanisms of actions.

Some specific actions may be more relevant and effective for specific conditions. Yet, even if the goal is to treat a specific condition, many, if not most, of these actions will be induced by the PEMF therapy to varying degrees. This is one of the phenomenal aspects of PEMF therapy. No one mechanism of action alone is likely to produce the best results. Rather, it is the combination of these actions that PEMFs stimulate which makes PEMF therapy so potent and valuable in helping with almost any health condition. And, because PEMF therapy is so safe, using appropriate application principles, it can be used across the entire age spectrum, from infancy to old age. Beyond the treatment of health conditions, where significant tissue or organ changes have already happened, PEMFs help cells that are minimally damaged or injured before the damage becomes cumulative enough to cause disease. This means that regular use of PEMFs can take care of the "cleanup business" in the body frequently enough that medications and medical procedures become significantly less necessary. Even if they are necessary, PEMFs continue to do their work along with them to produce even better and faster results. For example, I once worked with an orthopedic doctor who had a significant drop in the number of surgical procedures he needed to do when he started working with PEMFs.

Intensity Matters

The degree of impact of these physical actions of PEMFs depends on the intensity of the magnetic field and the depth of penetration into the body. Within the last ten years, PEMFs have become available at higher levels of intensity that enable them to not only penetrate deeper in the body but also to impact wider areas of the body at the same time. Prior to that, most of the whole-body PEMF systems were very-low-intensity and were not as strong in many of their physiologic actions.

Following the introduction of the very-low-intensity, whole-body PEMFs, we began to see medium-intensity PEMFs covering wider areas and now the high-intensity, whole-body PEMFs that provide high-intensity local or regional coverage. By local, I mean treating the hand, elbow, shoulder, heart, brain, knee, foot, etc. By regional I mean the ability to treat the chest, abdomen, the whole lower back, thighs, lower legs, pelvis, etc.

Whole-body PEMFs are further differentiated into when a single pad or mat is able to be run, or a dual-applicator system when two applicators can be run simultaneously. I call this approach a "magnetic sandwich." (See Appendix C for a more extended description.) This approach allows more uniform and higher-intensity magnetic fields to penetrate deep throughout the body, to help heal deeper tissues and organs. In scientific terms, it acts approximately like a Helmholtz coil setup. Some PEMF systems allow a whole-body pad that can be run at the same time as a local or regional pad, or a combination of these. The "magnetic sandwich" approach has become increasingly important in my work with PEMFs and I recommend it often to get the best therapeutic results, whether for health maintenance, anti-aging, or treating specific conditions.

In discussing the specific physiologic effects of PEMFs, let's consider each one separately and to what extent the specific physical action can be affected. I'm assuming that local and regional treatments are with medium to higher magnetic field intensities. These are seen in the table below. The scale being used is from 1X to 3X, with 1X being the lowest likelihood of activation of that activity and 3X being the highest likelihood of stimulation of that activity. I have further divided whole-body PEMF systems into low-intensity (because they are the most commonly used at this time in the community) and whole-body, high-intensity PEMFs, which are now available as well.

You might ask why I make these distinctions. The reason is that people ask my advice for a vast range of health conditions and no one device will solve all problems. You'd want to have a selection of devices, each of which could solve as many needs as possible. While you may be concerned about one particular health condition, it's quite possible that you may have multiple health conditions. And, when you own a PEMF system, other family members can benefit as well. As a result, you would want to consider a system that will give you the most flexibility, not only for needs you have now, but also for future, unexpected needs, as well.

As an example to help you understand this table, the size of the PEMF physiologic effect on acupuncture points and meridians is going to be larger on specific (local) acupuncture points, slightly less so for treating a larger area (regional), very little for whole-body, low-intensity magnetic systems, and very significantly for whole-body, high-intensity systems. The size of the physiologic effect is largely dependent on the magnetic field intensity of the applicator. Most low- and medium-intensity PEMF systems have higher intensities with local applicators compared to regional sized applicators. Usually, the magnetic field intensity is the weakest for the whole-body applicators in these PEMF systems. But local treatment affects smaller areas of tissue, compared to regional effects versus whole-body effects. If whole-body or regional PEMFs are used, many more acupuncture points and meridians will be activated at a lower intensity, expecting to produce a stronger overall physical effect, although a less focused effect. As a result, there will be more general health benefits produced by exposing many more meridians and points but less benefit to a specific organ. So, if one is intent on getting general acupuncture benefits, higher-intensity treatments would serve best. PEMFs may not produce as strong an acupuncture effect as using a needle, especially if the needle is attached to electric current (called electro-acupuncture). The same concepts would apply to all of the other physical actions.

Let's take another example, using PEMFs for treating infections. A local application of a PEMF is going to help a local infection more than it will benefit a more widespread infection. So, using a local applicator is not likely to help very much with a lung infection and even less so for infection that has spread into the bloodstream. Likewise, treating a lung with a regional applicator is not going to be as helpful for a systemic infection.

Likelihood of Physiologic Effects by Treating Locally, Regionally and/or Whole Body

The table below shows the probable strength of impact of PEMFs on various physiologic or physical actions at local, regional and whole body areas of stimulation. It further breaks down whole body stimulation based on low intensity or high intensity PEMFs. The level of physiologic effect on the different physical actions is graded from x to xxx. For example, acupuncture stimulation would be expected to have most of its effects with locally applied PEMF stimulation, by virtue of stimulating specific acupuncture points. Using a larger magnetic field applicator covering a larger area (regional; for example, over the lung, liver, back, etc.), the effects would be expected to be lower because larger applicators tend to have lower magnetic field strength than local applicators, given the area of the magnetic field. This can be compensated for by using a stronger regional applicator. Low intensity whole body PEMFs would have very weak actions on acupuncture points and meridians. To produce a strong acupuncture effect on acupuncture points and meridians, a high intensity PEMF would be required.

There is more detail provided below the table for each physical action of PEMFs.

It is important to again emphasize that all PEMFs produce multiple actions and one can't really "dial up" a specific action. By considering the type of magnetic field that is used, one might be able to see a larger emphasis for that particular action. However, as can be seen from the above table, there is much crossover in actions being activated based on the area being treated and the intensity of the PEMF. Regional treatment will include local actions, and whole-body treatment will affect regional and local areas, as well. Focused local action will produce the strongest effects locally, along with some general systemic actions. Often, the most efficient treatments will be stronger, higher-intensity whole-body PEMF systems. The trade-off is that these higher-intensity, whole-body systems tend to be more expensive.

What follows is guidelines for applying PEMFs for each of the physiologic actions they provide.

Acupuncture Stimulation: PEMFs interact with acupuncture points and meridians and numerous studies have demonstrated that acupuncture points and meridians are actually part of a comprehensive whole-body electrical system. So, in effect, PEMF therapy acts as a form of milder electrical acupuncture. Whatever

Specific physical actions	Size of physiologic effect			
	local	regional	whole-body low intensity	whole-body high intensity
Acupuncture Stimulation	xxx	xx	x	xxx
Antibacterial, Antifungal, and Antiviral Actions	xxx	xx	x	xxx
Anti-coagulant Effects	x	xx	xxx	xxx
Anti-Edema Activity	xxx	xx	x	xxx
Anti-Inflammatory Response	xxx	xxx	xxx	xxx
Anti-Spasm Activity	xxx	xx	x	xxx
ATP and Mitochondria	xxx	xx	x	xxx
Autophagy	xxx	xx	x	xxx
Circadian Rhythms	xxx	xx	x	xxx
Circulation	xxx	xx	x	xxx
Collagen, hyaluronic acid, and GAGs	xxx	xx	x	xxx
Detoxification	x	xx	xxx	xxx
Endocannabinoid system	xxx	xxx	xxx	xxx
Growth factors and nitric oxide	xxx	xx	x	xxx
Healing and regeneration of tissue	xxx	xx	x	xxx
Heart	xxx	xx	x	xxx
Immunology	x	xx	xxx	xxx
Nerves and Nerve Conductivity	xxx	xx	x	xxx
Oxygen	xxx	xxx	xxx	xxx
Pain	xxx	xx	x	xxx
Psychological and Cognitive Function	xxx	xx	x	xxx
Red Blood Cells	xxx	xxx	xxx	xxx
Skin	xxx	xx	x	xxx
Stem cell stimulation	xxx	xx	x	xxx
Stress	xxx	xxx	xxx	xxx
Water	xxx	xxx	xxx	xxx

the form of stimulation, individual acupuncture point and meridian stimulation eventually cascades to stimulate the entire body over approximately 24 hours. Even local acupuncture point and meridian stimulation will eventually impact the entire body.

From this perspective, it makes sense that local high-intensity treatment will have the strongest effect on local acupuncture points and their downstream meridians. The least impact will be with low-intensity systems, but, because low-intensity, whole-body systems stimulate many acupuncture points and meridians at the same time, the systemic benefits and effects can be strong. Clearly, whole-body, high-intensity PEMFs will have the most impact on the overall acupuncture system. It is not within the scope of this book to go into detail on either the actions of acupuncture stimulation or the specific impacts of treatment of specific points and meridians. There are many books available on the impact of treatment of specific points and meridians and the reader is directed to seek these sources for more in-depth knowledge, if desired.

The bottom line is that every time PEMF therapies are administered, acupuncture stimulation is happening at the same time, thus providing the benefits of both types of therapies.

Antibacterial, Antifungal, and Antiviral Actions: Bacterial, fungal, viral, and even parasitic infestations, all have both local and systemic aspects. Local and systemic involvement can include the organisms themselves; for example, sepsis is a whole-body infection, but can also cause major immunologic and inflammatory reactions that then involve the whole body. The focus of the use of PEMFs is to impact the infecting organisms both directly and indirectly.

I rely on PEMFs less as acting as an antibiotic or antiviral drug than to help the body to deal with the infection and its after effects, which can be more devastating in the long run than the initial infection. The use of PEMFs is important to help the body to be healthier and to resist infections, but also to help the body deal with the infection itself and to repair, heal, and recover.

Since most infections are usually local, local PEMF treatment is going to produce stronger results than whole-body treatment, unless the whole-body treatment is done using a high enough intensity magnetic field to effectively equal higher-intensity local treatment. Because local infections can rapidly move into the body and cause whole-body inflammation and immune changes, whole-body, high-intensity PEMF treatment is the most effective across the spectrum of impact of any infection, helping to heal local infection and protecting the rest of the body from the infection spreading.

Anti-Coagulant Effects: The coagulation system of the body is intended to decrease or stop bleeding and to prevent clotting. Most of the time, bleeding is local from vulnerable tissues (for example, a cut or wound.) However, the entire coagulation system needs to be balanced and prepared to respond to even a threat in a small area of the body. Likewise, a coagulation system that is overly aggressive and primed to clot will initiate undesirable clotting locally. In this situation, it is necessary to treat the whole coagulation system as well as the local problem. An example of this is somebody with diabetes or autoimmune disease where the blood is thicker (more viscous), often associated with inflammation, and when blood flow is reduced or interrupted, making undesirable clots more likely to form rapidly. This is often seen with clots in the legs, called venous thrombosis, which can form when someone is bedridden short-term (for example, a leg fracture) or long-term (for example, recovering from hip surgery in a rehab center).

This is why whole-body PEMF therapy often is preferred to local therapy. Higher-intensity whole-body PEMF therapy is more likely to impact the overall vascular and coagulation system, as well as acting locally. Local therapy can be applied to a local clot, to reduce pain, swelling and the possibility of spreading the clot, but the goal really is to reduce the likelihood of clotting anywhere in the whole vascular system. As a rule, it is not recommended to do PEMF therapy to a local area of bleeding—for example, immediately after surgery—until the bleeding is controlled, because PEMF therapy is very effective in improving circulation and reducing clotting.

PEMF therapy has been shown to act equivalent to the use of aspirin. If PEMF therapy is used at the same time someone is using aspirin, the risk of bleeding or bruising can possibly increase to double over that of just aspirin alone. Likewise, if someone is taking anticoagulants like Coumadin or other anticoagulant drugs longer-term, there is an increased risk of bruising when both PEMFs and these medications are used at the same time. That doesn't mean they shouldn't be used together; it is just that caution should be taken and increased vigilance for bruising or other evidence of bleeding. One strategy would be to lower the dose of Coumadin, aspirin, or nonsteroidal anti-inflammatory drugs, under the guidance of a physician, if one is going to continue to use PEMF therapy for all its other benefits.

Anti-Edema Activity: There are essentially three types of edema (swelling)— local, regional, and whole-body—along with another category, lymphedema. The first three types are due to fluid coming out of the blood vessels into the tissues. Lymphedema involves the backup or blockage of lymph flow. Most of the time lymphedema is regional. The underlying cause determines which type of edema will occur. Improving edema/swelling is important for tissue healing and recovery and pain reduction.

All cells and tissues develop some degree of swelling with "injury" whether a bruise, muscle sprain or strain, cut, burn, insect bite, puncture, etc. Usually, this damage and swelling is local, wherever the injury occurs. PEMFs applied locally will produce rapid results, often within 24 hours. For localized swelling, medium- to high-intensity PEMF therapy can be very helpful, regardless of the cause.

Overall, however, PEMF treatment should be directed to the whole-body to improve the general health of the tissues, combined with a regional treatment. Even more importantly, PEMF treatment should be directed at the failing organ, if that is the cause. For protein deficiency and allergic reactions medical therapies are more necessary. Whole-body PEMF therapy in this case would be best managed by higher-intensity, whole-body PEMFs.

Anti-Inflammatory Response: There is significant research demonstrating the effects of PEMFs on inflammation, both acute and chronic. PEMFs of almost any kind will help with inflammation in the area of application. Smaller PEMFs may be used locally, larger PEMF devices may be needed regionally, and certainly whole-body PEMFs would be necessary for whole-body inflammation, especially with autoimmune conditions. Recent research has shown that the optimal magnetic field intensity to help chronic inflammation is 15 gauss (1.5 milli-Tesla). This is dealt with in much more detail in this book's Appendix A.

Another important aspect of the intensity of the PEMF field needed to optimally manage inflammation is the physical principle of magnetic fields dropping off in intensity with distance from the applicator. This principle is known as "the inverse square law." This law dictates that the intensity of the magnetic field needed to heal inflammation with the optimal magnetic field intensity needs to be calculated based on the distance away from the applicator the target tissue for treatment will be. For example, the intensity would only need to be 15 gauss in the skin. If treatment is needed deeper in the body, for example, to treat inflammation in the kidney, one has to consider the depth of the kidney in the body for the magnetic field intensity to be adequate. Since the back of the kidney is about four inches deep into the average human body, the maximum PEMF intensity would need to be 182 mT (1820 gauss). This means that a PEMF system would need to deliver at least 1800 gauss to adequately target the kidney. This type of calculation would need to be made for any part of the body where PEMFs are used to target inflammation. Fortunately, these calculations have been done and are presented in Appendix A.

Whichever PEMF device is chosen to treat inflammation, the right intensity field is important to achieve the best results, whether treating locally, regionally, or systemically. Treatment times and how often they are applied will vary, depending on the problem and the cause, as well as the intensity of the PEMF field being used. Generally, the stronger the magnetic field, the more likely the results will be better and happen faster. The most common error in choosing a magnetic field is that it is too weak to work well or quickly. Fortunately, if a stronger than optimal PEMF magnetic field is chosen, there is very little risk of harm to the body. Healthy cells essentially ignore magnetic fields, even strong PEMF magnetic fields. A stronger than necessary magnetic field is simply wasted energy. It may still be useful for you for all the other actions that may be needed at the same time.

Even if a problem is local, treatment with a whole-body PEMFs system is not wasted. Since PEMFs have so many different actions, helping other parts of the body that do not have inflammation will likely be beneficial even to the local problem. Inflammation anywhere in the body is a drain on the body's health maintenance resources. Helping the rest of the body during this time of inflammation stress will likely speed up healing and shore up good health that helps the body anywhere else as well.

Anti-Spasm Activity: PEMF research decades ago showed that magnetic fields cause muscles to relax. If they are strong enough, they can also cause muscles to contract. All magnetic fields improve circulation, which is caused by opening up the blood vessels, improving blood supply to any muscles treated with PEMFs. Even local PEMF treatments can somewhat improve circulation away from a local area of stimulation. The strongest effect on the muscle will of course happen where the stimulation is applied.

When a muscle is injured, strained, torn, lacks blood supply, or is not properly balanced by the nervous system or body chemistry, it frequently goes into spasm. Applying a PEMF to the muscle will help it to relax. But healing the cause is important for making the benefit last. The length of time that the PEMF needs to be applied depends on the extent of the injury, the strength of the magnetic field, and how much of the area of the muscle is affected by the magnetic field.

Muscle spasms and tension can be treated with a local PEMF of sufficient intensity. Sleeping on a PEMF whole-body pad of sufficient intensity may also help prevent muscle cramping, among the other benefits that sleeping on a whole-body PEMF pad can provide.

ATP and Mitochondria: PEMFs have been found to increase of the number and size of mitochondria that promote cellular and intracellular regeneration. In addition, PEMFs not only increase the amount of ATP produced but also cause the ATP to release a phosphate molecule, thus producing energy. This whole process is then regenerated over and over again. It is unknown how long the benefits of PEMF stimulation of ATP will last after treatment is completed. Because of the constant recycling of ATP, it's possible this benefit may be short-lived, requiring frequent treatments, depending on the problem.

To affect mitochondria and ATP production, PEMFs can be applied locally, regionally, or systemically. Lower-intensity and medium-intensity PEMFs are likely to do this at a more superficial level in the body. High-intensity PEMFs will stimulate mitochondria and ATP better at all levels of the body. Repeated stimulation daily would likely produce the best results until the goals of stimulation are realized. For health maintenance purposes daily treatments would likewise be needed to optimize the body's health. PEMF stimulation before physical activity or athletic training and competition will increase the amount of ATP available to the muscles and the nervous system for the period of the training and competition. Likewise, PEMF treatment following competition will rapidly restore the ATP that was consumed during activity and competition.

As an example, a colleague of mine who was working with PEMFs during the Olympics more than 20 years ago observed that Eastern European athletes rebounded the next day from tryouts and competition as if they were robots. American athletes took several days to recover. He went past their training area and discovered that they were laying in PEMF devices. So, the Eastern Europeans knew about PEMF therapy for this purpose over 30 years ago.

Autophagy: Autophagy is the natural, around-the-clock process of cellular debris cleanup. It is very important for maintaining cellular health and longevity.

Cells that are choked with cellular debris have shorter life spans, leading to inflammation and increase the risk of cancer development. Autophagy efficiency decreases as we age, especially when we suffer major illnesses and with poor lifestyle factors. Several studies have shown that PEMFs improve autophagy at a basic level, indicating another reason why PEMFs help to maintain health, have an anti-aging benefit, and improve poor health conditions. Autophagy can be affected by application of PEMF fields locally, regionally, or systemically. Lower-intensity and medium-intensity PEMFs are likely to have a more superficial level in the body, whereas high-intensity PEMFs will stimulate autophagy at all levels of the body. Repeated stimulation daily will produce the best results.

Circadian Rhythms: Circadian rhythms are important to maintain the natural rhythms and cycles of most of the functions of the cells and the body. This includes our sleep rhythms. In people with dysregulated circadian rhythms, PEMFs applied to the brain at about 10 Hz have been found to reestablish rhythm. Since 10 Hz may be somewhat stimulating to people, even though it is the alpha, or relaxation, rhythm, it may be best to use this frequency during the day rather than in the late evening.

This 10 Hz stimulation can be especially helpful in avoiding the uncomfortable circadian rhythm changes associated with jet lag. A portable, medium-intensity PEMF system with 10 Hz can be used while in the airplane to help to maintain the circadian rhythms before reaching one's destination. Regular use at the new destination for several days will help to rebalance the circadian rhythm to the new normal.

Other than application to the brain, a medium-intensity PEMF system oscillating at 10 Hz applied regionally or to the whole-body will also be beneficial for aiding the natural clocks of the cells throughout the body controlled by genes, so that these genes operate normally again.

Circulation: Good circulation is critical to providing adequate nutrition and oxygenation to all the cells of the body. As discussed above, PEMFs cause blood vessels to dilate, thereby increasing circulation. In general, whole-body applications produce the best results, although local applications can also help.

PEMFs improve circulation in multiple ways, with the best results determined by how much of the body is stimulated and the depth of stimulation. Local PEMF treatment, even with lower-intensity PEMFs, would produce the most noticeable response locally and a mild systemic response as well. Higher-intensity and whole-body treatments provide the best general benefits to circulation, especially deeper in the body, unless the cause and the problem are very local.

Collagen, Hyaluronic Acid (HA), and GAGs: Collagen, hyaluronic acid, and GAGs form all of the connective tissue and support structures of the body. They can be positively affected by application of PEMF fields applied locally, regionally, or systemically, depending on the target tissue desired to be stimulated. Lower-intensity and medium-intensity PEMFs applied locally or regionally are appropriate for stimulating collagen, hyaluronic acid, and GAGs in superficial levels in the body, for example, the skin, fascia, most joints, tendons, and ligaments. Deeper structures in the body, such as bones and spinal discs, require higher-intensity PEMF fields for adequate stimulation. High-intensity PEMFs will also stimulate collagen, HA, and GAGs better at all levels of the body. Repeated stimulation daily will produce the best results until the goals of stimulation are realized. For health maintenance purposes, daily treatments would likewise be needed to optimize the body's health. Regular stimulation is needed to prevent or reduce the natural progression of aging effects on the skin, joints, tendons and ligaments, bones, and spinal discs.

Detoxification: We not only build up cellular debris, but also metabolic waste. The body needs to adequately and efficiently metabolize most of the molecules in the body, primarily through the liver. Removing this metabolic waste is called *detoxification*. In general, PEMF stimulation of the liver, the intestinal tract, and the kidneys facilitates the detoxification process. PEMFs in relation to the liver can be done with medium- to high-intensity PEMFs. High-intensity PEMFs may be needed to do this efficiently throughout the whole liver because of the size of the liver and the natural loss of intensity of the magnetic field with distance from the applicator. The same applies to facilitating the natural functions of the bowel in eliminating waste. Any waste processed through the kidneys would also be helped by PEMF stimulation of the kidneys using higher-intensity PEMFs.

Endocannabinoid System (ECS): The endocannabinoid system (ECS) is a widespread tissue control system that plays important roles in central nervous system (CNS) development, brain adaptability, and the body's responses to internal and environmental stresses. The ECS is comprised of cannabinoid receptors, cannabis-like molecules (endocannabinoids), and the enzymes responsible for making them and breaking them down. Research shows that PEMFs have a positive effect on the ECS receptors in the brain. PEMF treatments result in neuroprotective effects against overactive nerve cells by acting on the ECS, and therefore play an important role in neuroprotection against stroke or traumatic brain injury. Likewise, higher-intensity PEMFs applied anywhere in the body are likely to have impacts on ECS receptors anywhere in the body. Research shows that PEMFs have a positive effect on the ECS receptors in the brain. PEMF treatments result in neuroprotective effects against overactive nerve cells by acting on the ECS, and therefore play an important role in neuroprotection against ischemic stroke or traumatic brain injury. Likewise, higher-intensity PEMFs applied anywhere in the body are likely to have impacts on ECS receptors anywhere in the body.

Many of the actions of the ECS can be enhanced by treatment of the brain through the local use of medium- to high-intensity PEMFs. Since ECS receptors are also located throughout the entire body, adequate intensity, whole-body stimulation may activate many of the other receptors throughout the body.

Growth Factors: Growth factors naturally produced by the body are necessary for tissue repair, regeneration, and anti-aging. The best-known growth factor is human growth hormone but there are hundreds of others throughout the body. PEMF stimulation fine-tunes growth factors in many ways, especially by increasing nitric oxide production, which improves growth factors. A NASA PEMF neural stem cell stimulation study using a 10 Hz square wave PEMF signal found increased production of over 160 different growth factors that may facilitate nerve regeneration. Another study on stroke showed significant increases in various nerve growth factors. Growth factor increases have also been shown by using PEMFs for bone stimulation. Increases in pituitary growth factors have also been seen. Evidence to date shows that PEMFs can significantly increase growth factors throughout the body, whether in the brain, nerves, bones, etc., all contributing to tissue regeneration and healing.

The release and production of growth factors can be enhanced by application of PEMF fields locally, regionally, or systemically. Lower-intensity and medium-intensity PEMFs are likely to do this at a more superficial level in the body, such as skin and joints. Medium- to high-intensity magnetic fields may be needed for stimulation of growth factors in the brain and central nervous system, for repair and healing of damaged brain and nerve structures. High-intensity PEMFs will likely stimulate growth factors better at all levels of the body. Repeated stimulation daily will produce the best results until the goals of stimulation are realized. For health maintenance purposes daily treatments would likewise be needed to optimize the body's health.

Healing and Regeneration of Tissue: Tissue regeneration and healing is an ongoing, daily, lifetime process. The body's cells and tissues are constantly affected by living, even healthy living, going through cycles of birth, degeneration, and death. This process needs to be maintained at an efficient level to reduce the development of chronic conditions, early aging, and death. Life is also full of minor, and sometimes major, assaults such as bruises, cuts, sprains, strains, and infections, such as colds and flu. All of these events require healing and regeneration to maintain and restore natural functions.

Natural tissue regeneration and healing is not always efficient, depending on whatever else is happening in the body. Augmentation and acceleration of tissue healing and regeneration can be produced by application of PEMF fields locally, regionally, or systemically. Lower-intensity and medium-intensity PEMFs are likely to do this at a more superficial level in the body, such as skin and joints. Medium- to high-intensity magnetic fields may be needed for stimulation of growth factors in the brain and central nervous system, for repair and healing of damaged brain and nerve structures. Since brain tissue and nerve cells take a long time to produce stem cells and regenerate, one needs a long-term perspective for significant healing to be seen. High-intensity PEMFs will likely stimulate healing and regeneration better at all levels of the body. Repeated stimulation daily will produce the best results until the goals of stimulation are realized. In addition, routine daily PEMF stimulation will facilitate natural tissue regeneration processes before significant tissue breakdown occurs. Thus, for health maintenance and anti-aging purposes, daily treatments would be needed to optimize the body's health.

Heart: The heart is constantly pumping 24/7 to provide circulation to the body. Maintaining healthy heart function is critical to healthy living. The main components of the heart that lend themselves well to PEMF stimulation include the muscle, the "nervous system" of the heart, and the heart's arterial blood supply. PEMFs improve the function of all the heart's components. Magnetic stimulation typically causes the heart rate and blood pressure to decrease and results in the cardiovascular system becoming less reactive to the stress of living.

Not only do PEMFs help with the natural functioning of the heart, including reducing effects of aging, but they will also help with many insults to the heart, including improving lack of blood supply, inflammation, aging of the heart's electrical conduction system, augmenting muscle function, and reducing the workload and repairing damage from infections, toxins, trauma, and reduced blood supply.

Because of the inverse square law, PEMF fields need to be chosen which will have adequate depth of penetration of the magnetic field through the whole volume of the heart. The heart length, width, and thickness of the average heart in males are 12 cm (4.7 in), 8.5 cm (3.3), and 6 cm (2.3 in), respectively. They are only slightly less in females. One also has to account for the distance of the heart from the skin of the chest, which is about 1.7 cm (0.7 in). So, to achieve a 15 gauss magnetic field intensity at 7.7 cm (~3 in), one would need to start with a magnetic field intensity of about 1100 gauss applied over the left chest. Also, the applicator of the magnetic field needs to be about 5 inches in diameter.

The most important treatment is local over the heart itself with a sufficient higher-intensity magnetic field. Whole-body, low-intensity PEMF stimulation may help the body in general to relax and improve circulation. These would have secondary and less intense benefits to the heart. Almost any conditions of the heart can be treated. The goals are to improve function, reduce symptoms and help with healing of the heart.

Immunology: The immune system is both local in the tissues and systemic through the various circulatory systems, including arterial, venous, and lymphatic. It is both naturally present constantly, especially in the tissues, and adaptive, usually systemically, to respond to acute insults or demands. An insect bite will create a local immune response. A viral infection like influenza will create a systemic adaptive response.

Immune function can be enhanced by application of PEMF fields locally, regionally, or systemically, depending on need. The same principles that apply to using PEMFs for inflammation can be used for immune function benefits. Local treatment will have mostly a local benefit (for example the insect bite) and a mild systemic benefit. Most of the time, when focusing on stimulation of immune function, there is the need to "go low and slow" (see Appendix B) to be sure overstimulation doesn't occur, regardless of the intensity of the PEMF system used. This is true even with low intensities.

Also, when immune-modulating drugs and other agents are used, it does not appear that PEMFs interfere with their function. In fact, there is the possibility that PEMFs may reduce the need for higher doses by helping the body deal with the background effects of the inflammatory process. However, PEMFs are contraindicated when immune suppression is happening on purpose in the setting of organ transplantation. PEMFs may interfere with immune suppression, thus increasing the risk of organ rejection.

Lower- and medium-intensity PEMFs are likely to improve immune function at a more superficial level in the body, such as skin and joints. Medium- to high-intensity magnetic fields may be needed for enhancing immune function at deeper levels in the body. High-intensity PEMFs will affect immune function more at all levels of the body. Repeated stimulation daily would likely produce the best results until the goals of stimulation are realized. For health maintenance purposes daily treatments would likewise be needed to optimize the body's health. **Remember that the "low and slow" approach should be used when focusing on improving immune function.**

Nerves and Nerve Conductivity: PEMFs have significant impacts on nerves and nerve conductivity, including nerves that are nonfunctioning, damaged, or overactive. Normal nerve function can also be augmented by the use of PEMFs, especially when it comes to muscle rehabilitation or enhancement for sports.

PEMFs also enhance the production of nerve growth factor lost after major nerve injury. The conduction of currents through nerves follows the same principles as an electric current. Any treatment that improves the cause of, or reaction to, nerve damage will improve nerve function. Inflamed or irritated sensory nerves tend to be hyperactive. PEMFs often help to resolve the underlying cause of the nerve problem and quiet the overactive nerves. PEMF therapy has been found to be helpful for any neuropathy, but especially diabetic neuropathy.

Lower-intensity and medium-intensity PEMFs are likely to improve nerve function at a more superficial level in the body, such as skin and more superficial muscles. Medium- to high-intensity magnetic fields may be needed for enhancing nerve function at deeper levels in the body, including the brain. High-intensity PEMFs will likely affect nerve function more at all levels of the body.

Repeated stimulation daily produces the best results, especially in neuropathy and nerve damage, until the goals of stimulation are realized. Nerves regenerate extraordinarily slowly. The greater the nerve damage and the longer the nerve is that is damaged, the longer it will normally take. For health maintenance purposes daily treatments would likewise be needed to optimize the body's health. **The "low and slow" approach should be used when focusing on improving nerve function, to avoid aggravations.**

Oxygen: Oxygen is critical to cell function. Energy cannot be created in the body without oxygen.

There are two main components to oxygen delivery: the lungs and the vascular system or circulation. PEMFs help significantly with both. Lower-intensity and medium-intensity PEMFs can improve oxygen delivery function at a more superficial level in the body, such as the skin, muscles, and joints. Medium- to high-intensity magnetic fields are needed for enhancing oxygen delivery at deeper levels in the body. High-intensity PEMFs will likely affect oxygen delivery more significantly at all levels of the body. Repeated stimulation daily will produce the best results until the goals of stimulation are realized. For health maintenance purposes, daily treatments would likewise be needed to optimize the body's health.

Pain: Pain management is one of the most common applications for PEMFs. Whether the pain is acute or chronic, inflammatory or vascular, musculoskeletal or in the nervous system, PEMFs help address both pain perception (pain blocking) and the cause of the pain itself (pain elimination), as well as pain's other related mechanisms, including inflammation, swelling (edema), apoptosis or necrosis, diminished circulation, decreased cellular metabolism, and impaired cellular repair processes.

Lower-intensity and medium-intensity PEMFs help pain at more superficial levels in the body, such as the skin and joints. Medium- to high-intensity magnetic fields are needed to reduce pain at deeper levels in the body. High-intensity PEMFs will help alleviate pain at all levels of the body. Higher-intensity magnetic fields generally produce results better and faster, as well, especially when dealing with pain perception by stimulating the brain. Repeated stimulation daily will produce the best results until the goals of stimulation are realized. Routine treatment, even after the pain is gone for some period of time, is needed to be certain the tissues have fully healed so the pain won't come back. For health maintenance purposes, daily treatments would be needed to optimize the body's health and keep the cause or source of pain from returning. (See Chapter 9 for more detailed information about the pain conditions PEMFs are proven to help alleviate.)

Psychological and Cognitive Function: As you learned in Chapter 3, PEMF stimulation impacts psychological and cognitive function both directly and indirectly. Indirect benefits are especially significant when symptoms are present in other parts of the body away from the brain and nervous system.

Lower- and medium-intensity PEMFs provide some benefit for psychological and cognitive function when applied anywhere on the body. But these results are likely to be very short-lived and need to be repeated frequently. Medium- to high-intensity magnetic fields are needed for helping psychological and cognitive function by stimulating the brain at deeper levels. Entrainment effects are stronger with higher-intensity fields, as well, and higher-intensity PEMF fields generally produce results better and faster. Repeated stimulation daily will likely produce the best results until the goals of stimulation are realized. Routine treatment even after symptoms are gone for some period of time may be needed to be certain the brain has sufficiently changed so the issues won't come back. For health maintenance purposes daily treatments would be needed to optimize the body's health and keep the cause or source of the psychological and cognitive dysfunction from returning.

Red Blood Cells (RBCs): Among their other functions, RBCs are critical to delivering oxygen to the tissues. Circulation, inflammation, edema, and immune actions all influence RBC flow.

PEMFs maintain the charges on the outside of RBCs so that they don't clump together. This separation of RBCs allows for a greater surface area for oxygen and nutrient exchange. In addition, PEMFs increase the release of oxygen from hemoglobin. A short period of exposure can increase the rate of oxygen release up to several hours.

PEMFs have a positive effect on reducing RBC clumping or sludging of flow. Treatment anywhere in the body will have an impact on RBC function. Even local treatments improve this benefit systemically, as the blood flows through the tissue over and over again in the area of the magnetic field. The longer and more frequent the exposure the greater the benefit. Increased RBC clumping can be local, regional, and systemic. Since local or regional treatments will have the most effect in those areas, the location of need and the targeting of treatment become important to know. Whole-body therapy would produce significant improvement, even with low-intensity PEMFs, because of the total area of exposure. High-intensity, whole-body PEMF therapy would have the strongest and longest acting action.

Lower-intensity and medium-intensity PEMFs provide benefit for RBC functions when applied anywhere on the body. But results may be short-lived and need to be repeated frequently. Medium- to high- intensity magnetic fields are needed for improving RBC functions by stimulating at deeper levels. Higher-intensity magnetic fields generally produce results better and faster. Repeated stimulation daily would likely produce the best results until the goals of stimulation are realized. For health maintenance purposes, daily treatments would be needed to optimize the body's health.

Skin: The skin is the largest and most superficial organ of the body. It is the most susceptible to PEMF therapy, even low-intensity treatment. The most important function of the skin is to protect our bodies from the external environment. As a result, environmental factors, such as heat, cold, sun radiation, etc., result in the need for treatment, whether with PEMFs or otherwise. The skin also routinely manifests an outward expression of many problems deeper in the body and is frequently in need of help because of these. But a less known function of the skin is respiration. Any stimulation that increases blood supply to the skin, such as PEMFs, also improves respiration. PEMF therapy can increase the respiratory rate of regenerating skin by as much as 70 percent, preventing skin breakdown.

PEMF fields also inhibit lipid peroxide oxidation, which destabilizes cellular membrane charge, inhibits respiratory enzymes, and generates damaging free radicals in the tissues, all of which are key causes of premature aging of the skin. In addition, PEMFs have a direct effect on skin wound healing rates, with the healing rates varying depending on the location, cause, and depth of the skin wound.

Other PEMFs benefits to skin include improving circulation; reducing edema and inflammation; resolving infections and the impact of insect bites; stimulating tissue regeneration, resulting in the healing of scars, cuts, and wounds, by increasing collagen production; improving cellular nutritional status; and much more. Whenever any part of the body is treated with PEMFs, the skin is also getting treatment because the magnetic fields have to pass with the skin first. Regular use of PEMFs will keep the skin younger-looking by slowing down the natural aging breakdown of repair processes. Clinical experience and feedback from people using PEMF therapy indicate that their skin feels and looks younger.

Lower-intensity and medium-intensity PEMFs provide benefits for healthier skin when applied at the skin surface anywhere on the body. Results may be short-lived and need to be repeated frequently, depending on the stressors that are placed on the skin.

Many people are mostly interested in the anti-aging effects of PEMFs on the face. For this purpose, PEMFs delivering a minimum of 15 gauss work best. Medium- to high-intensity magnetic fields are needed for healthier skin by stimulating at deeper levels. For whole-body PEMF therapy, the magnetic field needs to penetrate at a sufficient intensity to maximize the benefits over the entire skin surface. For example, when laying on one's back and doing whole-body PEMF therapy, the magnetic field intensity on the other side of the body, due to the inverse square law, is dramatically weaker. Unless one uses higher-intensity whole-body magnetic fields that would provide at least 15 gauss on the other side of the body, a PEMF mat may have to be applied on both sides of the body. Hence, the "magnetic sandwich" approach (see Appendix C.) with higher-intensity magnetic fields would work the best for whole-body skin therapy. Higher-intensity magnetic fields generally produce results better and faster. Repeated PEMF stimulation daily produces the best results.

Stem Cell Stimulation: One of the goals of PEMF therapy is to help stem cells differentiate themselves into specific tissues needed for regeneration and healing. Stimulating stem cells with PEMFs not only increases the production, differentiation and survival of the stem cells, it also increases the growth factors needed for the stem cells to do all these things and provide the benefits of regeneration and healing.

Not only can PEMFs be used as a therapeutic modality to address an injury or disease state, they can also be used as a health maintenance modality. By encouraging existing stem cells to maintain their regeneration capabilities, you ensure they are available to differentiate or reproduce at the first sign of damage or breakdown. PEMF therapy is to be able to stimulate stem cells that are already present in tissues to keep those tissues healthy. It takes less energy to keep tissues in a constant state of good health than to repair or regenerate tissues after injury. Either way, health maintenance or repair/regeneration using PEMFs has been found to be possible and effective.

As with so many other actions of PEMFs, intensity matters. PEMFs create an environment for stem cells to grow and flourish. As I've said many times, "you can't grow a garden in the swamp." When trying to stimulate stem cells, the environment in which you want to stimulate stem cells has to be conducive to not only producing the stem cells but also encouraging their survival and function. The same PEMFs that would be considered for stimulating stem cells would have all the other actions described in this chapter as well.

Lower- and medium-intensity PEMFs provide benefit for stem cell stimulation and differentiation when applied superficially anywhere on the body. Results may be short-lived and need to be repeated frequently, however, depending on the stressors that are placed on those tissues. Medium- to high-intensity PEMF fields are needed for stem cell stimulation and differentiation at deeper levels. Higher-intensity magnetic fields generally produce better and faster results, especially deeper in the body. Repeated stimulation daily produces the best results and helps maintain and optimize the body's health.

How long PEMF therapy needs to be done for stem cell stimulation depends largely on the tissue type. The same applies to any other healing and regeneration treatments. Some tissues simply take longer and are more challenging to regenerate. The work is not done when the stem cells have regenerated because our goal, after all, is not to stimulate stem cells but to regenerate the tissues being treated. This is one of the reasons that stem cell therapy should not be done without the use of PEMFs, not only while trying to grow and implant the stem cells but also to make sure they regenerate the goal tissues.

Stress: Stress has at least two components, the brain and the body. The brain perceives the stress and responds to it. The response is both local in the brain at first and then in the rest of the body. The response of the rest of the body, in the short-term, is physiologic. If this continues long-term it may reset different organs and tissues to become chronic. So, treatment of stress responses with PEMFs should concentrate both on the brain and on physiologic functions in the rest of the body. Focus on the brain is the most important aspect.

Lower- and medium-intensity PEMFs may provide some benefit for stress when applied anywhere on the body. But results are likely to be very short-lived and need to repeated frequently. Medium- to high-intensity magnetic fields may help reduce stress by stimulating the source of stress reaction, the brain, at deeper levels. Positive, stress-reducing entrainment effects are stronger with higher-intensity PEMF fields, as well, which also generally produce better and faster results. Repeated stimulation daily to the brain and body will produce the best results until the goals of stimulation are realized. Routine treatment, even after symptoms are gone for some period of time, may be needed to be certain the brain has sufficiently changed so the stress response issues won't come back. For health-maintenance purposes, daily treatments will be needed to optimize the body's health and keep the cause or source of the stress-related dysfunction from returning. The goal of PEMF therapy is to reduce the physical aspects of stress reactions. The stress triggers are most often psychological catalysts mediated through the brain. So, PEMF therapy is not going to be as effective in the long run if not combined with dealing with the cognitive/psychological factors involved in the stress precipitant and response.

Water: Our bodies are composed of 75 to 80 percent water. We eliminate several liters per day through excretion, evaporation, and respiration. Our bodies also make water through their own metabolic processes. Our G.I. tract can produce as much as 10 liters of water per day, which is then mostly reabsorbed in the colon. Our bodies are very inefficient in their use of externally provided water. The water molecules produced by our bodies are much more efficient in their ability to be absorbed, utilized, and excreted. PEMF therapies change the bond angles of water molecules to make them more usable by the body. Even seeds and plants given magnetically treated water have been found to significantly grow better.

Lower- and medium-intensity PEMFs, when applied anywhere on the body, can provide some action on the body's water content. Medium- to high-intensity, whole-body PEMF fields are needed for stimulating body water at deeper levels throughout all of the cells of the body, with higher-intensity PEMF fields generally producing better and faster effects. PEMF water treatment effects are short-lived, typically lasting only about eight hours. So, whether treating water for intake directly or treating the body's water content, daily treatment is needed. For health-maintenance purposes, daily treatments with a sufficiently strong PEMF would be needed to optimize the body's health, as water is continually consumed by and produced in the body.

Summary

As this and the previous chapter make clear, PEMFs have a myriad of positive actions in the body. Because this is so, PEMFs can be used to treat individual health conditions to great effect. PEMF therapy will have some degree of benefit for almost any health condition because most conditions have many overlapping components that PEMFs address.

When we accumulate a certain set of undesirable physical signs, symptoms, and functions, we see patterns and apply a medical label to the condition— for example pneumonia, arthritis, heart disease, cancer, hypertension, or inflammatory bowel disease. The practice of medicine evolved over the centuries by discovering one malady after another, defining it and then proceeding to ascribe treatments specific to that malady. This process discounts the complexity of the human body's reactions and the complexity and interactions of the harms that befall the body. Many doctors are beginning to recognize that this approach is inadequate in dealing with complex systems and the need for new and more effective comprehensive therapies.

The future of medicine lies in developing complex, coordinated, complementary and integrated strategies to deal with these complex problems. PEMF therapies have that potential and have been shown by research to provide multiple health-enhancing benefits. The scientific evidence clearly shows that PEMFs have many actions in the body, all of which coordinate together to help the body to deal with various health conditions. This is why I consider PEMF therapy, of itself, to be such a worthwhile approach for maintaining and improving health, both within a clinical setting and as a home self-care tool. I also consider PEMF therapy as a safe and effective approach, to be necessary to make most other therapies work better. No single therapy can do it all. But PEMF therapy as a single therapy can do more and more efficiently than most other therapies, and has the most enduring value, to be able to be used day after day, in the convenience of the home setting.

In addition, PEMF therapy can also be used in conjunction with other therapies to create synergistic effects that increase the effectiveness of those therapies and PEMF. (You will learn how and why this is so in Chapter 6.)

Additional Guidelines for Using PEMF Therapy

Once you have access to a PEMF system, you need to apply PEMF correctly to get the most benefit from it. This is very important. PEMF treatment outcomes are largely dependent upon directing the magnetic field therapy to the correct area or areas of the body. Treatment parameters for doing so are made up of location, duration, and programming. This chapter provides further information about how you can most effectively use PEMF therapy.

Where to Direct PEMF Therapy

At the most basic level, applying PEMFs is as simple as directing the applicator (mat, pad, pillow, or coil) on or near the area of your body that requires treatment. This is easy when you have an obvious health problem. For example, if you have a broken bone, place the applicator over the break area. If you have a digestive problem, place the applicator over your belly. If you have a dental problem, treat the area over the tooth.

Your body is a complex organism, and while it is made up of many moving parts, it is still one interconnected whole. It is the philosophy of integrative medical practitioners to treat the whole person. To that end, it is often preferable to treat the entire body when using PEMFs, even if what you identify as needing treatment is only a small area of your body, such as a localized pain or swelling. Whole-body stimulation can also be augmented by local treatment. Whole-body stimulation by PEMFs tends to provide the most benefit in terms of preventative care as well.

Even in my early days of working with magnetic fields, I knew that PEMF therapy stimulates acupuncture points and meridians. Traditional Chinese medicine holds that there are as many as two thousand acupuncture points on the body. These are connected by twenty meridians, which are highways of communication and energy exchange. These meridians are not only connected to one another, but also to the body's internal organs, the senses, and the supporting tissues. Treating the entire body at once stimulates all of these acupuncture points and meridians, all augmenting each other, resulting in a more complete therapy.

This level of stimulation cannot be done using acupuncture needles. This is another reason why I strongly emphasize whole-body PEMF stimulation.

If you are working with a whole-body PEMF system, I recommend that you do at least one treatment per day on the whole-body mat. Twice a day whole-body treatment is preferred. The morning treatment is to "shake off the cobwebs" from the night before. The end of day treatment is to "shake off the stress" that we all accumulate as we go through our daily lives. You can then do other local treatments (either immediately after a whole-body treatment or later in the day or night) with the smaller pad that most whole-body PEMF systems include, directing it towards any specific problem areas of your body. If you own a whole-body system that allows two applicators to be used at the same time, treatment with a whole-body pad may be combined with local treatment simultaneously.

If your goal is general health maintenance, whole-body treatments are ideal. When you expose any portion of the body to a PEMF signal, you affect many different chemical, functional, electric, and magnetic processes. Exposing the entire body at once both simplifies and amplifies these effects.

Sometimes, when there are problems such as an ache or pain, the location of where the pain is felt is not necessarily where the problem itself originates in the body. Sciatic pain is a common example of this type of referred or trigger point pain. You may experience the most pain in your leg, but the cause originates from the base of the spine. Were you to treat only your leg, you likely would not achieve the best results from your PEMF device. I recommend getting clinical advice on the source of your pain so that your PEMF treatment can be most appropriately targeted. Armed with that information, if you treat the entire body, you'll be covering all your bases. Whole-body PEMF therapy takes the guesswork out of knowing where on the body to direct treatment. Particularly in cases of pain, I often recommend treating both the painful area and the spine directly. This way, you are treating both the area where the pain is felt and the area where the pain may be originating.

Whole-body PEMF systems always include a mattress applicator and usually also include a smaller pillow pad applicator as part of a standard package. The mattress applicators vary in weight, size, appearance, and portability, but all contain some configuration of copper coils embedded within them. If you have time, it's a good idea to first use the whole-body pad for a session, and then follow that up with a treatment using the smaller pillow pad, if you have a local area on your body that needs more attention.

If you are using a localized PEMF device, often your biggest challenge will be knowing where to direct the magnetic field. This is easy in the case of an obvious injury like a broken bone, but more difficult when dealing with a systemic or complex health concern.

Localized PEMF devices have all of the same components of many of the whole-body systems on the market, they just tend to come in a smaller package with a smaller applicator. Most of the time, they tend to be stronger than whole-body pads. Some localized PEMF devices are battery-powered and portable, making them convenient to use while on the go.

Whether you work with a whole-body system or a localized device, the PEMF treatment process is virtually the same. In both cases, you power your unit on and apply the PEMF field to your body. This means you will either lie or sit down on a mat (in the case of a whole-body system) or hold, strap, or wrap the applicator to a chosen body part (as is often the case with portable devices).

General Rules for Application of PEMF Fields

I recommend the following approaches for achieving the best results with PEMF therapies and to avoid any significant adverse effects.

- Applicators should be located as close as possible to the body. Using a system over a shirt or jacket versus directly on the skin makes no difference.
- Other therapies may still be used and considered in a complementary approach (see Chapter 6).
- PEMF therapy should be applied as soon as possible after a problem begins. PEMFs typically influence and resolve acute issues more rapidly than chronic or pathological problems.
- Treatment sessions must be long enough and repeated regularly. Consistent use provides the best results.
- Do not stop PEMF therapy until a sufficient number of treatments have been performed or rebound may occur.
- Individualization of the approach is necessary, especially in painful conditions.
- As with any other self-care approach, consult your doctor or other health care professional before beginning any new treatment.

How Long to Use PEMF Therapy

One of the most common questions people have before starting PEMF therapy is about how quickly they will see results. The answer depends on a variety of factors. Once the nature and severity of your health concern is understood, expectations can be reasonably set and an estimate can be made as to when and what improvement may be anticipated.

PEMF treatment times vary based on the system you are using. As a general rule, I recommend a minimum of 30 minutes of treatment applied twice per day, but your individual health circumstances and the intensity of the PEMF system you use will determine your actual needed treatment time.

You also need to have a good understanding of the intensities of the system you are using. Most of the time, smaller applicators are significantly stronger than the whole-body pads. While whole-body pads may be effective for local problems, extra attention with a higher-intensity local applicator may be better.

If you have a portable system, you can also do continuous treatments. If you have an extremely high-intensity system, as little as five minutes of treatment may be all that is required for some problems. Some PEMF systems, both portable and whole-body, can also be run overnight while you are sleeping, both to help with sleep and also to help with chronic, stubborn problems.

If you have had a health problem for a long time, or if your health issue is severe, you will get better results from longer treatment times. You needn't be concerned if longer treatment times are required because, unlike pharmaceutical drugs, you cannot be harmed by therapeutic magnetic fields because PEMFs pass completely through the body.

Another factor to consider when applying PEMF treatments is how long you should continue to do so over time. In general, I find that continuing treatments at least twice as long as the time it takes you to feel better is optimal. For example, if you have a painful condition that resolves after six weeks of daily PEMF treatments, I recommend continuing your daily treatments for up to another six weeks (12 weeks total). Just because you managed your pain symptoms does not mean that you have fully healed their underlying cause. The additional six weeks of daily treatments will help ensure that the underlying cause is resolved, as well, reducing the likelihood that your pain will recur at a later date. There are some, if not many, cases where you may have to apply daily treatments indefinitely. This is particularly true for chronic or degenerative issues, especially those with mechanical causes. Mechanical causes would include scars, discs or bony protrusions pressing on nerves, incompetent valves in the heart veins, implanted hardware, among others.

Because PEMFs are so excellent for preventative and anti-aging care, I also recommend that if you own a PEMF system, you never stop using it.

Managing Treatment Expectations: Having proper expectations is important when applying PEMF therapies. If you are depressed or anxious, for example, small health improvements may seem inadequate. To set realistic expectations, you must first understand the nature of your health problem, the depth of the damage or dysfunction associated with it, the types of tissues involved and their respective regeneration potential, and your age and overall health status.

Everybody is different, and every health condition is unique. Many people experience tremendous results within the first week or two of using their PEMF system. For other people, results may come more slowly. The progress of your healing can be enhanced by fine-tuning your treatment protocol.

Even when it is given the appropriate signal or stimulus, the body takes time to heal. A fracture, for example, will take eight to twelve weeks to heal to a point where the bone can be used. This does not mean the healing process is complete, only that the bone is usable once again. PEMF therapy can speed the healing rate, but it does not typically cause instantaneous healing. Illness rarely, if ever, occurs instantaneously. The same is true of healing. If we did not get to our current health state overnight, we are unlikely to heal overnight. You should be suspicious of anybody who tells you that you can expect miraculous results from your PEMF system, especially overnight.

Truly acknowledging the damage present in your body is a critical piece in solving the healing timeline puzzle. Gauging a specific tissue's degree of involvement in the given health concern is important to understand the amount of time it will take for that tissue to heal. Problems in the body have various degrees of involvement, and different tissues are involved in any given condition. Understanding what level or levels of the problem or problems you are treating will help you better determine how quickly healing responses will likely occur.

Most people starting PEMF therapy feel more relaxed and sleep better relatively quickly.

Pain reduction often happens to a significant degree early in the process, as well, and then gradually improves even more with continued use over time as tissue healing progresses. Even for tissues that do not have the capacity for full regeneration, PEMFs are valuable in reducing pain and swelling, improving circulation, and stimulating whatever regeneration may be possible.

As with all other types of therapies, PEMF therapy will not work adequately or completely for everyone, however. In research studies, there are always a percentage of participants that experience little to no benefit from the therapy. Though it is often possible that these participants would have found improvements with different parameters (more time, higher-intensity, or different frequencies), PEMF therapy is not a panacea, and there are circumstances where no benefit will be found. I often tell people that PEMF therapy does not raise the dead, whether bodies or tissues. A scar is still a scar. It may be a better-looking scar with PEMFs, but it is still a scar. To learn more about why PEMFs don't always work well and what can be done about it, please see Chapter 11.

How to Program PEMF Treatments

Instructions for programming your PEMF treatment is difficult to address in general terms. User manuals for PEMF systems are technically simple and vague and cannot possibly address every health condition. Even if they could, everyone is different and has a different body composition, vitality, mentality, and availability, making blanket statements rarely reliable.

I usually have people start off using their system in a "low and slow" fashion (for more on this see Appendix B) on a low- or medium-intensity setting to lessen the risk of any initial adverse reactions they may experience. It's best to work your way up to using the highest possible intensity the system you use will allow. Some people will reach the highest intensity in a few days, while others will need to progress more slowly. Rarely will people not be able to tolerate the highest intensity.

Since there are so many frequency options and program options in available PEMF systems, it is not possible to make specific types of program suggestions here. The following guidelines are still useful, however. (**Note:** If you choose to purchase a PEMF system from DrPawluk.com, you will receive personalized recommendations for appropriate use directly from my team and from me.)

Selecting Treatment Parameters: Mild problems that don't have deep levels of pathology, such as a mild muscle or ligament strain, a superficial burn, cut, insect bite, bruise, or puncture, will heal rapidly. In these situations, a minimum amount of PEMF stimulation may be all that is necessary. If you use your system for just five or ten minutes, or use it at a low-intensity setting, and do not get the results you want, you may need to increase your treatment time or intensity level. Trust your body to tell you what it needs.

In some cases, the best results will be achieved with 24 hours a day of use for a few days. After that, less time will usually be appropriate. Of course, this isn't usually feasible unless your PEMF system runs off batteries. Most PEMF systems limit treatment time cycles. If longer treatment times are required, you can apply several back-to-back treatments to extend the total amount of treatment time. PEMF systems that run continuously can be used for as long as you wish without having to reset them after each treatment run.

The bottom line is that there is no hard and fast rule as to the maximum treatment time that is needed. PEMF manuals may recommend specific treatment times, but remember that you cannot be harmed using the PEMFs I recommend if you choose longer treatments. By listening to your body, you will know when you have received enough treatment each day. Body signals indicating that it's time to end your PEMF session vary significantly from person to person and may include feelings of jitteriness or a feeling of excessive energy.

Selecting Treatment Locations: The best place to conduct a PEMF treatment is wherever you are most likely and comfortable to use it. Whole-body systems will require a reasonably flat, preferably firm surface. This can be either a bed, floor, massage table, recliner, lounge chair, or couch. Local system applicators can be applied lying down or sitting, even at a work desk. Small, portable PEMF systems can be used even while being active. Some people relax, nap, read, listen to music, or watch TV or movies while they do their treatments. Since most PEMF treatments tend to promote relaxation, you may find reading can be challenging while a treatment is happening.

Most PEMF systems—except for the high-intensity ones—will usually not interfere with electronic devices, meaning you can usually do work on a computer, laptop, or mobile device without problems. However, with high-intensity PEMF systems, I have personally blown two remote control units and had my laptop freeze, fortunately without any damage. It's usually advisable to remove electric watches and cards with magnetic strips. It's also best to follow the precaution recommendations in the user manual, especially for electronics implanted in the body, including pacemakers, defibrillators, pain modulators, insulin pumps, cochlear and hearing aids implants, among others. The rule of thumb for high-intensity PEMF systems is that electronic devices should be kept two to three feet away from them. Always follow manufacturer instructions.

Using Low- Vs. Medium- Vs. High-Intensity Systems: Every PEMF system has limitations or characteristics for treatments. These will determine how you use your device and how you will see benefits happen. The time that you have available for treatment is another major factor to consider. Deeper, more involved, complicated, and severe problems will take longer to heal and require more treatment time. Low-intensity systems typically take the longest time to produce notable benefits, especially with those problems needing deep healing. There are always exceptions to this rule, however.

Even if you want to use a high-intensity system for healing, the ways that tissue can respond might still be a limiting factor. PEMFs cannot make tissues do anything they aren't naturally capable of doing. Higher- intensity levels and more time do not always get the job done faster or better. While little harm can be done from extended exposure, your results may not happen any faster or as fast as you may hope. Finding the right balance of time and intensity is an important determining factor in the success and timing of your healing.

Treatment Consistency: It's always preferable to do daily treatments with your chosen PEMF system as opposed to infrequent, high-intensity treatments or an increased intensive number of treatments back-to-back to speed things up. The dynamics or momentum of your underlying problem will often determine the level of intensity or density of the number of treatments you require. Understanding the "momentum" or aggressiveness of the particular negative process of the tissue will tell you how often you have to receive treatments. For example, if you are treating pain and the PEMF reduces the pain significantly but it returns in four hours after you finish your treatment, then it may be best to repeat your treatments every four hours. Over the ensuing few days, it may take six to eight hours before the pain returns. With continuing treatment, the time before pain returns usually gets longer. In such cases, the interval between treatments would then increase gradually as the healing process of the body progresses and takes more permanent hold.

I see people who achieve pain relief for weeks after a single treatment and then, as the problem seems to return, they do another treatment, with relief then also lasting for a few more weeks. Other people do not achieve pain relief until two or three weeks after they've begun their treatments. Consistent daily home treatment then becomes much more important to keep up with the frequency of treatments the body needs to continue to maintain relief and achieve more permanent healing. In time, the hope is that the pain-relieving treatments are not needed at all, after which time the PEMF system can simply be used for health maintenance or until a new problem arises. Thankfully, your PEMF system will have you ready to deal with it.

Special Considerations: Referred Pain and Trigger Points: Referred pain presents in an area of the body different from its source and must be treated differently than traditional acute or chronic pain. There are numerous areas in the body where pain is felt remotely away from the actual area in the body that is causing the pain. Knowing whether you have referred pain or not is important, since it will change the approach you take for the treatment.

A problem in the back may lead to pain being felt in a hip, groin, or in the lower extremity. Treating the back will provide a better pain solution than treating the area where you feel the pain. Similarly, neck problems can cause referred pain in the shoulders, upper chest, upper back, or down into the arms and hands, in which case treating the neck area as well as the area where the pain is felt will be necessary.

In addition to typical neurological referred pain, that follows dermatomal patterns, you can have very different referred pain patterns associated with trigger points. These are also managed similar to referred pain approaches. Finding the trigger point and treating it is critical to dealing with this type of pain. Other information resources or clinicians can guide you on referred pain or trigger point patterns.

Using Magnetically Treated Water

Science shows that magnetically treated water is more usable by the body and the cells. Rather than relying upon expensive specialty waters to obtain the benefits that magnetized water provides, once you own a PEMF system, you can create your own "activated" water.

There are no hard and fast rules with this process. Some Russian literature states that 25 minutes on a medium-intensity PEMF device structures a two-liter bottle of water. Low-intensity PEMF systems may have less of an effect or may take longer to create an effect on restructuring water.

I do not recommend using plastic or metal containers when magnetically treating water. Glass containers with plastic caps are preferred because PEMFs may be able to dislodge plastic molecules into the water, particularly if lower-density plastic containers are used.

If you are using your whole-body system and are lying on your back, simply place the glass container between your legs and expose the water to the magnetic fields for about 25 minutes. Minerals in the water will magnetically structure the water faster because of resonance and ion charge production effects. It's better not to use distilled water without adding trace minerals.

Water activated by externally applied PEMF fields may not hold the restructuring for a long time. Therefore, it needs to be consumed the same day it was produced. A fresh batch will need to be produced every day. There is no rule regarding how much water should be consumed for optimal benefits. What is most important is to drink the amount you need to stay hydrated.

Magnetically treated water can be consumed like normal water. It can also be added to smoothies, to brew teas and make coffee, and for soups. It can also be used as the water you give your pets and to water plants.

Safety Concerns and Dealing with Potential Adverse Reactions

As mentioned, the risk of adverse reactions when applying PEMF therapy is not common. In some instances, though, they can occur. The best way to deal with potential adverse reactions is to anticipate them. Because PEMF therapies have such a wide array of actions within the body (see Chapters 3 and 4), you may experience some discomfort, especially when your treatment has just begun. It is my experience that these reactions happen about 5 percent of the time, and tend to be more common when the entire body is treated, as opposed to local treatments. They are also more common with higher intensities, and less so with increased time. To reduce the risk of uncomfortable reactions, see the directions in Appendix B, for "low and slow" protocols.

Most adverse reactions, if they occur, are mild and temporary and can be managed by simply continuing the therapy. These reactions are more common and more uncomfortable in individuals with electrical and electromagnetic hypersensitivities. Yet even in these cases, rarely does PEMF therapy have to be discontinued.

As you learned in Chapter 3, PEMF therapies can affect circulation, stimulate cell and tissue repair, stimulate nerve cells, cause relaxation, affect blood pressure and heart rate, alter the absorption of medications and nutrients, affect acupuncture energy movement, and stimulate vision changes, among many other actions. Because of this, overreactions by the body, whether just perceived or actually measurable, do happen. The two most common types of adverse reactions that some people experience when first applying PEMF therapy are related to circulation and nerve cells.

Sudden increases in circulation, especially in ischemic tissues (areas with restricted or reduced blood flow) and highly inflamed areas, might cause uncomfortable increases in circulation for a short time after PEMF therapy has been applied. This increase in circulation, while usually a desirable effect, can in some cases lead to a surge in oxidative stress. Therefore, it is desirable to have adequate antioxidant support in the body before beginning treatment.

Sudden improvements in circulation may also lead to aggravations of existing extensive or severe inflammatory processes, typically in the skin. Aggravation of hives is likewise possible and should be considered before starting treatment if there is a history of hives.

When nerve cells are suddenly stimulated, pain may be temporarily aggravated due to the increased signal traffic in the nerve and/or improved circulation to the nerve(s). We see this in individuals who have had prior fractures or scars in the area of injury. Even PEMFs applied away from the fracture site or scar may temporarily cause pain at the fracture site. If there are multiple pain-producing blockages along the body, PEMF treatment may cause the phenomenon of "chasing the pain." This process becomes like peeling the layers of an onion, to get to the deepest layers of a problem.

Contraindications

The major caution or contraindication for use of a PEMF device is placing an active applicator over implanted electrical devices such as pacemakers, cochlear implants, intrathecal pumps, etc. PEMFs, as well as other magnetic fields, can shut these devices off or otherwise interfere with their function. This is very important if somebody with an implanted electrical device has been told that they cannot do MRIs. More recently, manufacturers are designing implantable electronics that are "MR conditional." This means that these devices can be used in MRIs under certain circumstances. Devices that are MR conditional are unlikely to be affected by PEMFs, even high-intensity PEMFs. Nevertheless, proceed with caution and obtain direction from the manufacturer or professional.

PEMFs are also contraindicated in organ transplant patients. This is because these people are on immune suppression medications to prevent organ rejection. We do not want to risk adversely affecting the immune suppression/rejection process. There is a chance that PEMFs may actually stimulate or activate a more aggressive rejection process by stimulating the immune system.

The safety of PEMFs has not been established in pregnancy, although there is no evidence of harm. Nonetheless, most manufacturers warn against the use of their device during pregnancy. PEMFs should also be used with caution in Grave's disease because of over-activation of the thyroid gland, and in the case of active bleeding, because PEMFs decrease platelet adhesion.

Extremely high-intensity PEMFs should be used with caution or under professional supervision in people with implanted metals, such as joint replacements, dental implants, mechanical heart valves, metal stents, or metal staples in blood vessels or the intestines. Most implanted metals are biologically inert, as opposed to ferrous metals which can be affected more by PEMFs. Any effect of PEMFs on metals is not due to risk of injury or harm, but because extremely high-intensity PEMFs may stimulate the nerves in the area of the metal, causing sharp pain. In the long run, PEMFs around metal help the metal to integrate better into the body and reduce the inflammation caused by the foreign body material. **High-intensity PEMFs may also add to the shear stress of metal clips placed in or near blood vessels. High-intensity PEMFs to these areas in these situations should be avoided.**

High-intensity PEMFs were previously thought to be undesirable for breast implants. However, recent medical recommendations are to do periodic MRI screening of breast implants for contractures and the risk of cancer. High-frequency PEMFs beyond 100 Hz are probably also not desirable for treatment durations longer than an hour at a time, given the risk of agitating the plastic or silicone in breast implants, resulting in possible thinning and risk of leakage.

Occasionally, when one area of the body is treated and improved, another area that may have been quiet might show pain or discomfort. Normally these problems are not a concern, but should be recognized as a normal consequence of PEMF therapy. In some situations, when PEMF therapy causes pain in an area of the body part that does not normally have pain, this may indicate an unidentified underlying problem in the body part, and medical evaluation should be considered. In this case, PEMF therapy serves as an early-warning process.

Overall, the risk of adverse reactions caused by PEMF therapy is very low in comparison to other therapies. As with any other therapy you may start for the first time, begin slowly and pay attention to what you experience during and after each PEMF session, following the guidelines I've provided in this chapter and in Appendix B.

Precautions

Despite PEMF's generally recognized safety, account must be taken of some possible actions that should be considered in using this therapy. While few of these are serious, they must be anticipated and people should be alert to their potential.

Precautions should be taken in introducing PEMFs with people with autoimmune disorders, particularly those with severe conditions. In those situations, our motto is to go low and slow. Use a low intensity to begin with, gradually progressing the time and intensity to tolerance.

Adrenal gland, hypothalamic, and pituitary dysfunctions that are clinically significant enough to be endocrinologically or physiologically symptomatic may be over-stimulated by PEMFs before the body is ready to deal with that level of stimulation. Again, the rule is to go low and slow.

Active infections, whether bacterial, viral, or fungal should be managed appropriately medically because PEMFs may not have a predictable or fully reliable benefit, especially in the early stages of more severe infections. However, once medical therapies are initiated, PEMFs may be used to help with the management of the infection.

Cancer is not a contraindication to the use of PEMFs. However, the sickest individuals who are the most depleted by their cancer therapies are going to be the most vulnerable to excessive PEMF stimulation. Go low and slow here as well. Current evidence appears to suggest that PEMFs can be an appropriate complementary and integrative approach to use in the management of cancer, along with behavioral management, nutrition, and lifestyle.

Individuals with psychoses or acute major psychological states should only be managed by experienced professionals in attempting the use of PEMFs. There is new and ongoing research exploring the use of high-intensity PEMFs to the head in these conditions, but there may be unpredictable results, unexplained relapses and, in combination with powerful psychotropic medications, PEMFs may cause significant reductions in blood pressure and destabilize patients under control. Appropriate use and understanding are required to prevent problems.

Based on available research, PEMF therapy appears to be useful in the management of neurological diseases with seizure disorders, but any expectation of stopping medication needs to be mindful of clinical and legal implications. PEMFs need to be applied in these situations with caution and careful consideration.

Excessive menstruation is similar to active bleeding and PEMFs need to be used with caution so that blood loss is not increased.

Caution should be exercised in people with known low blood pressure, or predisposition to it, as well as people with severe or accelerated hypertension since sudden, significant blood pressure decreases may occur, causing vertigo or fainting. This reaction usually disappears within thirty minutes after the exposure and adaptation usually begins after five exposures.

In those with significant cardiac arrhythmias, proceed with caution and consultation with a physician. While PEMFs may be helpful to reduce the sensitivity of the heart to whatever is triggering the arrhythmias, they may activate the electrical activity of the heart, potentially temporarily aggravating an arrhythmia. There is also a possibility that PEMFs may make medications used to control arrhythmias be much more effective, creating the possibility of increased risk of reactions from the medication.

High-intensity PEMF muscle stimulation without adequate preconditioning of the muscle or prolonged stimulation may increase the risk of muscle soreness or bruising. Muscles that are already sore are likely to be helped by PEMF therapy but gradual increases in intensity should be used to determine the level of discomfort. Likewise, other areas of significant tenderness in the musculoskeletal system, such as over bones or joints (for example, tennis elbow, shoulder bursitis, etc.) should be approached using a low and slow protocol. Highly inflamed nerves, in the case of radiculopathy, also need to be managed with a more low and slow protocol.

Electrohypersensitivity (EHS) is a concern for many people. It is most likely caused by excessive mast cell activation or histamine hypersensitivity and is more likely to be caused by EMFs or frequency-based PEMFs, especially higher-frequency PEMFs, for example, greater than 100 Hz. This seems to be less of an issue with the impulse-based systems. PEMFs are less likely to initiate an EHS episode than to aggravate an already active process. While PEMF therapies may be helpful to reduce the inflammation in a body that may be an underlying cause, there is a balancing process needed between aggravation and treatment. One of the first steps in managing EHS is to remove as much EMF stimulation from the environment as possible to reduce precipitating, initiating, aggravating, or compounding effects before successful PEMF therapy may be used.

Using PEMF in Combination with Other Therapies

In this chapter, I am going to provide you with what you need to know to create and maintain an overall healthy foundation for yourself using diet and nutrition. This is vitally important, because without such a foundation, you won't have enough "charge" and cellular building materials for PEMF therapy, or any other therapies for that matter, to work with. Lacking these fundamentals to work with will make the benefits of PEMFs more difficult to achieve.

Then I am going to tell you about other useful therapies that can be used with PEMF therapy to enhance its effectiveness and vice versa.

Dietary Guidelines and Nutritional Supplements

While PEMF therapies provide a large array of actions that support health and reduce the problems associated with many health conditions, these actions produce better results when PEMFs are part of a more comprehensive wellness approach, including optimal nutrition support and, as necessary, various nutritional supplements.

A healthy diet is a vital cornerstone of optimal health. The foods you eat supply the fuel your body needs—in the form of vitamins, minerals, enzymes, amino acids, essential fatty acids, and other nutrients—to perform its vast number of daily functions. It is estimated that every cell in the body has thousands of chemical processes per second that need to be supported. The better your fuel supply (the foods you eat) is, the better able your body will be to generate energy, repair itself, and resist disease. Conversely, poor eating habits diminish your body's ability to maintain optimum health. They also reduce the degree of benefit you will gain from PEMFs and any other type of therapy. As Hippocrates, the Father of Western Medicine, advised many centuries ago, "Let food be thy medicine, and medicine thy food."

The key to eating well is to eat foods that will provide your body with what it needs to maintain your health. In general, since inflammation is a significant component of most health conditions, an anti-inflammatory diet is usually most helpful. A diet which consists of more raw vegetables and fruits is generally the most anti-inflammatory and is what I recommend to my patients.

It's also a good rule of thumb to eat foods as nature provides them so that the essential nutrients they contain are most available to you. This approach includes consuming whole fruits, especially with their rinds, rather than commercial fruit juices because of the sugar content of juices. When you drink a glass of orange juice, for example, you are getting the sugar equivalent of up to six oranges. You would never eat six oranges at a time. When the sugar is liberated from the fiber of the pulp, it becomes much more readily and rapidly absorbed into the blood. That rush of sugar into the bloodstream is never good and can be inflammatory. Poisoning yourself with sugar and then trying to treat yourself with PEMF therapy is like trying to put out the fire of inflammation while continuing to pour gasoline on the fire. That's not very smart and rarely effective. Were you to instead eat the whole orange, you would not only avoid this sugar rush, but also get the health benefits of the fiber and bioflavonoids that oranges contain.

Another important aspect of healthy eating is nutrient density. This has to do with how much nutrition there is in a food in comparison to how many calories it contains. Colorful foods tend to have the most healthful qualities, not only in terms of their vitamins and minerals, but also in antioxidants and cofactor phytochemicals like carotenoids that work synergistically with those nutrients, helping to make them more bioavailable.

The debate surrounding vegetarian and vegan diets versus an omnivore diet that includes meats, poultry, and other flesh foods is not one to put much stock in since it is possible to be very healthy or very unhealthy eating either way. If you choose to be vegetarian, be sure to supplement nutrients where needed, and consume plenty of sources of vegetarian protein. If you choose to eat meat, make it lean and not overcooked. It is generally accepted that fried or cooked fats derived from animals (meat, dairy, seafood) are strongly inflammatory in the body. To offset the free radical or oxidative stress caused by these foods, once again, raw fruits and vegetables eaten at the same meal are the answer.

If possible, also eat organic foods. Organic fruits and vegetables have been shown to have a higher nutrient content, compared to non-organic produce, and are also free of harmful pesticides, preservatives, and other chemicals used to grow non-organic, commercial food crops. Similarly, your meat and poultry food choices should ideally be free-range and free of the hormones and antibiotics that are commonly found in commercially harvested animal products.

Other healthy eating practices include eating plenty of fiber-rich foods (raw fruits, vegetables, and complex carbohydrates), and eliminating sugars and simple carbohydrates, "junk" foods, and unhealthy fats, especially trans-fatty acids and hydrogenated fats.

Finally, it is incredibly important to drink plenty of water, especially when using PEMF therapies, because energy transfers more easily in a body and tissues that are well-hydrated, with blood that is less viscous (thick). The magnetic signal will be the most robust in a body with adequate hydration levels. Drinking magnetized water can also be helpful, as was explained in Chapter 3.

The above nutrition information and throughout the book are not intended to be comprehensive, and there are many competing nutritional recommendations. For more individually suited recommendations it's important to work with a well-trained nutritionist.

Supporting Your Diet With Nutritional Supplements: Even if you eat fresh, organically grown food for all of your meals—something that is not easy to do for many people—such foods, although certainly richer in nutrients than non-commercial foods, are most likely still incapable of meeting all of your nutritional needs.

There are a number of factors that explain this, starting with the fact that the soil in which food crops are grown contains significantly reduced levels of vital minerals, compared to the level of soil minerals a century or more ago. Because of the commercial farming methods used by today's agricultural industry, much of the minerals that had been abundant in our topsoil prior to the early 20th century have been greatly depleted. To compensate for the poor condition of the soil, current nonorganic farming methods rely on substantial quantities of synthetic chemical pesticides, herbicides, and fertilizers to help crops grow. These commercial farming methods have not only resulted in significant declines in the mineral content of crop soil, but also declines in the overall nutrient content of the foods grown under such conditions.

Compounding the problem is the fact that much of our modern-day food supply, after it is harvested, takes weeks and even months before it reaches us. Comparatively few of us eat locally grown food these days. Instead, the food that we consume, even if grown organically, is shipped from other parts of the country, frozen, stored, and warehoused along the way. This further reduces the nutrient content of food. For all of these reasons, it makes good sense to augment your diet with various nutritional supplements. Because of our usual dietary habits and the quality of the food, as well as the normal stresses and demands of daily living, you never know on a day-to-day basis what essential nutrients you're missing from your food. You often hear doctors say that supplements and vitamins only make for expensive urine. I say, better to have expensive urine than cheap urine! You absorb what you need and eliminate what you don't. So, daily nutritional supplements and basic vitamins are necessary for almost everybody.

Supplement quality is directly related to supplement efficacy. The better the quality of your supplements, the better the job they will do for you.

To help ensure that you provide your body with sufficient amounts of the nutrients it needs to function at optimal levels, a good multivitamin/mineral is important. It will act as a security blanket, covering common diet deficiencies. In addition to a good multivitamin/mineral supplement, I recommend that most people take a basic foundation of nutritional supplements. These will support the body's general health regardless of underlying health conditions.

Basic foundation supplements I recommend to my patients include:

- Purity's Perfect Multi 2 twice a day or a similar quality multivitamin
- Vitamin D3 (2,000 – 5,000 IU daily)
- Omega-3 fatty acids (1,000 – 3,000 mg twice per day)
- Vitamin C (either a sustained-release formula of 1,000 mg twice per day, or general vitamin C 1,000 mg three times per day)—these are minimums
- Magnesium (any form other than magnesium oxide) 350-500 mg/day
- Curcumin, 500 mg twice a day to reduce inflammation (optional)
- Green tea extract, 500 mg twice a day for general well-being and prevention (optional).

When using PEMF therapies, maintaining proper levels of magnesium in the body is vital because PEMFs cause a great deal of calcium ion movement in the body. Magnesium is what calcium latches on to as it moves in and out of the cell, so a magnesium deficiency may undermine the effectiveness of PEMF treatments. Most good multivitamins, including the one recommended above, will provide adequate magnesium levels. Since most of us could use more magnesium, supplementation with it is recommended, especially when PEMF therapy is employed regularly.

In addition to the foundation supplements above, I recommend various other supplements to support detoxification and healthy sleep, as well as easing pain and pain-related conditions, and for managing stress. Certain supplements can also help people suffering with osteopenia and osteoporosis, and possibly prevent their occurrence.

Additional, more specific supplement recommendations are given in Chapter 10 for each specific condition discussed.

Detoxification: Supporting detoxification is an important component of healing, whether or not PEMF therapies are used. PEMF therapy facilitates detoxification. Toxicity can be present in the body from a number of factors: environmental toxins, old viral infections, fungal infections, dental amalgams, insecticides and pesticides, heavy metals, etc. The use of nutrition and supplements improves the detoxification process, allowing the body to go through a healing process so that it can recover.

When toxins are released by cells they usually end up in the gastrointestinal tract. The major detoxification pathways in the body include the liver, gut, kidneys, and skin. When toxins are processed by the liver they end up in the gut and may recycle back into the circulatory system through the veins in the gut. Trapping toxins in the gut after excretion by the liver is an important part of removing them from the body. Otherwise, they just keep recycling in the body without removing the total body burden.

The following nutritional supplements aid the body's detoxification system:

- Chlorella pyrenoidosa, a freshwater green alga, 10 grams daily, can be used for inflammation and detoxification.
- Chitosan – 1 to 2 with each meal, when there is fat with the meal.
- Beta sitosterol – standard dosing per the label instructions on the bottle.
- Selenium – 200 to 400 mcg twice a day.
- EDTA – as recommended by your practitioner.
- DMSA – as recommended by your practitioner.

Sleep: These supplements can be used individually or in combination at bedtime as needs arise and results determine:

- Melatonin 3-12 mg at bedtime (some suggest taking one dose at about 4 p.m. and the rest at bedtime). If there is trouble staying asleep as well,

1-3 tabs of regular melatonin can be taken at dinner or up to 2 hours before sleep and 1-3 tabs of sustained or extended release melatonin at bedtime.

- 5-HTP capsules, 50-200 mg with meals or at bedtime (do not mix with SSRI anti-depressants or anti-Parkinson drugs).
- St. John's wort 300 mg (use caution with some medications).
- Kava: as dried root, 450 mg 1 or 2 capsules at bedtime or up to twice per day.
- Valerian: as extract, 400 to 900 mg 2 hours before bedtime.
- German chamomile: As tea, steep 3 grams of dried flower heads in 150 ml boiling water for 5 to 10 minutes and strain; take 1 cup up to 3 times daily. Caps 2-3 times a day. Drops – two to five times per day take 30 to 40 drops in a little water.
- L-theanine, 100 mg-200mg.
- GABA, 500-1,000 mg at bedtime.
- Magnesium, 600 to 750 mg daily (any form other than oxide)

Pain: Since pain is caused by so many different problems in the body, the specific treatment approach needs to be tailored to the cause. Inflammation is probably the most commonly associated cause and is likely present most the time. In injury, when nerves are bruised, crushed, or cut, pain management is more related to pain suppression with over-the-counter medications such as acetaminophen (like Tylenol), salicylate (like aspirin) or other nonsteroidal anti-inflammatories (NSAIDs, like Ibuprofen). Supplements that help ease pain symptoms include:

- Vitamin E (mixed tocopherols only – not the cheaper dl-alpha tocopherol) 400 to 1600 IU daily.
- Calcium 1.5 g daily.
- Magnesium 600 to 750 mg daily (any form other than oxide).
- Curcumin 1000 to 4000 mg twice a day.
- Ginger: As dried root, 1 g 2 to 3 times per day to start, increased up to 4 g daily.
- Willow Bark extract and Boswellia – usually found in combinations of supplements for pain and inflammation.
- Bromelain – 500 mg three times a day.

- Samento (Uncaria tomentosa or uña de gato) 1 capsule or 15-30 drops of liquid extract twice a day.
- SAM-e enteric-coated 400 mg two to three times a day.

For inflammatory soft tissue conditions such as arthritis, bursitis, and tendonitis, add the following supplements to the list above. Such conditions should also be treated with a combination of therapies, including PEMFs.

- Glucosamine sulphate (not hydrochloride) 500 mg three times daily.
- Chondroitin 400 mg three times daily (alone or in combination with Glucosamine).
- Capsaicin cream (Zostrix) – thin film of cream (0.025 to 0.075 percent) applied to the joint/s four times a day.
- MSM, 3000 mg/day as a powder, mixed in water.
- Hyaluronic acid, 100-500 mg/day (a good combination may be found in Ultimate HA).
- Collagen joint support – Dose per label directions on bottle.

Stress: Stress, especially cumulative stress, can cause long-term damage to our health. These supplements can help prevent that from happening:

- Adaptogen combination preparation – for example, Vital Adapt Siberian ginseng – as powdered root, 0.6 to 3 g 1 to 3 times per day, or ethanolic extract, 0.5 to 6 mL 1 to 3 times a day; use for 2 to 8 weeks, then abstain for 2 weeks.
- Gotu kola: As dried leaves, 600 mg 3 times per day; as tea, 600 mg dried leaves steeped in 150 mL of boiling water for 5 to 10 minutes and strain; take 1 cup 3 times per day.
- Valerian: as extract, 400 to 900 mg 2 hours before bedtime

Osteopenia/Osteoporosis: The following supplements should be used in combination with walking on hard surfaces up to seven days per week, and may be further benefited by going on an alkaline-producing diet. PEMF therapy is key to helping osteopenia/osteoporosis.

A good bone building formula, such as, OsteoPlus, Bone Health Take Care, Osteosheath, or Bone-Up, taken as directed on the bottle label.

- Hormone replacement with bio identical hormones (see your healthcare practitioner).
- DHEA 25-50 mg/ day, estrogen supporting supplements such as Estrovera or HRTPlus.
- High dose K2, such as Ultra K2.

Complementary Therapies That Can be Used With PEMFs

There are usually multiple factors that combine to cause and exacerbate most chronic health problems. For healing to be achieved, each of these factors must be addressed and resolved. Similarly, there are multiple factors that need our attention if we are to create and maintain good health. In addition to the dietary and nutritional recommendations above, being healthy requires adequate amounts of restorative sleep, regular exercise, cultivation of positive emotions, and stress management, among other things. Healthy people pay attention to all of these areas, as do the most effective physicians.

Unfortunately, not all physicians are trained to address all of the factors that support optimal health, nor are they trained to consider and rectify the multiple causes of disease, which are often lifestyle-related. Knowing how to do so simply isn't part of the education they receive in medical school, which is almost entirely devoted to teaching medical students how to diagnose disease, prescribe and use drugs, and in some cases, perform surgery, with little attention given to anything else that is lifestyle- and wellness-related.

Further compounding this problem, most medical students then train to become specialists in treating only one system of the body, such as the cardiovascular system (cardiologists), the GI tract (gastroenterologists), or the brain (neurologists). As a result, their medical training becomes reductionist, meaning it focuses on one body system at the expense of all the others. This explains why so many doctors, while being able to manage the symptoms of their patients' diseases, often are incapable of making a significant impact on the course of diseases or curing them.

Take the issue of chronic pain, for example. All too often, the best that many physicians can offer for pain is pain medications. While such drugs can certainly lessen pain, they do nothing to address what is causing it. As a result, pain patients are reduced to having to rely on pain meds on an ongoing basis, potentially risking serious side effects and even death. (As I pointed out in this book's Introduction, every year in the U.S., over 16,000 people die as a result of taking popular pain reliever drugs like ibuprofen. Add in deaths caused by taking other pain meds, including opioid overdoses, and that toll is much higher.) In addition, many of these pain medications negatively impact the body's microbiome and the immune system.

Pain medications temporarily reduce the body's pain signals, lessening pain symptoms. But the goal is not just to reduce the pain. The goal is to heal the cause. If all you are doing is suppressing the pain, you're not finishing the job. What's required is a more comprehensive approach that eliminates the root cause of the pain. This is a really important issue that I had to come to grips with as a doctor, and which led me to go far beyond my conventional medical training in order to become capable of treating my patients most effectively and completely using integrative, or "whole person," medicine.

As another example of what I am talking about, consider antibiotics and infection. An antibiotic drug is prescribed to help reduce infection from harmful bacteria. It might kill the bacteria, or at least slow their growth, or it might not. It gives the body a fighting chance to recover from infection. When doctors prescribe antibiotics, they hope that their patients will get better, without side effects, and that the antibiotics will shorten the time of infection and reduce symptoms and damage. But if, for example, you have a kidney infection, pneumonia, or meningitis, do you want to leave that to chance?

I wouldn't think so. Because if you leave it to chance, the body may not be strong enough to heal itself. And if all doctors do to help support the body to heal itself is prescribe an antibiotic, the patient may not improve and may even become worse. And most doctors will not even give nutritional supplements and other things to help the body to be stronger and more vital to repair the damage that's caused by the infection.

We should not be treating people with antibiotics alone for any type of serious infectious disease because, by doing so, we're leaving things to chance. If the antibiotics don't work, the patients' health might become permanently damaged, and they will suffer for the rest of their life.

This is why I do not rely on pain meds or antibiotics alone to treat pain conditions or infections. I take a broader approach, incorporating multiple therapies, so that I don't leave anything to chance. This includes PEMF therapy because of the wide range of benefits it is proven to provide. Based on my experience, PEMF therapy can and should be combined with other therapeutic approaches in order to maximize patient recovery, especially since it is uncommon for complementary therapies to interfere with one another.

However, it can be difficult to find advice about combining therapies, primarily because physicians tend to have specialties. Practitioners of any discipline who only practice one discipline, even with excellence, tend to know little about other therapeutic options. The integrative medicine that I am trained in urges physicians and patients alike to know as much about health as possible, and to explore a wide range of therapeutic options to achieve optimum treatment results and well-being. This includes proper nutrition and the other elements of healthy lifestyle mentioned above.

Because PEMF therapies work on such a basic level, their effects are almost always enhanced with the use of other modalities, and vice versa. That being said, there is usually a best practice in terms of sequence of use, duration of treatment, and time between applications. In addition, you should always consult your physician or other health professional before beginning a new therapy.

What follow are some of the therapies that work well with and complement PEMF therapy. Because of space limitations the descriptions below are fairly short and not in-depth and serve mostly to highlight the relative aspects of these therapies and PEMFs.

Acupuncture: PEMF therapy can be used at the same time that acupuncture is being used. PEMF and other magnetic fields have been found to stimulate acupuncture points and meridians. Although acupuncture needles are temporarily stronger in action than magnetic fields, when the needles are applied along with PEMF, the therapeutic effects are even stronger.

Conversely, other acupuncture-related therapies, such as acupressure, cupping, and moxibustion, are not typically as strong in their actions as PEMF fields are. PEMF therapy is also an excellent alternative to acupuncture when acupuncture treatments are indicated for people who are not comfortable with the needles.

Since magnetic fields act more directly on cells and tissues through which they pass than acupuncture, acupuncture and PEMF can be used together to provide patients with the benefits of both modalities. For example, in the case of spinal arthritis, a deep joint problem that causes significant pain, multiple tissues are often involved. Edema can be, as well. PEMF therapy can effectively treat any edema in muscles, ligaments, or nerves, as well as relax muscles and start cellular repair of both joints and other soft tissues. At the same time, acupuncture will help reduce pain almost immediately and help a person relax. The secondary actions of acupuncture on the immune system and other hormone and repair mechanisms take more time to take effect and can easily be overwhelmed or reversed by other events in a person's life or processes happening in the body after an acupuncture treatment. Combining both therapeutic systems will often result in the primary actions of both acupuncture and PEMF therapy being more active and more effective than waiting for the secondary actions of either therapy to kick in.

Based on my clinical experience as a practitioner of both therapies, I recommend that PEMF treatment be administered first, followed by acupuncture. However, many acupuncturists find benefits in doing both therapies at the same time. PEMF therapy will act on the body's tissues directly, and rebalance all of its cells, while the acupuncture's systemic actions will correct any blockages or imbalances in the body's energy pathways (meridians) and organ systems. When the secondary effects of both therapies kick in, the overall therapeutic action of each therapy is greatly increased.

Chiropractic, Massage, and Physical Therapy: Chiropractic manipulation and massage work directly on muscles, superficial soft tissues, and ligaments to reduce tightness, spasms, strains, and subluxations of the spine. These forms of bodywork help to stimulate acupuncture points and meridians, improve circulation to tissues, and relax muscles. Secondarily, massage works to flood the body with endorphins. Since many toxins and wastes are stored in muscles, along with a great amount of tension and related blockages of circulation, regular treatments with these therapies can help provide rapid structural relief and help most people to maintain better health.

These therapies and PEMF therapy significantly improve the benefits of each other. As with acupuncture, when PEMF therapy is used in combination with these therapies, the greatest benefit will likely be achieved from using PEMF therapy first, followed by chiropractic manipulation, massage, or physical therapy. On the other hand, when there are mechanical problems, these may have to be resolved first before PEMF will be helpful to complete the work needed. For massage, PEMF therapy helps relax both patients and their muscles before massage is started, thereby requiring less work on the therapist's part to get deeper into tissues for much deeper stimulation.

Regular (ideally, daily) use of whole-body PEMF therapy at home decreases the need for manipulation or massage by helping tissues remain detoxified and relaxed, while also keeping the cumulative physical effects of stress to a minimum. Even so, massage has more direct physical action on the muscles themselves than PEMF therapy, which is why the combination of regular local and/or whole-body PEMF therapy and chiropractic care, massage, or physical therapy treatments keep the body from aging as quickly and help to prevent musculoskeletal problems from developing or worsening. A growing number of chiropractors and other bodywork practitioners now offer PEMF therapy for this reason.

I would place osteopathic manipulation alongside these other therapies in terms of potential PEMF therapy use and how to think about it as discussed above.

Infrared Therapy: Infrared is invisible radiant energy and is part of the electromagnetic spectrum. Its wavelengths are longer that those of visible light, but significantly shorter than the wavelengths used in PEMF devices. The discussion below is a limited review of a growing area of interest.

The three types of infrared (IR) therapy are far infrared (FIR), mid-infrared (MIR) and near infrared (NIR). Infrared is primarily used to generate heat in tissues. In addition to generating heat, IR also introduces high frequency EMFs into the body. Infrared does not typically penetrate the body deeply, with an IR signal usually dissipated within one to two inches into the body because of the natural drop-off of the intensity of these high-frequency stimuli. High frequencies dissipate into the body very rapidly, while heating the tissues along the way. This is one of the reasons why IR is used in saunas to detoxify the body, primarily through the skin.

There are both passive and active FIR devices. The active infrared systems are driven by using electrical line current and tend to create more dynamic action in the body than the passive systems. Active systems are most commonly used in health practitioners' offices. The passive systems are usually designed for personal or home use, and radiate FIR signals using either ceramic or fiber materials. FIR systems have been designed for whole-body applications, including in saunas, blankets, covers, clothing, and other items. Active FIR, especially applied to the whole body, tends to generate more heat in the tissues than passive FIR. ELF PEMFs usually penetrate the body more completely without loss of signal, as opposed to higher frequency IR, which get absorbed by the tissues.

IR in all formats can be used alongside PEMFs to obtain additional health benefits. The person is essentially going to be getting a broader spectrum of frequencies and intensities when these modalities are combined. IR will help local, superficial musculoskeletal problems more dynamically and quickly than many PEMFs, especially low-intensity PEMF systems. This means that if someone owns a whole-body PEMF system, they can still use an FIR sauna or a local IR treatment device.

For cases of acute arthritic or musculoskeletal problems I am more inclined to use IR to start with for several treatment sessions, followed by longer-term PEMF management, especially if I think the underlying problem is, or is likely to become, more chronic.

Some IR systems use red colored diodes for their IR signals. In order to generate current to the diode, AC current may be modulated in such a way as to introduce ELFs as well as the diode frequencies into the body. This makes such a device a dual treatment system that uses IR and ELF simultaneously. This type of system would be expected to be even more dynamically acting than simple IR by itself, especially if it's higher-intensity PEMF.

As with many other therapeutic approaches, I recommend using PEMFs before using IR if they are going to be used on the same day. However, IR may help superficial acute problems more quickly than PEMF therapy, so in the case of an acute injury, I recommend using IR first and following that with PEMF treatment.

Laser Therapy: There are two types of laser therapy systems. One system is tissue-destructive and used for ablation and to treat and remove skin lesions and the like. The other system is tissue-healing enhancing. There are two types of this latter system, high-intensity and low-intensity. The low-intensity systems are known as low-level or cold laser. The high-intensity laser equipment tends to be very expensive and mostly affordable by practitioners. Most very effective, low-level lasers are also expensive and tend to be used by practitioners. There are some less-expensive home-based systems available, which unfortunately also tend to be very low intensity and less effective.

Low-level lasers are often used in a similar way to IR. Their beam is very narrow and focused. Because of this level of intensity, they are able to penetrate the body more deeply than IR and can often even pass through less dense, superficial areas of the body, such as the hands. More expensive professional models with much higher laser intensities are more likely to penetrate deeper, thicker body parts, such as the abdomen or lung. Lasers may be used with different colors and therefore have the combined benefits of the laser frequencies along with the color benefits. Most therapeutic lasers emit red.

Unlike IR, laser therapy is used primarily for local area applications and most typically have to be applied by professionals. PEMFs can be used alongside laser therapy. Because of the intensity, very high frequency, and focus of the laser beam, PEMFs are useful for wider and deeper areas of treatment and will interact with tissues at lower frequencies. Low-frequency PEMFs penetrate the body completely, but lasers tend to be more superficial in their depth of penetration. In addition, lasers cannot be used safely around certain body structures, such as the eyes and brain. For the most part, PEMFs do not have these limitations. PEMFs can be used simultaneously with low-level laser therapy, or before or after.

Light Therapy: Active light therapy can include lights or lamps that radiate specific colors, have colored crystals applied, use natural spectrum lighting, and so on. Light therapy is most typically a whole-body treatment approach. Specific colors are used to generate specific actions and reactions in the body. Lighting systems, like with laser and infrared systems, are limited by the thickness of the tissues exposed. They are also often blocked by clothing.

When light therapy is administered, there is a significant amount of attenuation, absorption, and diffraction of light as it moves into the body. Many of the light's resonant effects are due to the stimulation of the optical nervous system and not the tissue directly. For these reasons, PEMFs would not be expected to interfere with light therapies and may be used concurrently with them. Some research also indicates that PEMFs may act like light therapy, even though their frequencies are considerably lower.

To avoid frequency interference, I recommend that PEMFs be used prior to light therapy if used on the same day. When combined, both therapies would be expected to have a beneficial, synergistic effect.

Hypnosis, Counseling, and Psychotherapy: I have worked with many practitioners who combine PEMF therapies along with psychological approaches. Most PEMF systems cause people to become relaxed. There are specific PEMF devices which have selectable frequencies that can be specifically used to tune the brain into different levels of relaxation, from light to very deep. PEMFs can be also used for stress reduction. Then, because PEMFs help make people more relaxed, they can more effectively participate in psychological therapy approaches. In this case, I recommend doing PEMF therapy before and/or during psychological therapies.

Ozone Therapy: Many of the effects of ozone therapy are comparable to effects of PEMF therapy. Deep ozone therapy usually requires a skilled professional. Ozone works internally to create the production of oxygen in tissues. PEMFs also improve oxygenation and circulation. Research done in Cuba found that combining PEMF with ozone therapy increases the benefits of ozone over standard therapy for arthritis of the knee.

To be effective, ozone has to be absorbed by the tissues, enter the circulatory system, then be distributed to tissues. By the time the ozone gets into the tissues, it may be diluted dramatically. Because PEMFs will assist in this dispersion, we recommend these therapies be combined to improve effectiveness.

Homeopathy: Homeopathy is based on an almost completely different set of principles than magnetic field therapy, although both can be resonance-based. Homeopathy relies on principles of similar resonance. To be effective, homeopathic remedies must resonate with the symptoms of the person being treated.

PEMFs produce frequencies or magnetic fields that could potentially interact with the frequencies of homeopathic remedies. In addition, PEMF frequencies are typically much lower than those of homeopathic remedies. This means that PEMF frequencies likely interact with homeopathic remedies as a result of harmonic resonance where their frequencies overlap. Even so, the likelihood of significant harmonic interaction is probably very low.

Since it is not known for certain whether homeopathic remedies can be canceled out by PEMFs, I recommend that homeopathics be used at different times. Preferably, patients should receive PEMF therapy first. In fact, several days of PEMF therapy use may very well help to clear the body's internal terrain and "static" before homeopathy is used.

Extracorporeal Shock Wave Therapy (ESWT): Extracorporeal shock wave therapy (ESWT) is a noninvasive treatment that involves the delivery of sound shock waves to injured soft tissue to reduce pain, reduce inflammation, improve circulation, and promote healing. One of the original uses of ESWT was for breaking up urinary tract stones. Now it is frequently being used to treat chronic tendon inflammation and wear-and-tear issues. These include tennis elbow, rotator cuff problems, plantar fasciitis (heel spurs), and more. Most of these structures are relatively superficial in the body and therefore accessible to a strong sound wave. They can be very effective especially for chronic superficial problems of the musculoskeletal system, some skin disorders, burns, and diabetic foot wounds but cannot be used very deep into the body. This therapy needs to be delivered by a skilled professional with specialized equipment. PEMF therapy can easily be combined with ESWT, especially when one is used superficially and the other is available for much deeper and continuing home use.

RIFE Therapy

Royal Raymond Rife (May 16, 1888 – August 5, 1971) was an American inventor best known for a claimed "beam ray" invention during the 1930s, which he thought could treat some diseases by "devitalizeing disease organisms" through vibration or specific frequencies. Rife did studies in a laboratory on Petri dishes, on cultures using "RIFE" frequencies. What might work in a petri dish on one organism may not work in a body setting, not to mention the issue of the intensity the magnetic field and the distance from the tissue being treated. While all molecules radiate frequencies, there is not enough credible, reproducible research knowledge to have any degree of certainty or dependability on the likely effects of frequencies. Frequencies can be constructive or destructive—that is, they may support or amplify a molecule or work to destroy it. Because I don't know what Rife frequencies are going to do, or whether it will work for you, I avoid Rife all together.

I have a very expensive Rife machine. I've done something called frequency specific microcurrent, which is equivalent to Rife, but using very-low-intensity electrical current. I've trained in it and I have the machines as well. There clearly are practitioners, users and manufacturers who swear by these devices.

You can use magnetic field therapy with Rife. If you do, I would do the magnetic field therapy first, followed by the Rife next.

In addition to the above therapies, PEMF therapy can be used with many other therapeutic, energetic, and resonance therapies. Generally speaking, PEMF therapy is safe for use with most other modalities and is usually best applied before any other resonance therapies are used on the same day. These may require application by a practitioner; some are available for home use. New uses and applications appear regularly.

In my own clinical practice, I regularly employed or recommended PEMF therapy along with the therapies discussed above, and consistently found that adding PEMFs to my patients' overall treatment plans improves the benefits of the other therapies. I also encouraged my patients to consider purchasing their own PEMF systems so that they can continue to obtain the benefits of PEMFs on their own, while also helping to sustain the benefits they receive from the other treatments they receive.

I hope that this chapter furthers your understanding of just how versatile and valuable PEMFs can be for improving your health. In the next chapter, you will discover more information about the types of PEMF systems that are available and how they work.

Types of PEMF Systems and How to Choose the Best System for Your Specific Needs

Since most problems for which people seek PEMF treatment are chronic and need long-term treatment, ideally, you should acquire your own PEMF system and begin using it in your home. For acute problems requiring short-term treatments, you could seek out a health practitioner who offers PEMF treatments. Many people will try out treatments in a professional setting first to see the impact of PEMFs for their problems before realizing or determining that long-term treatment is needed. Long-term treatment in a professional setting can be quite expensive and would not likely occur frequently enough to have the most impact, so, from a cost-benefit perspective, the investment in an effective home system can make more sense.

Determining which system is the best one for your individual needs requires educating yourself about the systems that are available and how they work. In this chapter, I will provide you with this knowledge so that you can make an informed decision about the PEMF systems that will offer you the most benefit, based on your specific health concerns. (In Chapter 10, I go into more detail about specific health conditions and, less specifically, the types of magnetic field systems that could or should be considered.)

My goal as a physician has always been to help people choose the right PEMF system for themselves, based on their present health status and any health condition(s) they may be dealing with, as well as their ability to use a particular system. I also consider any budgetary constraints they may have, and continuously gather information from scientific studies so that I can be as informed much as possible about the most current treatment options. Please know that I would never recommend a PEMF system that I have not used myself. Every system that I work with and which is covered in this chapter has its advantages and disadvantages, with each system treating some problems better than others. The information that follows will help you determine what you should focus on while as you research which PEMF system to choose.

Peak Intensity

The peak intensity is one of the most important considerations when selecting a PEMF system. There is much debate online about the value of intensity of pulsed electromagnetic signals, with manufacturers and distributors on both sides of this debate. Some claim that low intensity is all that is needed and that higher intensities are unnecessary or even dangerous. Some claim that only high intensities are effective. The truth is that both work, and will have different effects and so do intensities in the middle of the range.

Much of the value of PEMFs in helping the body is based on Faraday's law, a basic law of physics. One of the major actions of PEMFs is to generate energy or charge in the tissues. Faraday's law dictates that the more charge that's needed to do the work, the higher the intensity of the PEMF signal needs to be.

This is represented with the equation dB/dT, where d means change, B means peak intensity, and T means time. We are talking about the change in intensity over the change in time. The higher the intensity reached in the shortest time, the higher the dB/dT value. The higher this value is, the greater the amount of charge produced in the tissues. Some of the highest intensity PEMF systems available on the market have dB/dTs high enough to cause nerves to fire and activate muscle contraction. PEMF devices with that level of intensity have been FDA-approved, indicating their safety and effectiveness.

In many cases, dB/dT needs to be higher to accomplish any real healing work. The PEMF signal needs to be able to pass deep enough into the body (or completely through the body) to do its work in increasing the charge in tissues at sufficient levels necessary to produce healing results. Magnetic fields themselves are unlimited as they pass through the body, but their intensity component decreases based on another basic law of physics known as the inverse square rule. As with any radiation source, including cold, heat, light, radio waves, and microwaves, magnetic fields are subject to the same rule. Magnetic field intensity drops off extremely rapidly with distance from the surface of the coil applicator of a PEMF system. Even though the field goes into the body with no resistance, the intensity drops off as it passes through the tissues. The side of the body closest to the coil applicator gets the maximum intensity. The other side of the body or limb gets a much lower intensity. If charge is necessary to produce healing results, and research tells us it is, then higher starting intensities are necessary to be able to reach the tissue being targeted.

At 6 cm (2.3 inches) away from the applicator, a 100 mT (1,000 gauss or 100,000 microTesla) magnetic field has dropped to around 2mT (20 gauss or 2,000 microTesla). This is a 98 percent drop in intensity in less than two and a half inches. This same ratio applies to all magnetic field strengths, whether one gauss or one thousand gauss. The table below shows the intensity of a 100 µT (microTesla) or 1 gauss (0.1 mT) PEMF up to 5 inches (13 cm) away (or into the body) from the surface of the applicator:

Distance		Intensity	
Inches	**cm**	**mT**	**µT**
0	0	0.1	100
0.5	1	0.025	25
1	3	0.0063	6.2
2	5	0.0028	2.8
3	8	0.0012	1.2
4	11	0.0007	0.7
5	13	0.0005	0.5

From this table you can see that at half an inch from the body, the magnetic field intensity drops to 25 microtesla/µT - (one quarter of the original intensity) and that 1 inch into the body that field has now dropped down to 6.2 microtesla/µT. In other words, at one inch into the body there is about a 94 percent drop in the magnetic field. You can see more examples in Appendix A of the degree of loss of magnetic field strength based on the starting intensity.

As you can also see, once you are five inches from the applicator, there is little magnetic field (only 0.5 percent) left in terms of the field's ability to generate charge.

Research evidence continually and consistently shows that the intensity of a therapeutic magnetic field is important, perhaps more so than any other component. Even the other components of a magnetic field, such as frequency or waveform, rely mostly for their effects in the body on the intensity of the PEMF signal at the tissue being stimulated.

However, PEMF systems must still be tailored to the unique needs of the individual in order to provide the most benefit. Most extremely high-intensity PEMF systems do not have adjustable frequencies. In some cases, they have no frequencies at all, and instead have a repetition rate or pulse rate. Technically speaking, a pulse rate is not a frequency, although many people mistakenly use the terms pulse rate and frequency interchangeably. Even if frequency is correctly described, thousands of studies have been done on PEMF systems using frequencies of many kinds to produce benefits. The majority of these studies are done using intensities ranging from 10 gauss to 1,000 gauss.

In research settings, "low-intensity" magnetic fields seem to be categorized as those at or around 15 gauss (1,500 microTesla). One study compared a 0.5 gauss (50 microTesla) PEMF with a 15 gauss (1,500 microTesla) PEMF system used for six hours per day for 90 days in the treatment of arthritis. They found that NSAID (nonsteroidal anti-inflammatory drug) use was 26 percent in the higher-intensity group compared to 75 percent in the lower-intensity group. At a three-year follow-up, the percentage of patients reporting complete recovery was also higher in the higher-intensity group.

In a "medium-intensity" study, researchers used a 35 mT (350 gauss / 35,000 microTesla) PEMF for 15 minutes over 15 treatment sessions and found the signal improved hip arthritis pain in 86 percent of the patients. This is a significantly shorter treatment course than for the lower intensity study reported on above. PEMFs of 40 mT (400 gauss or 40,000 microTesla) for 20 minutes per day over 25 days gave relief or elimination of pain in between 90 and 95 percent of patients with lumbar osteoarthritis.

In one "high-intensity" study, PEMFs reaching up to 1.17 T (11,700 gauss) were used for recovery after injury in post-traumatic postoperative lower back pain, reflex sympathetic dystrophy (RSD), neuropathy, thoracic outlet syndrome, and endometriosis. Pain was reduced by more than 10 times with active PEMF versus sham treatments for each of these conditions.

My many years of experience using PEMFs of various intensities has shown me the same thing that research supports: low-intensity PEMFs may require treatments to last a very long time or may need to be continuous. By contrast, medium- to high-intensity PEMF systems provide symptom relief benefits in less than a month with just minutes per day of treatment.

This does not mean that increased treatment time can always eventually make up for a lack of intensity, however. If the tissues you need to treat are not being reached by the magnetic field, then benefits may never be achieved, or the PEMF treatment may only provide modest benefits at best. Let's take the hip joint for example. If you assume the depth of penetration needed is 12 centimeters (4.7 inches), then a 200 gauss intensity magnetic field would be delivering about

1 gauss to the target tissue. Given the shape of the hip joint, the calculated "dose" would vary throughout the joint. When considering using extremely low-intensity magnetic field devices, such as one that produces just 1 gauss (100 microTesla), the dose at the hip would be just over 1 microTesla.

There is little research to support that PEMFs will be active at this level of intensity in tissues. You may still receive some passive benefits, but given that most research points to the generation of charge in tissues as being the most obvious reason PEMF therapy works, intensity may well matter more than any other single factor.

System Parameters

The first and perhaps most important thing to know when deciding which PEMF system to use is that there is not one best system that is ideal for everyone. There are dozens of PEMF systems on the market and each one is unique. Some are intended for daily use, others for use in a clinician's office. Some treat the entire body at once (whole-body systems), while others treat only a small portion of the body (local application systems). Of course, each manufacturer believes they have created the optimum system, and each will have a slightly different philosophy about what PEMF parameters offer the most benefits in the body.

All the patients I've worked with and treated taught me a bit more about how PEMFs work and what PEMFs work the best for specific circumstances. As a physician, I've concluded that there is no such thing as one-size-fits-all or even one-size-fits-most PEMF system.

As I discussed in Chapters 2 and 4, PEMF therapies have a multitude of simultaneous actions on the body due to their combination of mechanical, chemical, electrical, magnetic, and tissue effects. Many problems, conditions, and health needs will be positively affected by almost any type of PEMF field, regardless of frequency, waveform, intensity, or coil configuration. While there are many PEMF brands and options with a variety of parameters from which to choose, the most important considerations you can make before deciding on a system are personal ones. Your health history, lifestyle, budget, and current health concern(s) or objectives must all be examined before making a purchasing decision. The advice of a physician or clinician knowledgeable about or trained in the use of PEMF therapy, if you have access to such practitioners, should also be considered when deciding on which system is most appropriate for a given condition. Most conventional physicians, however, have almost no information or knowledge about PEMFs and cannot really guide in decision-making.

When I work with people to help them decide on a PEMF a system, the discussion always begins with a lot of questions. Are you always on the go, or is your lifestyle more stationary? Are you an athlete? Is your health condition chronic, or do you have a new, localized injury? If you plan on purchasing a PEMF system, is this purchase for yourself, or do you want to treat friends, neighbors, or the family with it? Are you going to be using the system in your home, or are you a healthcare practitioner? What kind of budget are you working with? The most important piece of information to guide your decision is usually about what you hope to treat and what results you are hoping to get. The ideal system to choose depends on that answer. Chronic health conditions require different PEMF stimulation than what is needed for health maintenance. If you have a lot of health concerns, or if you're hoping to treat multiple people with one system, the recommendations change again.

If your goal is to maintain your overall health, then a full-body system with a reasonable range of frequencies, a medium intensity, and a comparatively lower price point may be most suitable.

If you are struggling with severe or chronic pain, a higher-intensity system (whether it's a full-body or local system) would be the best choice.

If you intend to treat a lot of different conditions, a PEMF system with a wider range of frequencies and somewhat higher, adjustable range of intensities will probably be best.

If you are an athlete needing to use the unit on the go or someone who travels frequently, a battery-powered device may be best.

If you have extreme sensitivities to medications, foods, smells, electrical equipment, or supplements, then a low-intensity system with multiple intensity levels should be considered.

If you are looking for something simple, I would suggest a unit with as few buttons or programs as possible, or a full-body unit with few options.

There are a variety of elements that make up the technical specs of each PEMF system. The most widely studied elements are frequency and peak intensity, but waveform, coil configuration, applicators, treatment time parameters, programs, if any, and application area also need to be considered. Knowing which parameters are most likely to affect your health concerns or objectives is important in when comparing similar PEMF systems to one another.

Frequency Range: Frequency range is always an important aspect of a PEMF system. Some systems produce a single frequency, others produce frequencies within a small range, and some have a wide range of optional frequencies.

Most full-body PEMF systems have at least one frequency that mimics that of the brain—roughly between 1 and 30 Hz. These frequencies are sometimes referred to as "Earth-based" frequencies, which is somewhat of a misnomer since there is a vast array of frequencies present on our planet and in our atmosphere. Most PEMF systems for therapeutic use that have frequencies are in the "Earth-based" ranges.

In addition to PEMFs system that produce only brainwave level frequencies, there are other systems that produce much higher frequencies—some into the kHz range. Both high and low frequencies have been studied extensively, and each range has its place therapeutically. The body itself produces a vast array of frequencies, and different cell types, organ systems, and pathologies all communicate in different ways, creating their own biological windows that create, or respond optimally to, unique frequencies.

While a wide variety of frequencies have been studied individually, little comparative research has been done. Though a particular study may find that a specific frequency is excellent for relieving arthritis pain, that does not mean that other frequencies will not work just as well or even better for providing arthritis pain relief, as an example. PEMF systems that allow you access to a wide variety of frequencies let you cover more ground in the body, since the body will tend to choose what frequencies it needs at a given time and ignore the rest. Additionally, what frequencies your body wants and needs at a given moment or even that day could be different tomorrow or next week.

Selecting a PEMF system based on its available frequency range is appropriate in certain cases. For example, if people have trouble sleeping, they will absolutely need access to the lower frequencies in which the brain operates during sleep. Consideration of frequency ranges is also important when people are dealing with a disease that presents itself in multiple ways, such as post-treatment Lyme disease syndrome. A broader range of frequency choices will be more helpful in such situations.

When more alertness is desired, higher brainwave frequencies will be more useful. If there is a lot of anxiety, EEG research shows that lower frequencies, especially in the alpha range (9-13 Hz) are best. To regenerate tissues, 10 Hz can be important, while musculoskeletal problems often require multiple frequencies, with 10 Hz, 50 Hz, or 100 Hz often proving to be the most useful. These frequency options may be available individually or as packages with built-in protocols, depending on the PEMF system you choose.

Intensity Options: You should always find out what the magnetic field intensity is of the PEMF system you're considering. It's amazing how often manufacturers or their representatives won't tell you what the peak intensity or the intensity range is of their PEMF system. You should insist on being told what the peak intensity is. If they're not willing or able to tell you, you have to ask yourself what they are hiding.

Intensity levels vary dramatically between PEMF systems. It's important to note that with consumer PEMF systems, "high-intensity" and "low-intensity" are relative. Just as a wide variety of frequencies have been studied, so have a wide variety of intensities. When relying on such research to help guide your decision, it's important to consider how the research was done. There is an often-cited NASA study, for example, that used very low intensities. Many manufacturers of low-intensity systems tout that research as proof that their system is going to be effective on stem cells. But what is left out of the conversation is that the research in that particular study was done *in vitro*, meaning conducted on a cell sample in a culture dish, not on a living organism and done for 24 hours continuously. Translating that into human use requires that intensities be made much higher. Very-low-intensity PEMF systems are only likely to affect stem cells within about a quarter of an inch into the body at the most, depending on multiple other factors.

Not many PEMF systems are available within what is considered a "medium" range intensity. They mostly provide either extremely low-intensity or relatively high-intensity levels. Manufacturers and distributors of low-intensity systems may claim that higher intensities are unnecessary or even harmful but this is not true. Manufacturers and distributors of high-intensity systems may claim that lower intensities are ineffective. This is also not true. Research supports success with a variety of intensity options when it comes to PEMF systems.

Choosing the most appropriate PEMF system and intensity levels all depends on what you need.

Are you seeking rapid relief from musculoskeletal pain? If so, low intensities aren't going to be your best option.

Are you over-stimulated by electro-sensitivities from harmful EMFs? If you are, then medium or high intensities may further aggravate you. Very low intensities may be better for you, at least at the beginning.

The choice of intensity of a PEMF system is often tied to how quickly you can expect to see results with that system. Again, higher intensities generally produce faster results, especially in terms of pain relief, musculoskeletal healing, injury recovery, and tissue regeneration.

Some PEMF systems use a philosophy called "graduated intensity" where the magnetic field intensity varies at different points on the applicator. For example, a PEMF system might provide a higher intensity at the feet than at the head. (I often recommend customers flip the mat around in this scenario so that the head gets a stronger treatment, depending on the condition or conditions being treated.) Or a system might produce a higher intensity along the center of the mat, where the spine would be, than on the sides. This isn't really a pro or a con, just a different philosophy from a given manufacturer. Regardless, long-term use of low-, medium-, and high-intensity PEMF systems are all considered safe.

Waveforms: Waveforms can be downright confusing for consumers, but they are an often-cited parameter when PEMF systems are compared to each other. A wide variety of waveforms exist in nature, in your body, and in PEMF devices. The most common waveforms are sinus, sawtooth, and "square" (which are really trapezoidal waves). Other waveforms include trapezoidal, rectangular, impulse, and triangular, among others.

It's important to note that within each loosely defined waveform there exists a huge range of variation. There is no cut-and-dry sine wave, for example. Some manufacturers say they use a NASA "square" wave. There is such a thing, but it's different from all other square waves and only existed in the original NASA research that was conducted years ago. While many PEMF systems produce a square wave signal, none produce the exact same NASA "square" wave (which, even in research subsequent to NASA by one of the original scientists, was tweaked further).

The main reason waveforms are important is because they either mimic (enhance) or counteract (diminish) natural processes in the body. Waveforms also tend to be tied to intensity. "Square" waves can produce higher intensities than sinus waves, for instance. The key once again is the intensity generated by the upslope of the waveform and the time that it takes to reach a peak (dB/dT). This is the only truly effective value to be able to compare PEMF systems properly.

Most PEMF systems produce a single waveform. Others produce one waveform on a full-body mat and another waveform on the pillow or probe applicator.

Still others offer the option of changing which waveform you're using for a given program. While this variety is an attractive feature, I recommend that waveform not be the deciding factor when considering which PEMF system will best suit your needs—not even if it's a "square" wave or sawtooth system. Just as little comparative research has been done on frequency selection, I am not aware of research directly comparing waveforms for given conditions. This is one area where I would like to see new research done.

Coil Configuration and Application Areas: Two other aspects of PEMF systems are their coil configuration and the application area they cover. All PEMF systems use copper coils to produce the desired magnetic field, but the configuration of those coils varies from system to system. Some systems have tightly wound coils that are all the same size. The number of "turns" of copper wire in a coil drives the intensity. Other systems have concentrically wound coils, and some have varying sizes of coils spread out in varying patterns within a mat. All of these configurations produce a magnetic field as designed by the manufacturer. Some configurations are designed to produce a higher-intensity magnetic field, some produce a more uniform field across the surface of an applicator, and others intentionally focus the magnetic field on one part of the mat or applicator. There are no right or wrong coil configurations, just differing objectives on the part of the manufacturer.

Application area refers to how much of the body is being treated with the PEMF field. There are two types of PEMF systems: full-body systems and local systems. Full- or whole-body systems usually come standard with a smaller applicator, as well.

Depending on the brand, the full-body mat usually produces lower intensities than the smaller pad. The reason for this is that the PEMF machine has a maximum energy output regardless of the numbers of applicators attached. The more applicators or the more widely spread out the coils are, the more dispersed the energy. Densely packed coils produce much more energy than loosely packed, wider area coils. That's why many local PEMF systems produce higher intensity in their applicators than full-body systems.

This is important, because you can stimulate a small group of tissues locally with more intensity than you can when you stimulate the entire body. Every time tissues are stimulated, there is some degree of amplification. The more cells that are stimulated, the more amplification there is. That is why lower intensities tend to be better tolerated with whole-body stimulation.

Other Considerations: In addition to the above parameters, when choosing a PEMF system for yourself, you also need to know if the manufacturer provides good customer service and support; the reliability of the manufacturer; and the experience and knowledge of PEMFs of the salesperson, distributor, or any other person recommending a particular PEMF system to you. In addition, PEMF systems are usually not covered by insurance, even if they are FDA-approved. Being FDA-registered is not the same as being FDA-approved. FDA registration simply allows a system to be imported into the U.S. Most home-use PEMF systems are not FDA-approved for specific health indications. They are considered wellness devices. The term wellness in this scenario describes complementary modalities that are not condition-specific. Even if a system is FDA-approved, it is often approved for only a specific condition (indication) or a very limited set of indications. FDA-approved PEMF systems tend to be much more expensive.

Primary Considerations for Choosing a PEMF System

The primary criteria to consider when choosing PEMF treatments, as well as choosing a PEMF system to purchase, are intensity, treatment area sizes, frequencies and programs, ability to self-design programs, program times, portability, and ease-of-use. Paying attention to these criteria will help you make the best choice for your own needs.

Intensity and Treatment Area: These are the parameters I tend to narrow down first. Intensities can be classified easily as extremely low (less than 0.5 gauss), low (0.5 gauss – 10 gauss), medium (10 gauss - 100 gauss), high (100 – 1000 gauss), and very high (greater than 1000 gauss).

Most commercial PEMF systems rarely get above 100 gauss. Most whole-body PEMF systems fall in this category, although a large number, including some of the most expensive systems, are less than 1 gauss. To put things in perspective, the Earth's magnetic field averages about 0.5 gauss. Most clinical research on PEMFs has been done on medium- to high-intensity systems. While some people do experience significant benefits from low- and very-low-intensity PEMF systems, in my experience, benefits tend to happen faster and better with medium- to high-intensity PEMF systems for individual health conditions. This is confirmed by a review of the evidence from the available research, and described across a range of health conditions in my book *Power Tools for Health*.

The size of the PEMF system's applicator or applicators determines the surface area of treatment. A long and wide pad applicator will typically treat the entire body. A regional applicator treats a specific area of the body, for example, the abdomen, the chest, the pelvis, hips, shoulders, or upper or lower back. Regional applicators are often called pillow applicators and come in various sizes, depending on the PEMF system.

Local applicators treat smaller areas of the body, such as a hand, knee, elbow, foot, or part of the shoulder. There are many different configurations for local applicators, including small flat pads, circular open coils, and paddles. Generally, the smaller the applicator, the higher the field intensity, even with the same PEMF system, because the control units will put out the same amount of energy whether a large area of coil is used or a smaller area. With smaller area coils, more energy is delivered to the coil, resulting in a higher field intensity. To be certain, check the manufacturer's intensity measurements, usually stated as maximum field intensity.

Whole-body PEMF systems are typically used for health maintenance and for when a number of local areas of the body need to be treated. This can be accomplished more easily and in less time by using a whole-body system. Systemic health conditions such as osteoporosis, autoimmune diseases, vascular diseases, arthritis in multiple areas of the body, or multi-area skin disorders normally also require a whole-body PEMF system in order to achieve the best benefit.

Frequencies, Waveforms, And Built-In Programs: Frequencies, waveforms, and built-in programs should also be taken into account when choosing a PEMF system. Some PEMF systems do not use frequencies. Instead, they emit only single EMF pulses that are repeated based on intensity. This repetition or pulsation rate is erroneously interpreted as a frequency, but it is not a frequency.

Other systems only have one frequency. This does not necessarily mean such systems aren't useful, but it does limit flexibility in the actions and benefits that specific frequencies have based on your treatment goals.

Still other systems have a broad capacity for selecting individual frequencies, while others only have a built-in, limited set of frequencies or frequency sets. A few systems have the ability to select individual waveforms, but this is rare, and not necessarily useful.

Other PEMF systems:

- allow for tuning or frequency selection for brainwave entrainment.
- have recommended frequency sets for specific conditions.
- have non-selectable background frequencies which can then be modulated with user selectable, specific frequency sets.

I'm not a fan of PEMF systems that recommend specific frequencies for specific health conditions. I've found that the manufacturers of these systems have not done an adequate amount of research to prove that those condition-specific selected frequencies are either the best or exclusive for a specific condition. In addition, many manufacturers do not provide the data on the actual frequency packets used to treat specific conditions. It's been my experience that, except for brainwave entrainment considerations, most frequencies have benefits for most conditions, though results will be variable if the optimal frequencies are not used. The science on which frequencies are best for which conditions is still far from satisfactory.

Often the frequency packets used in the preset programs are counter to brainwave entrainment considerations. For example, if a condition-specific packet has 30 Hz as one of its frequencies and people using it are anxious, this treatment could potentially make them more anxious, or interfere with their ability to fall asleep if used near bedtime. Also, if a condition-specific packet has a low-frequency, such as 5 Hz, this may not be desirable if one is about to drive, operate machinery, or function in a work setting, since such low frequencies tend to slow down brain waves and make a person more tired or less alert. That said, it is often unpredictable how people will respond, with some paradoxically reacting the opposite of what would be expected.

Many magnetic frequencies have been studied and proven to be effective for a variety of health conditions. Based on these studies, it cannot be said that a specific frequency will only do certain things or that specific conditions can only be treated with specific frequencies. Rarely is a selection of frequencies an all-or-none process. Any individual frequency will cause its own biological effects and have additional effects on brainwave entrainment. Biological effects do not specifically equate to the management of any particular condition, but to the biological state of the tissues as part of the health condition, whether local, regional, or systemic. Clearly, local treatment has systemic effects and systemic treatment has local effects.

Program Times: Most, but not all, PEMF systems have time limitations for their programs. Some only run for 15 minutes, others for an hour, and some can be run continuously. Often, PEMF systems require the user to re-run the program, possibly multiple times, if longer treatment times are desired or recommended. The amount of time needed for treatment will vary based on the individual or condition being treated, as well as whether it's for health maintenance or otherwise.

PEMF system sales representatives that claim only eight minutes a day is necessary are ignoring the available research and biologic actions, as well as misleading people into thinking that this is all that is needed to achieve results.

Portability: Except for battery-operated PEMF systems, access to an electrical outlet is necessary to operate most PEMF systems. That can be a major constraint for people, depending on the amount of time necessary for treatment, and particularly for people who need to treat multiple areas of the body in a given treatment session or in a given day. A battery-operated system will allow an individual to carry on daily activities, including driving, thus allowing for extended treatment times. Even medium-intensity PEMF systems may sometimes need to be used for hours at a time for best results. In this situation, battery operation is essential. It's important to choose a PEMF system that will fit your lifestyle or work habits, if available.

Ease of Use: Certain applicators for PEMF systems are challenging to use because of their bulk, size, awkward configuration, or complex set up. It is necessary to understand how one is going to use a system to be sure that the right system is chosen for one's needs and ease-of-use.

Return Periods: All reputable PEMF manufacturers allow you to return the system within a specified window of time after the purchase, usually between 30 and 90 days, depending on the device and the manufacturer. Devices purchased internationally may be more likely not to have return periods. There are some exceptions to this rule, however. Hygiene, for instance, can be a concern with some PEMF devices, like those intended for prostate or pelvic issues. Return periods nearly always have a restocking fee, as well, so it's important to understand the cost of a return before you make a purchase decision.

Be Aware of Myths About PEMFs That Can Impact Your Decision

There are a lot of bold claims and conflicting information on frequency, intensity, and waveforms. Many of these claims are myths, having either very weak or no research behind them. They range from "this specific frequency is all you need" to "high intensities are physically harmful," and everything in between. The most common myths and misconceptions about PEMFs are addressed below:

Only Earth-Based Frequencies Are Safe: This claim is untrue, because the Earth produces all sorts of frequencies, and you're exposed to a huge range of them every day. The light that surrounds you is made of frequencies, and these different frequencies are what enable you to see color. Sound waves hit cilia inside your ears at different frequencies that enable you to hear music, voices, and other sounds, some of which are produced by the Earth. The bottom line is that the Earth produces a plethora of frequencies that are all around you, even if you were entirely unplugged and isolated. To claim that frequencies above 30 Hz are dangerous implies that your ability to see the color red, which has a frequency of 400-484 THz, is also somehow dangerous.

Some PEMF systems range up to 250 kHz and are scientifically proven to be safe. For example, there are multiple studies showing that 1000 Hz PEMF treatment can be effective for treating anxiety, depression, anorexia, OCD, and many other disorders.

The Schumann Resonance Is the Most Important Frequency: The Schumann Resonance is, in fact, multiple bands of frequencies, not just the 7.83 Hz that we so often read about. One of the Schumann Resonances, for example, is above 60 Hz, which is well outside of what some consider "Earth-based," yet is obviously safe since we are continuously exposed to it just by being on Earth.

Only Wound Coils, Not Mesh Coils, Can Produce a 'Pure' Magnetic Field: It is indeed correct that copper coils are the only way to produce a magnetic field, which is why all PEMF systems have copper coils. The layout of coils is a little different in almost every PEMF system, however. Some have eight coils distributed evenly throughout, and other systems have one single coil that is large enough to loop your arm through, and they do not come with a mat. All PEMF systems produce a true and "pure" magnetic field. As long as they are copper, the way coils are laid out does not affect the fact that each system is putting out a pulsed magnetic field.

The NASA 'Square' Wave is Essential to Getting the Best Healing: The NASA "square" wave was a specifically designed "square" wave. There is no way to exactly replicate this "square" wave, so the only time the "NASA "square" wave" was used was in the specific NASA study it's referenced in. Even subsequent NASA research using a similar signal does not use the original waveform. It's been tweaked and refined dozens of times by the NASA researchers. In any event, a "square wave" is not technically possible to produce. It is actually a form of trapezoidal wave.

There is also no way to know that the "square" wave is the best waveform. There are numerous PEMF studies that have been performed with great benefit using "square," rectangular, sawtooth, sinusoidal, and other waveforms. Waveforms simply mimic naturally occurring processes inside the body, and that isn't limited to just "square" waves.

Certain Intensities Can Be Dangerous for Humans: The research refuting this myth is overwhelming. There is an enormous amount of research demonstrating that high intensities can be not just beneficial, but also necessary for treating some health conditions. Even for preventative purposes, there is no reason to believe that high intensities are dangerous. MRI machines operate safely at 4-7T, and the highest intensity available among the PEMF systems that I recommend is <2T. The amount of research done on intensities above 30 G all way into the tens of thousands of gauss has shown no negative side effects whatsoever.

Keep in mind that PEMF intensities may be infinitely high, but their drop off is significant. This means that if you choose a low-intensity unit, about five inches from the applicator, the field all but disappears. For deep-seated issues, by the time the field penetrates all the way to reach the tissue that requires treatment, it may be so weak that it creates no change at all. This is also one of the most common myths about PEMFs, that all intensities have equivalent effects.

Microcirculation Is Only Affected by Certain Systems, Intensities, Or Frequencies: Circulation is positively affected by any PEMF system, no matter the intensity or frequency. Even local systems will affect circulation in the area where applicators are placed on the body and will have benefit in other parts of the body away from the local area of stimulation. Microcirculation is affected equally as well as macrocirculation, and all PEMF systems can claim that benefit. Even slight increases in intensity can positively affect blood oxygenation, however.

Biofeedback Is an Essential Part of a PEMF System: The systems that come with biofeedback systems are so low-intensity that the heart rate barely changes, if it changes at all. And that is what a biofeedback sensor is, essentially: a heart rate monitor. There are many heart rate monitors available that are inexpensive and can be worn while doing a PEMF treatment, though this isn't necessary to gain the benefits of a PEMF treatment. Some people find it of value to monitor their heart rate while doing PEMF therapy, but this is not an indicator of how well the PEMF is actually working in the tissues.

Hormesis Is a Phenomenon that Pertains to PEMFs: Hormesis is defined as the random phenomenon that some small amount of a stressor promotes the body to perform better, while too much of the stressor is dangerous. This can pertain to too much exercise, too much fasting, and even too much electrical stimulation. But there is not one peer-reviewed, substantial scientific study that shows that PEMFs can damage the body. In fact, there is a significant amount of research that shows people exposed to hundreds of thousands of high-intensity pulses directly to the head did not experience one single negative side effect. It has also been shown that small amounts of PEMF therapy usually underperform higher, right, amounts.

If your body doesn't require PEMF treatment, it simply lets the field pass completely through it, leaving cells and tissues unharmed and unaffected. The most you might feel is a little jittery, like you have excess energy. Taking a break from treatment and drinking plenty of water usually makes people feel better quickly.

The Best Treatment Protocol Is Eight Minutes Twice a Day: There is no research to show that eight-minute treatments twice per day would be beneficial, making this one of the most common myths about PEMFs. Every single person who needs a PEMF system will also need a slightly different treatment protocol. Some people will need hours of treatment per day, while some will need 30 minutes twice a day. Like any other treatment, treatment protocols will vary based on the person and cannot possibly be simplified to this level of only eight minutes twice per day.

Given these and other myths about PEMFs, be sure consider the actual factors that this chapter discusses in order to make an informed decision when it comes to choosing a PEMF system.

Examples of PEMF Systems

The following chart is of PEMF systems I recommend. They are by no means the only systems available for people, but they are the only ones I endorse based on my extensive testing of, and research into PEMF systems over the past 25-plus years. I have used many other systems and didn't include them for a number of reasons, including the fact that:

- they could have had similar attributes to systems I was already using
- their construction was faulty or shoddy
- access to service and parts was not reliable
- the companies have not been in operation long enough to establish a strong track record
- they were too complicated for most people to use
- they were intended more for professional use only
- their cost was too high for the probable value
- their marketing was too aggressive
- the warranty periods were too short
- they didn't have the right applicators
- they were part of multilevel marketing companies with prohibitive participation contracts.

There are other PEMF systems available in Europe and Asia that are not available in the U.S. and Canada, so I have omitted them as well. I have also not listed PEMF systems that are FDA-approved, and therefore require prescriptions and need to be ordered by doctors. The typical medical indications for these systems include healing nonunion fractures, bone fusions, treatment-resistant depression, wound healing, and edema. Because of FDA restrictions, these systems are not typically available for use for reasons other than their FDA-approved indications.

With all that said, here are the PEMF systems I consider most effective and suitable for consumers.

PEMF Device Comparison Table

PEMF Device Name	PEMF Device Picture	Price*	Max intensity	Applicators	Frequency range	Number programs	Waveform	Rental option	Warranty
Almag		$599	200 Gauss	4 Coils on string	7.8 Hz	1	Sinusoidal	No	1 Year
BioBalance		$2,590	Full Body Mat: 5 Gauss Pillow: 10 Gauss	Mat, Pillow	.5 – 1000 Hz	6	Sinusoidal	Yes – 8 weeks	2 Years
EarthPulse		$699-$1,199	1,100 Gauss	1 Coil	1 – 14.1 Hz	10	Trape-zoidal	No	5 Years
HUGO Intense		$8,999	7,500 Gauss	Dual Full Body Mats, 60' Cord Coil	1-50 pulses per second	1	Nano-second pulse	No	3 Years
HUGO Pro		$25,990	12,000 Gauss	Dual Full Body Mats, 60' Cord Coil	1-50 pulses per second	1	Nano-second pulse	No	3 Years
FlexPulse		$1,290	200 Gauss	2 Coils	1 – 1,000 Hz	6	Trape-zoidal	No	2 Years
MediThera		$2,450	0.75 Gauss	Mat, Pillow, Pen	.3 – 250 Hz	3	Sawtooth	Yes – 8 weeks	2 Years
MicroPulse A9		$429	200 Gauss	2 Coils	10/100 Hz	1	Trape-zoidal	No	1 Year
Parmeds Home		$3,575	Full Body mat: 70 Gauss Pillow: 200 Gauss	Mat, Pillow	1 – 50 Hz	10	Square-gated Sinusoidal	No	3 Years
Parmeds Pro Special		$6,450	Full Body mat: 150 Gauss Pillow: 1000 Gauss	Mat, Pillow	1 – 50 Hz	10	Square-gated Sinusoidal	No	3 Years

(Continued)

PEMF Device Name	PEMF Device Picture	Price*	Max intensity	Applicators	Frequency range	Number programs	Waveform	Rental option	Warranty
Parmeds Super		$7,190	Full Body mat: 150 Gauss Pillow: 1000 Gauss	Mat, Pillow	1 – 50 Hz	10+100 in software	Square-gated Sinusoidal	No	3 Year
Parmeds Ultra		$13,950	Full Body mat: 500 Gauss Pillow: 1600 Gauss	Mat, Pillow	1 – 50 Hz	10 + 70 in software	Square-gated Sinusoidal	No	3 Years
Parmeds MutiFlash		$5,250-$5,975	4,000 Gauss	Coil, Pad, Mat	<1-5 Pulses per second	1 with 10 intensity levels	Impulse	No	3 Years
Parmeds Premium Flash		$7,700-$8,850	7,200 Gauss	Coil, Pad, Mat	<1-5 Pulses per second	1 with 10 intensity levels	Impulse	No	3 Years
Parmeds UltraFlash		$7,700-$8,850	>10000 Gauss	Coil, Pad, 2 Mats	<1-5 Pulses per second	1 with 10 intensity levels	Impulse	No	3 Years
PEMF 120		$19,900-$20,800	9,360 Gauss	Straight Rope, Loop Coil, Butterfly Coil Paddle, Mat	1-10 pulses per second	1	Impulse	Yes – 90 days	3 Years
Pulsed Harmonix A2500		$4,950	~2500 Gauss	Mat, Mitt, Pouch	1-27 pulses per second	1	Impulse	No	3 Years
Sota Magnetic Pulser		$380	6,000 Gauss (slow), 2,500 Gauss (fast)	Paddle	1 Hz	2	Impulse	No	2 Years
TeslaFit Plus V2		$6,950-$8,195	3,990 Gauss	Loop Coil, Butterfly Coil Paddle, Mat	1-10 pulses per second	1	Impulse	2	3 Years
TeslaFit Duo		$11,700-$13,500	5,220 Gauss	Loop Coil, Butterfly Coil Paddle, Mat	1-10 pulses per second	1	Impulse	No	3 Years
TeslaFit Pro		$19,900-$20,650	8,290 Gauss	Loop Coil, Butterfly Coil, Paddle, Mat	1-10 pulses per second	1	Impulse	Yes – 90 days	3 Years

* Prices are subject to change. These prices are meant to give a sense of approximate cost.

Examples of PEMF Systems I Use and Recommend by Intensity and Area of Coverage

When looking at the disease/condition chart and device types best for those conditions in Chapter 10, I specify using PEMF devices that are local or whole-body and of low, medium, or high intensities. Throughout the discussion of each condition, I may refer to *very-high-intensity devices*. Very-high-intensity devices were not specifically mentioned, so I have added a column in the table below for those devices that are very-high-intensity.

The purpose of this table is to give you a reference point for specific PEMF devices. These devices are available on DrPawluk.com, where there is more specific information about them. There are also numerous, condition-based blogs with more extensive information, videos, and other resource material available for review on DrPawluk.com.

There is other more in-depth information on the research evidence for the use of PEMF treatment for 50 health conditions in my book *Power Tools for Health*.

The PEMFs in the table below are devices that I routinely use and recommend. There are many PEMF systems available today that were not available 10 years ago. Many of them overlap in their characteristics with those in this table. PEMF systems that are not in this table can still be very effective.

When purchasing a PEMF system it is very important to know what the peak intensity is. There are many ways of measuring magnetic fields, which can lead to a lot of confusion. This is why peak intensity is frequently mentioned. Actually, the range of intensities in the device is also important, so that one may know what the lowest and highest intensities are. Knowing the lowest intensities can be very important for developing your own "low and slow" protocols. There is a possibility that the lowest intensity in the system may create a need to go even "lower and slower" than the system allows. For ways to deal with "low and slow" protocols, see Appendix B.

Intensity is the product of the applicator as well as the voltage output of the control unit. So, the configuration of the applicator and the layout of the coils in the applicator is important to know where the magnetic field is the weakest and the strongest. In many cases the applicator will work best when the edge of a coil, the strongest area of the coil, is placed over a target area of the body. Generally, the weakest part of a coil is in the center of a circular applicator or center of the coil.

As a rule, whole-body PEMF applicators have lower intensities than their local PEMF applicators. This is usually because the coils have to be distributed through a much larger area, causing the electrical voltage produced by the control unit to be reduced across that larger area. PEMF systems that only have local applicators are designed to maximize the possible magnetic field of that system. There is always a trade-off between using whole-body stimulation and local stimulation. Ultimately, whole-body stimulation is more efficient and produces possibly even more effective health results than placing stronger local applicators over multiple areas during a treatment session.

PEMF Devices by Local vs Whole-Body and Intensity Level

PEMF DEVICES BY LOCAL VS WHOLE BODY AND INTENSITY LEVEL

PEMF Device	Local Intensity - in Gauss				Whole body Intensity - in Gauss			
	low	medium	high	very high	low	medium	high	very high
Almag	0.1-10	10-100	100-1000	>1000	0.1-10	10-100	100-1000	>1000
BioBalance		x	x					
EarthPulse	x				x			
FlexPulse			x	x				
Hugo Devices		x	x					
Medithera				x				x
MicroPulse A9	x				x			
Parmeds Home			x					
Parmeds ProSpecial/Super		x	x			x		
Parmeds Ultra 3D			x	x			x	
Parmeds Multiflash			x	x			x	
Parmeds Premium Flash				x			x	x
Parmeds Ultra Flash				x			x	x
PEMF 120			x	x			x	x
Pulsed Harmonix			x	x				
SOTA				x				
TeslaFit Devices			x	x				

Note: The above table may be used to guide device selection based on the conditions being treated in Chapters 9 and 10.

It is important to know the applicators that are available for a given system. The applicators emit or project the magnetic field needed to do the work for PEMF therapy. They can be broadly classified into whole-body, regional, or local. Regional applicators cover larger areas of the body while not being whole-body. The following are some sample applicators for several PEMF systems.

Sample Applicators

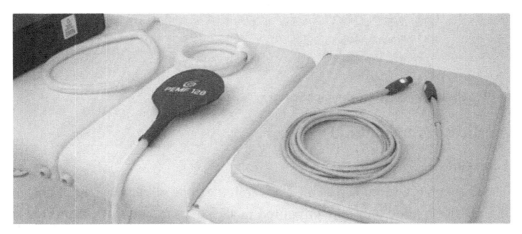

PEMF-120 and TeslaFit Applicators

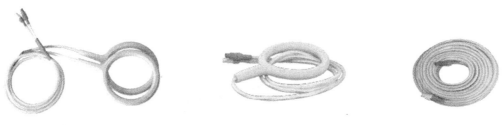

Hugo Applicators

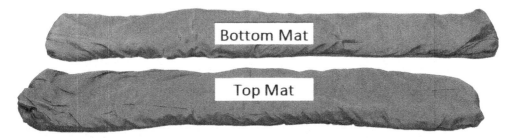

Parmeds Flash Applicators

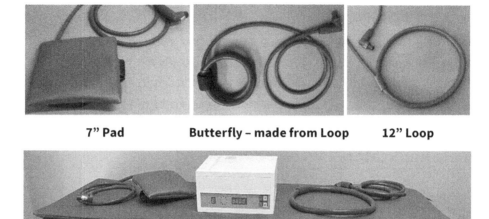

7" Pad   **Butterfly – made from Loop**   **12" Loop**

Whole-Body Mat plus other applicators

Applicator Placements

Loop coil

The loop coil is also known as the lasso coil. It can be placed over the abdomen to treat the gut and lungs or configured in such a way as to direct treatment at the pelvis or hip. It can be placed over the head like a necklace so that it rests on the shoulders. However it is configured, the loop coil is durable and used more regularly than the other coils. It can also be configured into ellipse form by compressing the sides. Ideally, the sides should not touch, since the magnetic fields may negate each other. This elliptical form may also be easily shaped around contoured areas of the body such as a hip, shoulder, knee, thigh, etc.

Placements on the head

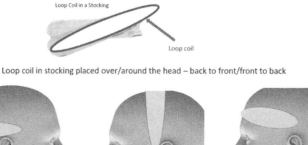

Loop Coil in a Stocking

Loop coil

Loop coil in stocking placed over/around the head – back to front/front to back

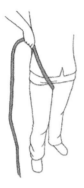 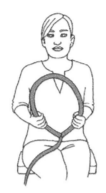 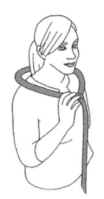 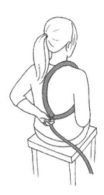

Butterfly Coil

The butterfly coil is also known as the figure 8 coil. It can be used in many ways. It can be configured around a joint like a knee or shoulder or made to open around the neck. It can be "closed" or left open and used for brain stimulation. The magnetic field from the butterfly coil is strongest at the "hinge" or center point of the figure 8.

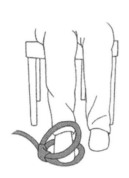 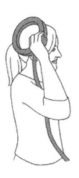 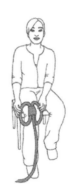 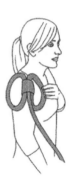

Straight (Rope) Coil

The straight coil is also known as the rope coil, must be manually "coiled" by the user. It can be used to treat an entire extremity – wrapped down a leg or arm, for example. It must be made to have at least 4 "turns" or coils, so if you are wrapping an arm, for example, you want to wrap the rope at least 4 times to get benefit. The closer the turns (as in the third example below), the stronger field will be. The rope coils can also be wrapped around the chest or abdomen.

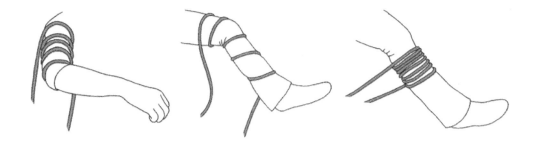

Small, Portable PEMF Coil

Below are example placements of a small portable PEMF coil. The small coils can be used one or two at a time. With many PEMF devices, when two coils are used at a time the total energy is divided equally between the two of them. For deeper PEMF work it may be best to use one coil at a time. Many support options are available including wraps, braces, bands, tape, etc. Remember, magnetic fields penetrate almost anything, except metal, completely. They can even be taped onto the outside of clothing, shoes, wraps, casts, etc.

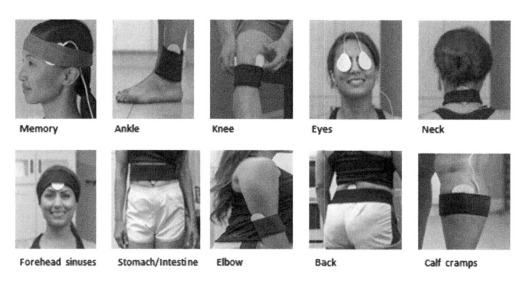

Memory	Ankle	Knee	Eyes	Neck
Forehead sinuses	Stomach/Intestine	Elbow	Back	Calf cramps

Coils may be secured to the body using a wrap or band (such as a sweat band or Ace bandage) or with athletic tape. Or, the coil may also be held in place by being tucked under snug-fitting clothing or in a pocket.

Summary

There are many potentially confusing choices when selecting an appropriate PEMF system for yourself, family, friends, and even pets, but I hope the above guidelines will help you to decide which type of system is best for you, whether or not you intend to purchase your own system for home use.

There are a limited but growing number of physicians and other health practitioner who are treating people in their offices with PEMF systems, but you should not be misled into thinking that office-care treatment is a long-term solution. Likewise, healing does not happen because of one or two treatments. You need to understand and respect the nature of your body and how it heals. The pharmaceutical and supplement industries understand this, which is why users of their products typically need to take them for the long-term.

I understand that PEMFs may feel like an expensive investment in the short-term, but in the long term, owning a system will provide you with the convenience and ability to treat yourself independently at your own pace and with almost no risk. Ultimately, the cost of your PEMF system, should you purchase one, might end up being only pennies per day, especially if you and other family members continue to use the system for years.

The guidelines and examples of PEMF systems presented in this chapter will help you evaluate any PEMF system you may be considering for your own health care and healing. Yet, do not be led into believing that any one system is a cure-all. There is no such thing as "one-size-fits-all." However, there is likely to be an ideal system for you that you will be able to find benefit from and afford.

If you still have concerns of questions about selecting a PEMF system, feel free to apply for a free consultation via my website. You can request one at www. DrPawluk.com/consultation.

Why You Should Consider Owning Your Own PEMF System

Based on my many years of researching and using PEMF systems and experiencing the many health benefits they provide, both for myself and for my clients, I've learned that owning your own PEMF system is one of the best things you can do to maintain good health and help resolve any health problems you may have. Going for professional help can be extraordinarily useful. However, owning your own PEMF system that is right for your needs and conditions gives you the most flexibility to own and control your own health care, not only for the short term but also for the long term.

People buy PEMF systems for specific needs that make sense at the time, but PEMF systems are likely to be useful for unexpected, or even expected, health needs long into the future. A PEMF system purchased solely from the perspective of a current problem(s) may not be adequate for future needs.

There are two major advantages of owning a PEMF system—convenience and cost savings over time.

As I've explained earlier in this book, the best results from PEMF therapy are achieved from daily treatments, ideally for at least 30 minutes twice a day. But as I've also pointed out, in some cases, treatments times may need to last much longer than that—in some instances, even 24 hours/day using portable, battery-operated devices—for meaningful and lasting results to occur. Having the ability to provide yourself with regular, ongoing treatments is simply not possible if you have to rely on your physician or other healthcare provider to administer PEMF treatments for you. Even scheduling treatments once a week with your provider may not be practical if he or she has a busy practice, as most clinicians do. Moreover, it is also unlikely that your scheduled appointment will last for the necessary amount of time required for a PEMF treatment to benefit you. In addition, when PEMF therapy is required for acute health problems that occur suddenly, such as a backache, sudden migraine, or an unexpected muscle or ligament strain, it may take days or more before your health care provider can even see you.

Then there is the cost factor involved in receiving professional PEMF treatments. Even if it were practical for your health care provider to provide you with daily PEMF treatments, the costs you would incur would be prohibitive over time, both because PEMF therapy is typically not covered by health insurance and has to be paid for out-of-pocket, and because of the fees providers charge for such treatments. Keep in mind that the expenses related to running a medical or health care practice are far greater than most patients and clients realize, often running to six figures or more per year before the practitioner sees a penny in profit. As a result, though monetary gain is not the primary reason motivating the vast majority of clinicians who enter our profession, if we are to be able to continue to serve those in need of health care, we need to charge accordingly for the services we provide. There simply is no other alternative.

We must also remember that conventional health services, broadly speaking, are designed for and cover a limited set of services primarily from a bureaucratic fiscal or political perspective. Bureaucratic and insurance services tend to have a short-term perspective on healthcare needs. This is because people change their insurance coverage fairly frequently or move. Once you shift insurance coverage, you are no longer their responsibility. So, why should they have an interest in your long-term health? To them, anti-aging is not a priority. That means that there is a huge unmet need for innovative services outside the scope of these conventional services. As a result, the costs of these often much more successful services are not covered, even though they are necessary and effective.

Like all other patient and client services, when it comes to PEMF treatments, pricing structures must be based so that they help meet the economic needs of the overall medical/healthcare practice. This means that, even if it was possible for you to achieve daily PEMF treatments at your practitioner's office, after a single month of five treatments per week, you would have paid at least $400.00, assuming a very low cost per treatment of $20.00. (In reality, the cost of a single professional treatment is likely to be double that, or more). At that rate, you could buy many of the various PEMF systems available for consumers in a matter of months.

Owning Your Own PEMF System Provides You with an Exceptional Price-Per-Day Value: As you saw in Chapter 7, there is a large difference in pricing for the various PEMF systems I recommend. Units intended for use at home can range from as little as a few hundred dollars all the way up to $20,000 and more. Whole-body systems are more expensive, but they are also more complex and treat more of the body.

The true value of owning your own PEMF system is that it is a one-time purchase that can be used by you and your entire family for a vast range of needs, known and unknown, in the comfort of your home for years to come. There are no refills, no co-pays, no fighting with insurance companies, no need for each family member to have a different system, and no need to take time off to schedule and travel to receive your treatments. Moreover, even your pets and plants, if you have them at home, can benefit from PEMF systems.

The bottom line is that when you factor in a lifetime of at-home daily, or at least regular, use of whichever system you might purchase, PEMF units are an exceptional value. And this value is made even better considering that multiple users in your home can receive regular benefit.

What you are paying for when purchasing a reputable PEMF system is quality construction and quality service. These factors are equally important. Often, people make purchasing decisions based on affordability, so the best PEMF system for their needs may not be considered to be affordable. It may be necessary, but not perceived to be affordable. Thinking only of affordability is not considering value, especially when it comes to health. Poor health is extraordinarily costly to the individuals suffering from it. If a more affordable, but less effective PEMF system is chosen, it will likely take longer for benefits to be achieved, resulting in increased frustration in their purchase because one's needs are not being met as expected. Patience is required in these circumstances, and greater value should then be placed on the amount of support your PEMF reseller or dealer is able to provide you.

Whole-Body System or Local PEMF System?

If you are considering buying a PEMF system to support and improve your health, the criteria I outlined in Chapter 7 can help you choose the system that is most appropriate for you. Because the purchase of a PEMF system is both a short-term and a long-term investment in your present and future health, it's important to consider not only what is motivating your decision now but also to consider and plan for how the system you consider purchasing might help you with your future health needs.

Since the PEMF system you buy will be available to you for years to come, it is worthwhile to think about getting a system with more features and options than systems you might consider just for the short term. In line with that, once you decide to purchase a system, your next need to decide whether you need a whole-body PEMF system or a local PEMF system. As we have covered, a local system will have applicators that are basically only useful for treating one small area of the body at a time, such as a hand, knee, elbow, foot, part of the shoulder, part of the back, prostate, bladder, or neck, whereas a whole-body system with a long and wide pad applicator will typically treat your entire body.

Whole-body PEMF systems are usually used for health maintenance and can provide more benefits more easily and quickly because they allow you to treat several local areas of your body at the same time. Systemic health conditions such as osteoporosis, Lyme disease, chronic fatigue syndrome, autoimmune diseases, vascular diseases, or multi-area skin disorders, also normally require a whole-body PEMF system to achieve the best results, and quite likely a higher-intensity system.

Another advantage of whole-body PEMF systems is that they have smaller, pad-type regional applicators that can be used separately from the whole-body pad. This allows you to treat a local area of your body, such as your abdomen, chest, pelvis, hips, shoulders, or upper or lower back. Regional applicators are sometimes called pillow applicators and come in various sizes, depending on the whole-body system you choose.

Deciding Which Magnetic Field Intensity Will You Need: After deciding on whether you wish to purchase a local or whole-body PEMF system, your next most important decision will usually be determining what level of magnetic field intensity you need. Lower intensities may work well for superficial problems in tissues that are not deep in the body, such as the hands, elbow, shoulder tendinitis, carpal tunnel, heel spurs, eyes, teeth, or TMJ. Higher-intensity local PEMFs are needed for problems deeper in the body, such as in the brain, spine, prostate, bladder, hips, knees, heart, lung, gallbladder, pancreas, kidneys, and bones. Local treatment PEMFs can range in maximum intensity from 10 gauss to around 10,000 gauss. If you want to do whole-body and regional treatments with the same PEMF system, intensity also becomes very important. Regional applicators can range in intensity from less than 1 gauss to 7,000 gauss.

Long, body-length pads that come with whole-body systems almost always operate on lower-intensity fields than local or regional applicators or pads. Knowing the intensity of each applicator is therefore important before you decide which type of system to purchase. There are several choices among whole-body PEMF systems ranging in intensity from < 1 gauss (< 100 microTesla) to 500 gauss or more. The general rule of thumb is that the higher the intensity, the faster the results, and the less the treatment time that will be necessary to achieve them.

Many people make their decision based on the cost of a PEMF system, often sacrificing results that might be better and more rapidly achieved by more expensive systems. Results are often promised by manufacturers and distributors of very-low-intensity PEMF systems that ignore the research studies showing that higher intensity is needed. (To learn more about these proven intensities, please review Chapters 4, 5, and 7, and also see my previous book, *Power Tools for Health* (see www.DrPawluk.com/product/power-tools-health).

General health maintenance may be reasonably effective with either low-intensity or higher-intensity PEMF systems when they are used daily. However, if there are significant health problems in multiple areas of your body, higher-intensity whole-body pads will be needed, preferably over 50 gauss(>5000 microTesla or >5 milliTesla). Generally, the higher the intensity, the more expensive the PEMF system will be.

After you have decided on what type of PEMF system you want (whole-body versus local), and the magnetic field intensity you need, other factors to consider to further narrow down your choice of a specific system include frequencies, applicator shapes, whether the system is portable or AC powered, and whether rentals are available (see below). Advice about the variety of PEMF options available to you are available by contacting my team and me at www.DrPawluk. com. We will be more than happy to help you sort out all the PEMF options on the market.

Beware of Scams and Outright Lies

Unfortunately, not all claims made by certain PEMF manufacturers and distributors are reputable. When people are misinformed, it is easy to be taken in by inflated claims and purchase PEMF systems that seem legitimate, but are in reality ineffective for the specific problem or problems that you may have. The truth is that any PEMF device is likely to have *some* benefit to health, but it may not provide the level of benefit you need or are looking for.

Even medical professionals have to do extensive research to really understand the science behind PEMF therapy. Conventional medical training simply doesn't include this information. If your only source of information about PEMFs is a general internet search, you probably won't have the knowledge you need to make the best selection. Empowering you with that knowledge is why I wrote this book, as well as *Power Tools for Health*, and created DrPawluk.com and my blog, videos and much other informative and educational material on that site that is regularly expanding.

What follow are the most common claims made by some PEMF companies whose primary interest seems to be making money, not helping heal as many people as possible.

FDA Approval Is Necessary/Best: Most manufacturers of PEMF devices actually choose NOT to seek FDA approval. Why? Because such approval is far too limiting. If a device is FDA-approved, there are strict parameters around what it can be marketed for. There must be clear research to support the claims and research is expensive to conduct. Moreover, if a PEMF device is FDA-approved for a particular use, its manufacturer can't claim it provides other benefits, even though most PEMFs do.

Also don't be confused by claims of PEMF systems being FDA-registered either. All that means is that the FDA knows the device is being imported into the U.S., and *all* imported PEMF machines have to be registered, whether that information is part of the manufacturers marketing plan or not.

Claims That a PEMF Device/System Is the Best One on the Market: The simple truth is there is no one best unit. You can't find a one-size-fits-all model, or even a model that is best for most people. The same applies to cars. There are many choices in cars because there are many needs or preferences. And a claim that a particular system helps with circulation does not mean that that is the only system that helps with circulation, or that that is really the only benefit of PEMFs that is important or most needed. The PEMF device or system that is best for you will depend on what you need it for now, and perhaps how you might use it in the future. Another consideration is whether other family members will use it as well. Manufacturers love to make claims that their machine is the best on the market. It might be, for specific purposes, but not for the broadest range of needs.

PEMF Machines Can't Be Used for Specific Conditions: PEMF devices are first and foremost wellness devices. Magnetic field therapies are safe for almost any application when used properly, even at very high intensities (such as an

MRI machine). Although some people or manufacturers/distributors might claim that you shouldn't use PEMF therapy in conjunction with certain medications or with certain health conditions (including cancer), there is very little evidence that PEMF therapy causes any significant adverse effects. In fact, the opposite is true. Ample evidence exists that shows that PEMF therapy can be a very effective complement to most other treatments, including medications, especially in the area of pain relief.

Only One PEMF Device Will Work for Your Condition: Again, some manufacturers will say almost anything to get you to buy their device. But the truth is, there are many devices available on the market, and if you understand what signal intensity and coil configuration you need, many different PEMF systems can offer relief for the same conditions. In making a purchasing decision, you may want to be made more comfortable by knowing whether a device has research behind it or whether it can be effective for specific conditions. Unfortunately, even though there are thousands of research studies about PEMF effectiveness, there is never enough research to satisfy all questions. Research is expensive and it's nearly impossible to find evidence for every PEMF system out there, which is why basically understanding frequency and intensity, as well as whether you need a whole-body system or a local, targeted system, is so important. I often say that whatever PEMF system you use will benefit your health at least to some extent, regardless of specific conditions. That's because the overall positive effects on your body will at least indirectly help you cope with most specific conditions. Your body will decide what benefits it will see, and how quickly. This will depend on the PEMF being used, the starting point in the disease process, how aggressively treatment is done, and many other factors. But you have to start somewhere.

Rental Options—Try Before You Buy

Higher-priced PEMF units, usually whole-body systems, sometimes, but not often, have rental programs that allow you to experience the unit before you purchase it. This way you can discover if the unit meets your specific needs before you purchase it outright. However, if you choose a rental option, make sure the rental program is a reputable one, and one that affords you enough time with the system to be able to make an informed decision. As mentioned, low-intensity systems will likely take a bit longer to produce results, so it would make sense that low-intensity units have longer rental periods.

Most of the time, rental programs are not long enough to see significant results. It takes time for the body to heal. You might notice some, likely limited, improvement in some aspects of your condition(s), but you can't expect significant healing. That takes long-term therapy, longer than the rental period.

Before deciding to rent, also be sure to compare and contrast rental programs to get an idea of what is fair. And always make sure that you rent the right equipment for your problem. If you rent the wrong equipment, usually based on lower-priced rentals, you may be disappointed with the results. Unfortunately, you would not likely be able to conclude that PEMFs won't work for you. It would be that just that particular equipment for that particular period of time would not work well enough for your particular needs. Rentals also do not usually allow adequate time to be able to proceed through a "low and slow" protocol, if there are issues with sensitivity and the risk of possible reactions at the beginning of starting a course of treatment. (See Appendix B for discussion about "low and slow" protocols.)

Working With a Trained Professional Is the Best Way to Find the PEMF Device that's Right for *You*

Although this book was written to help you better understand why PEMF therapy can be such an important solution for maintaining and improving your health, and to help guide you in understanding the complexities of choosing the best PEMF device for your specific needs, even after reading it, you may still find you need more information before you make your purchase and begin applying PEMF therapy on yourself and your loved ones. You can find more help on my website, including my blog articles, both of which are designed solely to help you make the right decision for the PEMF treatment benefits you desire.

But because there are so many factors involved in selecting the best PEMF device, I always recommend that you work with a physician or medical team that is broadly well-versed in PEMF therapy. I have studied PEMF therapy for years, and I am always happy to help you make the right selection. Call my office or apply for a complimentary consultation if you are considering purchasing a PEMF device. (Visit www.DrPawluk.com/consultation.)

My team and I can help you make the best choice for *you*.

PART TWO

Health Conditions That Can Be Helped by PEMF Therapy

CHAPTER 9

PEMF Therapy for Pain Relief

Pain relief is the number one reason so many people seek out PEMF therapy—*because it works!* And it works more effectively and safely for most pain conditions than any other therapy I've come across in my 50 years of serving patients and clients as a physician.

The prevalence of pain is an extremely urgent public health and socioeconomic problem. In the U.S. alone, chronic pain affects at least 116 million American adults, more than the total affected by heart disease, cancer, and diabetes combined. At least 17 percent of people ages 15 and older suffer from chronic pain to such a degree that it interferes with their daily life. Pain, in acute, recurrent, and chronic forms, is prevalent across age, cultural background, and gender, and costs North American adults an estimated $10,000–$15,000 per person annually. At any given moment, at least one in four adults in North America is suffering from some form of pain. More than 26 million American adults suffer from frequent back pain, one of the most common locations of chronic pain.

What Pain Is at a Biological Level: Pain is both normal and necessary in acute situations. The pain you feel when you sprain an ankle, touch a hot stove, or are fighting off an infection is a message from your body to your brain, signaling your brain to send help.

Acute inflammation is a physiological response to cell damage. It begins at the exact location of the problem, and, in addition to being felt through pain sensations, is often visible through redness, swelling, and heat. Acute inflammation makes your blood vessels dilate and increases blood flow, sending white blood cells to the injury site to aid in healing. Certain chemicals are released, calling immune cells, hormones, and nutrients into action. All of this promotes the healing process, and, as the body heals, inflammation is reduced.

Chronic inflammation, on the other hand, means that there is a steady, low-level of inflammation in the body even when there is no obvious injury or infection. While there is still a lot that remains unknown about chronic inflammation and what causes it, research has shown that it can lead to a wide range of health issues, including chronic pain. When the immune system is activated with nothing to heal, those white blood cells can begin attacking apparently healthy organs, tissues, and other cells. As noted above, chronic pain is a major health issue that can take a toll on daily life, both individually and on the whole of our society.

As I gained experience as a practitioner of holistic/integrative medicine, I was not confident in the success of pain reduction approaches that relied solely on using nutrition, supplements, lifestyle changes, or psychological/emotional/cognitive approaches. For the more significant pain problems that typically resulted in reliance on narcotics, I felt that something else was needed. Even though I was trained in acupuncture, I found that it was not always helpful enough in mitigating more significant pain.

As I explained in this book's Introduction, it was my search for a more effective solution to pain management that led me to research and then use PEMFs for that purpose. I soon discovered that PEMF therapy can be a pain treatment *par excellence*, whether in a practitioner's office or for home use. Most significantly, PEMFs don't just help to relieve the symptoms. They also address the underlying causes of the pain, particularly inflammation. Addressing pain's causal factors is more likely to produce a lasting response, eventually offering the possibility of healing the dysfunction. In my experience, almost everyone suffering from pain, even severe chronic pain, benefits from PEMF therapy, and they are frequently able to avoid surgical procedures and decrease or avoid the use of pain-relief drugs. Research has shown that PEMFs work for numerous pain-related conditions, including:

• Abdominal pain	• Intermittent claudication	• PMS
• Angina	• Ischemia	• Post-workout aching
• Arthritis	• Muscle spasms and tears	• Postoperative pain
• Bruises	• Nerve entrapment	• Reflex sympathetic dystrophy
• Burns	• Nerve pain	
• Bursitis	• Neuroma	• Sinus pain
• Carpal tunnel syndrome	• Painful shoulder	• Sprains
• Cervical disc injuries	• Pelvic pain	• Strains
• Dental pain	• Peripheral neuropathy	• TMJ
• Fibrocystic breast disease	• Phantom pain	• Tendonitis
	• Plantar fasciitis	• Tennis elbow
• Fibromyalgia		• Trauma
• Fractures		• Whiplash

The Problem With Conventional Pain Management

The default treatments for management of chronic pain are often medications, surgical procedures, or physical therapy. Unfortunately, these treatments are often ineffective and sometimes dangerous, causing their own side effects and complications.

Medications simply cover up the pain, while not addressing the actual problem. And they can sometimes cause serious side effects, including permanent damage to your kidneys or liver, stomach bleeding, and addiction. The risks of complications with surgery are also great. I've seen far too many patients come to me after surgical procedures have failed them, and in many cases, made their problems worse. Rarely will conventional doctors refer patients to alternative modalities like acupuncture, massage, or chiropractic therapy, let alone PEMFs. But PEMF therapy for pain should always be considered.

Physical therapy is another commonly prescribed therapy for treating pain. It also can be expensive and time-consuming. While it can be a good and proper short-term solution for an acute problem, it's not practical for treating chronic conditions. Other alternative treatments, like chiropractic care and acupuncture, can also provide some relief, but the underlying problem is still there. Cold laser and shockwave therapies, which rely on being provided by professionals, have the same limitations. When these treatments wear off, the pain returns, sending you back for treatment again and again.

Medical specialists tend to have tunnel vision. When you go to a specialist for a problem, that specialist has a single approach to dealing with your problem. I refer to these specialties as "parlors"—parlors of neurosurgery, orthopedics, pain management, natural medicine, massage, etc. Every doctor has a parlor, or specialty, as do other healthcare professionals. If you end up in the wrong parlor, your problem may be addressed in the wrong way. That's not to say that the specialists are not well-meaning (they almost always are), but that they cannot see beyond their own parlor. Only a well-informed consumer (or well-rounded, holistic practitioner) can see past the parlors and find out what other options may exist.

In addition, most doctors don't always tell their patients that the problem will linger and require lifetime management. This becomes a huge disservice to chronic pain patients. They are given false hope that this approach to treatment (whether it's surgery or an injection) is going to truly resolve their problem. Yes, people may temporarily feel better, but within a few weeks or months or even a year after the treatment, the problem returns, sometimes more severely, because the underlying cause was not dealt with. Truthfully, not all causes can be eliminated. Sometimes this is obvious. More often, trial and error reveal that the problem cannot be removed and the goal of treatment changes to pain management. When this happens, the safest and least risky approaches become paramount.

This helps explains why most people only find PEMFs at the end of a long search for an answer to their pain. Almost everyone I speak with who comes to me in pain has tried both conventional and other alternative medical approaches for their pain before they consider PEMFs. It's only once these other treatment options have failed (or presented dramatic side effects) that many people do their own research and learn about PEMF therapy.

Most of the time pain management should be directed first at the cause or the specific area with the pain problem. Conventional pain management primarily depends on what I call "numbing and dumbing." Numbing is accomplished by using a topical or injectable numbing agent such as lidocaine or Novocain. Numbing is also accomplished by cold therapy, such as placing ice over a painful site or taking ice baths. "Dumbing" can be considered anything that makes the brain less perceptive to pain, such as opioids, antidepressants, anticonvulsants, and sedatives and tranquilizers. These "numbing and dumbing" approaches are very short-lived and need to be continually repeated. Hence the need for a more complete and long-lasting solution.

Steroid injections are the most commonly used procedures in conventional pain practice. The primary goal of steroids is to reduce inflammation. The downside of steroid injections is that they tend to weaken the connective tissues into which they are injected. For example, steroids injected into the skin will leave pock marks in the skin where the tissues have "melted" away. Because of this complication, there is also a limited number of time steroids can be injected into a given area in the body that could be causing pain.

The "dumbing" approach mentioned above involves changing the brain's perception of the pain through the use of pain medication. Theoretically, this is a reasonable way to deal with chronic pain. However, such an approach can often result in side effects, dependency and addiction issues, and the major challenges in withdrawal, even from the non-opioid medications.

People who suffer from chronic pain are sometimes also prescribed selective serotonin reuptake inhibitor drugs (SSRIs) to help them cope with the associated depression and anxiety pain can cause. Users of SSRIs can sometimes become "lifers," developing lifetime dependencies, because withdrawal from these agents can take a long time and be very uncomfortable. Because these drugs change brain receptors, the receptors become dependent, just like somebody would become dependent on using crutches.

When these conventional approaches don't work or stop working, there is an escalating cycle of more aggressive attempts at pain management that could end up resulting in implanted pain modulators, surgical or radio-ablation rhizotomy (killing nerves), cutting the spinal cord, or brain surgery. All of these procedures have significant side effects and complications. Some people have even been recommending intravenous ketamine, as one injection or even given via IV over 24 hours, which have to be done in a hospital setting. Ketamine has a long history of use as an anesthetic for operations. IV ketamine only provides short-term pain relief in those with chronic non-cancer pain, with increased risks of nausea, vomiting and even longer-lasting, neurological effects.

As you can see, conventional pain management approaches are limited in scope, have significant side effects and complications, and are often ineffective. That is not the case with PEMF therapy for pain.

Using PEMF Systems to Manage Pain

PEMFs have major advantages over most other pain management approaches because of their pain-relieving capability, and their documented effectiveness for reducing inflammation, decreasing swelling, improving circulation, helping with tissue regeneration, decreasing nerve irritability, improving nerve recovery, decreasing overactive immune responses, and many more benefits. The body reacts to the PEMF signal to produce all these actions. Moreover, the body decides how it will respond, which is why PEMFs are so safe and work in so many different ways to help with pain management. In addition, PEMFs work synergistically with almost all other treatment approaches to help with pain and heal tissue.

The side effect profile of PEMFs is very limited, particularly if basic rules of application are followed, especially with a "low and slow" approach (See Appendix B). On the other hand, as they say in sports training, "no pain, no gain." The goal is to decrease discomfort caused by "training" the tissues with PEMF stimulation by increasing the stimulation only as tolerated.

When PEMFs are used to address the cause of the pain and help with the symptoms, improving the symptoms is more often a byproduct of helping the tissues to be healthier. The pain improving effect, called antinociception, as is true with pain medications and steroids, is short-lived and will return if the underlying cause is not dealt with. This is why PEMF therapy often has to be long-term to help with tissue healing and regeneration. Tissues don't regenerate right away. For example, a fractured bone may be usable within two to three months, but it is still vulnerable to break down for a year or two, until a solid union of the fragments is completed.

Chronic pain and severe acute pain create changes in the brain that sensitize the brain to any other sensory stimuli entering the brain. This is called centralization. High-intensity PEMFs applied to the brain change the way the brain receives signals from the rest of the body, combating centralization. In this capacity, PEMFs provide antidepressant, anti-anxiety, stress-reducing, circadian rhythm-restoring, sleep-enhancing, relaxation, and other healing benefits.

PEMFs deal with the brain in very different ways. And, unlike the drugs, they do not stay in the brain. But, like the drugs, PEMF therapy has to be repeated multiple times until the brain resets itself. Any sense of dependency on PEMFs is the result of the fact that they have not finished their work. Once the brain has been reset, called remodeling, the PEMF treatments can be decreased or even stopped. However, being able to stop PEMFs also depends on the healing of the cause of the pain signal, such as from bone-on-bone arthritis, spinal stenosis, amputations, or other injuries. Because of this, PEMFs may be necessary long-term, possibly even for a lifetime. Some tissue injuries just cannot be healed, but only maintained.

The goal of PEMF therapy is to not only treat the local area causing the chronic pain problem, but also the pain-reception area, the brain. The treatment of the brain for pain conditions is essentially the same as other conditions where the brain is the target of treatment, such as chronic fatigue syndrome (CFS), fibromyalgia, migraine, concussion, depression, and traumatic brain injury (TBI). See Chapter 10 for further discussion of chronic pain management with PEMFs for these and other conditions.

Numerous studies document the ability of PEMFs to both relieve pain symptoms and address pain's underlying causes. However, it is important to realize that the best PEMF system for pain depends on the specific pain problem to be treated. As I've pointed out throughout this book, low-intensity PEMF systems typically require longer courses of treatment to achieve effective pain relief. Depending on their severity, for some pain conditions high intensities are necessary to adequately reach the source of pain deep within the body (see Appendix A). Even after symptoms have resolved, continued treatment can help heal the source of the problems so that they won't recur.

Frequencies and intensities are other important considerations, as I explained in Chapters 4 and 5. Each PEMF device is designed with specific frequencies and intensities, with many devices available for clinical and home use providing extremely low frequency, ranging from 3 to 1000 Hz. These include familiar frequencies from delta (1-4 Hz), theta (5-8 Hz), alpha (9-13 Hz), beta (14-25 Hz) and gamma (26-100 Hz). Overall, the intensity of therapeutic PEMF devices ranges from 0.1 mT (1 gauss) to 800 mT (>10,000 gauss). While some conditions require high intensity to be most effective, even very-low-intensity PEMFs can still have some impact on the perception of pain. Neuroimaging research has revealed changes in specific areas of the brain with pain stimuli that were modified by low-intensity PEMF exposure (Robertson et al., 2010).

What follow are the main reasons why PEMF therapy can be so effective for managing and resolving pain, even after other types of therapies, both conventional and alternative, have failed.

PEMFs Treat Pain Where It Begins: Damaged nerve networks stuck in a constant state of inflammation send pain messages to your brain. In response, your brain responds with its own messages that are intended to help. Unfortunately, sometimes these help signals can actually perpetuate the pain because the associated nerves remain inflamed. PEMF therapy calms those nerves, finally allowing them to recover.

The majority of pain sources treated with PEMF therapy are musculoskeletal disorders such as arthritis, sprains or strains, factures, osteoporosis, neuralgias, neuropathies, and many more. While inflammation is crucial to the healing process, when the body overcompensates, tissue swelling (edema) can cause pain and delayed healing. With soft tissue and musculoskeletal issues, as well as post-traumatic wounds (such as after surgery), edema reduction must occur to speed healing and achieve pain reduction. PEMFs help accomplish this by changing the local tissue where the pain originates, reducing edema and thus reducing pain. Studies have shown these tissue changes in numerous conditions, including acute ankle sprains, whiplash injuries, and chronic wound repair, when PEMF therapy is used.

Since pain is communicated through nerve signals from the point of origin to the brain, often, with more severe or chronic pain, this pain "centralizes" in the brain. In such cases, PEMF treatment to the brain is the best option. Pain can also be transferred to other parts of the body, however, so determining the actual source can be tricky. For such cases of referred pain, I recommend working with a knowledgeable health practitioner to establish the cause and the source of your pain to determine the most effective treatment protocol.

PEMFs Stimulate Change at the Cellular Level: PEMFs heal tissues deep within the body when the correct intensity is applied to the source of the pain. In PEMF therapy, low-frequency pulses of electromagnetic stimulation are used to relieve pain and heal damaged tissues. These pulses activate energy at the cellular level to stimulate natural repair processes. Adenosine (see Chapter 3 and Appendix A) is a molecule that has been called a "guardian angel" in human disease. Working through the adenosine receptor (AR), adenosine plays a key role in controlling inflammation. A2A receptors have a complex relationship with immune and inflammatory processes. Under normal conditions, acute inflammation-producing molecules naturally stimulate the A2A receptor to prevent or decrease inflammation. Low adenosine production means these receptors don't work as they should, and chronic inflammation can result. PEMFs increase ARs and stimulate A2A receptors which, in turn, increase production of adenosine and allow for its more efficient functioning. The end result is a larger anti-inflammatory response than pain medications are capable of achieving, without side effects, desensitization, or receptor resistance.

Neutrophils, which make up 40 to 70 percent of white blood cells in the human body, have an abundance of A2A receptors in their membranes. These neutrophils are called to the site of inflammation very quickly after trauma. In a lab study, PEMFs of the right intensity applied at the surface of neutrophils significantly increased the binding of adenosine to the A2A receptor. This research clearly showed that having the proper intensity is critical to effectively reduce inflammation anywhere in the body.

PEMF Therapy Reduces Pain for Both Short- and Long-Term Relief: Because of how effective they are at reducing inflammation, PEMFs are an effective treatment for both acute and chronic pain. In acute situations, treatment with PEMFs can speed tissue healing and reduce pain quickly, without the risk of side effects of the medications often used to treat acute pain.

With chronic conditions, PEMF therapy is even more valuable. Animal studies show that PEMFs reduce the pain receptors in the brain. Some studies found that the relief was equivalent to 10 mg of morphine. This relief, in addition to the natural healing responses that PEMF therapy creates in the body, makes PEMF therapy an ideal option for the management of chronic pain and its causes.

One of the great things about PEMF therapy is that it can be done in the comfort of your own home. The initial investment is often less than ongoing professional treatments would cost, and when you own a PEMF machine, multiple family members can make use of the therapy as needed.

FDA approval is not required for devices that are used or marketed primarily for wellness. This has resulted in a dramatic proliferation of relatively lower-cost, easily accessible, commercially available "wellness" PEMF systems. This position of FDA most likely results from the perspective that low-intensity, low-frequency PEMF systems are generally regarded as safe (GRAS).

PEMFs Reduce the Need for Pain Medication: PEMF therapy is frequently performed along with the use of pain medications. Clinically, PEMFs have been shown to not only decrease pain, but to also reduce dependence on such medications. In one study using very-high-frequency PEMFs for the treatment of cervical dorsal root ganglion pain, the need for pain medication continued to be significantly reduced in the active group after six months. A study on knee pain found that even after follow-up at one year, 85 percent of the study's participants reported pain reduction beyond the time of stimulation. Medication consumption also decreased by 39 percent at eight weeks and by almost 90 percent in the follow-up period after eight weeks. The study documented a 2.2-fold reduction in narcotic use by PEMF-treated, post-surgical patients.

PEMFs Benefits for Pain Are Backed by Science: Several researchers have reviewed the benefits provided by PEMFs in Eastern Europe and elsewhere and provided a synthesis of the typical physiologic findings of practical use to clinicians, resulting from PEMF and other magnetic therapies. Animal studies have shown that PEMFs reduce pain perception in the brain. And, as mentioned, other research demonstrated that pain relief from PEMFs is equivalent to 10 mg of morphine.

Research has also established that PEMFs' mechanisms of action when treating pain conditions include, at a minimum, reduction in inflammation, edema, and muscle spasms/contractions; enhanced tissue repair; and improved pain tolerance, because PEMFs act as a natural form of antinociception, meaning they block the detection of painful stimuli by sensory neurons, and are capable of doing so longer than narcotic analgesic drugs. In addition, PEMFs affect pain perception both directly and indirectly, positively impacting neuron firing, calcium ion movement, membrane potentials, endorphins, dopamine, nitric oxide, and nerve regeneration. Indirect benefits of PEMFs can also improve circulation, cellular metabolism, tissue oxygen supply, and prostaglandins. (For research and references on more than 20 mechanisms of PEMF action, please see the October 2020 issue of *Townsend Letter*.)

The bottom line is that PEMFs offer physicians a tool that amplifies other treatments they are already providing (see Chapter 6). PEMF therapy not only expands the range of indications physicians can treat successfully, it also deepens the benefits of the other therapies they are applying.

At its most effective, PEMF therapy benefits from informed supervision and guidance by the practitioner. In the clinical setting, the fact that PEMFs penetrate clothing, casts, or bandages without attenuation means that PEMF therapy can be applied without having to expose or come in direct contact with the skin or target tissue. This allows simple focused application to organs within the body, usually without concern for harm or negative effects to intervening tissue.

Using PEMF Therapy to Treat Specific Pain Conditions

Research reviewed by myself and others has shown that PEMFs are effective for treating a wide variety of pain-related conditions, including, but not limited to abdominal pain, arthritis, bursitis, carpal tunnel syndrome, cervical disc injuries, fibromyalgia, fractures, muscle spasms, nerve pain, peripheral neuropathy, phantom pain, plantar fasciitis, PMS, postoperative pain, sinus pain, sprains and strains, and pain caused by trauma. (These and many other conditions and how to treat them with PEMFs are addressed in Chapter 10.) PEMF therapy is also effective for treating the classes of pain conditions that follow below.

Note: For best results, I always emphasize the need for good nutrition and the use of appropriate nutritional supplements. PEMFs work synergistically with supplements, as I discussed in Chapter 6. Supplements and nutrition need to be individualized. This is especially true when it comes to recovery from pain, as well as all other health conditions. As a result, I recommend consulting with a professional skilled in nutrition and supplements to assess your nutritional status and guide you on the supplements that are most appropriate for you. Unless they are trained in the use of nutrient supplements, doctors rarely make recommendations for supplements. The recommendations I make for them in this chapter are based on my own clinical experience, as well as the supplement recommendations from the authoritative book *Nutritional Medicine* by Alan Gaby, MD (Concord, NH: Fritz Perlberg; 2017).

In addition, for certain of the conditions below, I suggest the use of a "magnetic sandwich" approach to applying PEMF applicators. For more information about this approach, see Appendix C.

Back Pain

Back pain is one of the most common musculoskeletal disorders, with more than 15 percent of the entire U.S. population experiencing lower back pain at any given time. Certain types of back pain caused by spinal stenosis and arthritis of the back, for example, are conditions that are not usually reversible. They frequently persist for the rest of a patient's life and are typically progressive.

Back pain is one of the most frequent issues for which PEMF therapy is sought. It is also one of the most gratifying conditions to treat. Success in treating back pain with PEMFs depends on the location in the back of the problem, and its severity (including how severe a nerve is involved), and whether it is complicated by surgery or other interventions, other health conditions and medications, and involvement of multiple levels. There are many causes of back pain, but the most common that we see are degenerative disc disease (DDD) and arthritis of the spine (DJD).

Back pain is complicated by the complexity of the structures of the back. MRIs can look very bad, but people may have no back problems. On the other hand, an MRI may look relatively normal and there could be severe back pain. Pinpointing the true source of the back pain (the pain generator) can be very challenging.

As a result, people with surgery will often have persistent back problems or the pain may go away after surgery only to return later. This is because of the potentially misleading nature of MRIs and back X-rays.

What looks obvious on an MRI or X-rays is not necessarily the cause. The challenge is always to figure out what the source of the pain is. Unfortunately, back surgery frequently creates new problems that have to be healed. Healing may not be adequate or there may be complications. PEMF therapy should be considered as a first-line therapy unless there is clear neurologic damage that could be very rapidly resolved by surgery, such as for a displaced disc fragment. A disc fragment is usually a clear indicator for surgery, called microdiscectomy. However, sometimes they will get better on their own since they break down and the body re-absorbs the disc fragment. The only real indication for surgical intervention, is significant neurological symptoms and signs.

In clinical practice, I recommend PEMF for back pain because the stimulation penetrates deeply into the body to heal the tissues. In contrast, a study using a static magnet pad found no relief for back pain, likely because it was too shallow in its application. Higher-intensity PEMF is often necessary in more severe or chronic back pain situations to support effective pain reduction.

A number of studies have been conducted on the use of PEMFs for back pain. The findings of these studies indicate that it is best to apply PEMFs on a consistent basis over an extended period of time to achieve the best results. When this is done, the studies showed that 95 percent of individuals found relief. Benefit was found for patients suffering from herniated discs, spondylosis, radiculopathy (spinal nerve compression), sciatica, spinal stenosis, and arthritis. PEMFs have also been shown to increase cellular repair in the spinal discs, meaning that PEMFs can be used not only to help heal damaged discs but may also be useful for preventing the breakdown of discs leading to lumbar disc disease. People who have tried other modalities and failed to find relief for such conditions will often find relief from PEMFs.

The goal of PEMF therapy is to reduce inflammation anywhere in the lower back. This includes the joints of the spine, the nerve roots, spinal cord, the disc, and the muscles of the lumbar spine. The magnetic field needs to penetrate these tissues at a depth of four inches, and possibly another one or two inches in cases of larger bodies.

Should back surgery prove necessary, PEMFs can be used leading up to surgery to condition and improve the health of the tissues so that they recover faster from the procedure. Then PEMFs can be continued during the recovery period and beyond until complete healing occurs. After healing is complete, the PEMFs can be used for other needs in the body, as well.

Chronic pain can be an unfortunate consequence of back surgery, and largely unpredictable. This is called failed back surgery syndrome (FBSS) or failed back syndrome. In these situations, PEMF therapy can make a huge difference in the patients' ability to recover and function. While PEMFs may not be able to eliminate the pain because of the degree of damage to the back, severe pain may become tolerable, mild pain. It may be best to continue the PEMFs after any kind of back surgery for at least a month after discharge from surgical follow-up to be certain the tissues are fully healed, even if all symptoms have resolved. Remember, discs and bone take a lot longer to heal. Muscles, skin, and fascia heal much faster, and most the time, this is all we notice. There may be deeper problems that previously led to the back pain in the first place that could still benefit from continued treatment, so that pain does not return.

Intensity of the PEMF: Since about 15 gauss needs to be delivered about four inches into the body, per the tables in Appendix A, this would best be done using a magnetic field intensity of between 2000-4000 gauss or higher. It is likely that multiple vertebral levels are involved. An MRI or CT scan of the spine would confirm this. That means, per the graph in the document in Appendix A, lower magnetic field intensities may be somewhat helpful, but the best results will happen with the higher-intensity magnetic field. Intensities higher than this would work very well although the extra energy is not needed. The extra energy doesn't create any problems in the body and would go deeper into the bowel and pelvis to potentially help any other issues in the path of the magnetic field, known or unknown.

Applicators: Local, high-intensity applicator should be about 10 to 15 inches in diameter or length. The width should be a minimum of three inches. Larger applicators will do the job as well, as long as the peak intensity of the magnetic field is at least 2000 gauss.

Treatment Time: 30 to 60 minutes twice a day. 60 minutes may be needed early in the course of treatments until symptoms are significantly reduced. After that, maintenance can be done for 30 minutes per day. The reduction of symptoms does not mean the tissues are normal. That is why maintenance treatment needs to be ongoing, preferably daily, at some level. The body will tell you if treatments are not strong enough or often enough. For mild-to-moderate problems, based on what the imaging studies show, treatment may only be needed once or twice a week for maintenance purposes. For more severe back problems, especially spinal stenosis, daily treatments for the foreseeable future will be required.

Supplements: Useful supplements for back pain include vitamin D3 5000 IU/day if less than 50 kg and 10,000 IU/day for those >50 kg., P5P (pyridoxal phosphate, the active form of vitamin B6) 100 mg/day, B12 5000 μg/day, thiamine 100 mg/day, vitamin C 2000 – 4000 mg/day, Chymoral, 1-2 tablets 4 X/day, curcumin 1000 – 3000 mg 2X/day, CBD 25 – 100 mg 1–3X/day.

Degenerative Disc Disease (DDD)

PEMF systems are extraordinarily helpful for relieving pain caused by degenerative disc problems. Nothing will fully correct this problem short of spinal fusion, however. Spinal fusion prevents the vertebrae from compressing the discs during movement, prolonged sitting or standing, coughing or sneezing, or carrying weight. Because of the risks of the surgery, spinal fusion is reserved for patients in the most severe circumstances. Sometimes surgery will remove a fragment of the disc if that is necessary. This can be extremely helpful. For most people the discs are not severe enough to warrant surgical procedures. Most of the time, the fundamental conventional treatments are going to be physical therapy, medications, and maybe chiropractic. Relaxing the back muscles is critical, since muscles that are contracted or in spasm pull the discs closer together, aggravating the problem. Degenerative discs are caused by dehydration of the disc and wear and tear. They are comparable to dried-out, jelly-filled doughnuts, losing their ability to be cushions between vertebrae. Unfortunately, current medical/surgical therapies do not correct the disc, they simply provide stabilization and pain management. Newer surgical therapies such as inter-vertebral cages, fail as well, and are not proven over the long-term. They have complication rates as high as 27 percent.

PEMFs help degenerative disc problems by reducing muscle spasm, relieving pain, reducing inflammation of the nerve being compressed by the disc, and improving circulation to the area. PEMFs allow for daily treatment in the home setting, reducing the need for medications, physical therapy, and chiropractic. With some patients the need for these services is completely eliminated. They also tend to reduce or eliminate the need for steroid injections into the back, which only provide temporary relief anyway.

Because of the frequency with which DDD problems happen, and the fact that DDD basically is lifetime condition, I recommend PEMFs to all of my patients with degenerative discs, as well as all other types of back pain, with great results. There is no perfect solution for this problem, but PEMFs in my experience are the best and safest solution available. A purchase of a PEMF system will provide lifelong benefit.

Intensity of the PEMF: Since about 15 gauss needs to be delivered about four inches into the body, per the tables in Appendix A, this would best be done using magnetic field intensity of between 2000-4000 gauss. As mentioned before, it is likely that multiple vertebral levels are involved. An MRI or CT scan of the spine would confirm this. That means, per the graph in the document in Appendix A, lower magnetic field intensities may be somewhat helpful, but the best results will happen with the higher-intensity magnetic field. Intensities higher than this would work very well although the extra energy is not needed. The extra energy doesn't create any problems in the body and would go deeper into the bowel and pelvis to potentially help any other issues in the path of the magnetic field, known or unknown.

Applicators: Local, high-intensity applicator should be about 10 – 15 inches in diameter or length. The width should be a minimum of three inches. Larger applicators would do the job, as well, as long as the peak intensity of the magnetic field is at least 2000 gauss.

Treatment Time: 30 to 60 minutes twice a day. 60 minutes may be needed early in the course of treatments until symptoms are significantly reduced. After that, maintenance can be done using PEMFs about 30 minutes per day. The reduction of symptoms does not mean that the tissues are normal. That is why maintenance treatment needs to be ongoing, preferably daily, at some level. The body will tell you if treatments are not often enough. For mild-to-moderate problems, based on what the imaging studies would show, treatment may only be needed once or twice a week for maintenance purposes. For more severe problems, especially spinal stenosis, daily treatments for the foreseeable future may they be required.

Supplements: D3 5000 IU/D if less than 50 kg and 10,000 IU/D for those >50 kg., P5P 100 mg/D, B12 5000 µg/D, thiamine 100 mg/D, vitamin C 2000 – 4000 mg/D, Chymoral 1-2 tablets 4 X/D, curcumin 1000 – 3000 mg 2X/D, CBD 25–100 mg 1–3X/D.

(For how to use PEMFs to treat arthritis of the spine see **Arthritis** in Chapter 10.)

Shoulder Pain

Shoulder pain is the third most common form of musculoskeletal pain, accounting for 5 percent of all visits to primary care providers in the U.S. each year. Despite the number of patients who seek care for shoulder pain every year, most don't receive effective treatment. In fact, as many as 40 percent of shoulder pain patients still have pain a full 12 months after they first seek help for the problem. Most of the problems in the shoulder area relate to tendons, the rotator cuff, the shoulder joint, and the acromioclavicular (AC) joint. The most common treatments for shoulder pain include ice and topical pain relievers, NSAIDs, rest, physical therapy, and even surgery, which aren't guaranteed to resolve the problem or relieve pain.

A study done on 46 patients with subacromial impingement syndrome (shoulder overuse) divided patients into two groups. Both received pendulum exercises and cold packs five times a day, restriction of shoulder movement, and NSAIDs daily. The test group also received PEMF treatment 25 minutes per session five days a week for three weeks, while the control group received sham treatment. Overall, both groups achieved similar results, likely because of the short duration of the study and the number of treatments and interventions applied. But the PEMF treatment group had an 85 percent reduction in pain-disturbing sleep versus only 41 percent in the sham group.

The value of PEMFs for the treatment of persistent rotator cuff tendinitis was tested in a double-blind controlled study in 29 patients whose symptoms didn't respond to steroid injection and other conventional conservative measures. The PEMF treated group (15 patients) showed a significant benefit compared with the control group (14 patients) during the first four weeks of the study when the control group received a placebo. In the second four weeks, when all patients were on active coils, no significant differences were noted between the groups. This lack of difference persisted over the third phase when neither group received any treatment for eight weeks. At the end of the study, 19 (65 percent) of the 29 patients were symptom free, and five others were much-improved.

Intensity of the PEMF: 100-2000 gauss, depending on the depth of the whole shoulder. The tendons and the AC joint tend to be superficial. The shoulder joint tends to be two to four inches deep.

Applicators: Local or regional applicators. Local applicators would be applied to the more superficial tendons, the AC joint, and the front and back of the joint. Regional applicators may be needed around the whole shoulder area. Applicators can include a butterfly coil, a loop coil, or paddle. A loop coil or butterfly coil can be used by placing the arm inside the coil and bringing the applicator up to the shoulder. The butterfly coil can also be opened out and the front part of the butterfly can be placed in the front of the shoulder and the other coil over the back of the shoulder. The butterfly coil and the paddle applicator can be placed over the front, side, or back of the shoulder.

Treatment Time: 30 – 60 minutes twice a day to begin with. As improvement is seen, the treatment time may be reduced to what works best. The most common mistake is to not continue treatment beyond the time when symptoms are gone. Even though symptoms are gone, healing may not have been completed. Resumption of activity too soon will cause symptoms to flare up again. A rule of thumb would be to continue treatment for at least a month after symptoms are gone.

Supplements. Curcumin 1000-3000 mg 2-3 times/day, hyaluronic acid oral 200-1000 mg/D, topical DMSO, glucosamine and chondroitin sulphate, vitamin C, hydrolyzed type 1 collagen (Col 1), L-arginine alpha-keto-glutarate, boswellic acid, methylsulfonylmethane (MSM), 3000-5000 mg powder, bromelain, Vinitrox and/or CBD gel or oral. Doses will have to be individually tailored. It is not recommended to use capsaicin or icy/hot creams to the shoulder while doing PEMF therapy because of the risk of chemical burns.

Musculoskeletal Disorders

Musculoskeletal disorders make up the vast majority of pain sources that are commonly and effectively treated with PEMFs. In addition to back pain, these disorders include arthritis, tendonitis, sprains and strains, fractures, post-op pain, osteoporosis, wounds, neuralgias, neuropathies, hip disorders, muscle spasms, spinal cord injury, and trauma, as well as burns, neuromas, heel spurs, phantom pain, carpal tunnel syndrome, headaches, tennis elbow, reflex sympathetic dystrophy (RSD/CRPS), and so on.

A series of 240 patient cases treated with PEMF in an orthopedic practice documented decreased pain in patients suffering from rheumatic illnesses, delayed healing process in bones, and pseudo-arthritis, including those with infections, fractures, aseptic necrosis, venous and arterial circulation, RSD (all stages), osteochondritis dissecans, osteomyelitis, and sprains, strains and bruises. The clinically determined success rate approached 80 percent. X-rays evidence of continued improvement confirmed cartilage/bone reformation and healing at the joint margin. Double-blind clinical studies have shown similar success rates when PEMFs are used for chronic wound repair, and to treat acute ankle sprains, neck pain, and whiplash injuries.

There are no specific treatment or supplement applications for musculoskeletal disorders. These can be addressed by reviewing the various conditions in Chapter 10 that relate to the musculoskeletal system.

Fractures

There are many kinds of fractures. Any bone in the body can be fractured. There are simple or complex fractures. There are fractures near or around joints, which create additional complexity in management. Fractures in children are different than fractures in the elderly. Fractures in small bones heal at different rates than fractures in large bones. Another type of "fracture" is called an osteotomy, where a surgical procedure is used to cut into the bone to reshape it. This is frequently done in podiatry. Osteoporotic bone will fracture very easily with little stress. These fractures would be best managed with PEMFs. Fractures that don't heal well are called delayed unions or nonunions. These are particularly helped by PEMFs.

It is very common in today's medical environment to use instrumentation to help stabilize fractures. This is called open reduction and internal fixation (ORIF). ORIF includes the placement of hardware in the area of the fracture, including plates, nails, or screws. Often these are removed later. In the meantime, they cause inflammation and irritation even while they stabilize the fracture and allow earlier return to function. PEMFs in this setting can be very useful in reducing the inflammation caused by the hardware and the surgery and facilitate even more rapid return to function, not to mention reducing swelling, inflammation, and pain.

In evaluating acute care, researchers assessed pain and swelling of distal radius fractures after an immobilization period of six weeks. In the study, 83 patients were randomly allocated 1) to receive 30 minutes of either ice plus PEMF, 2) ice plus sham PEMF, 3) PEMF alone, or 4) sham PEMF for five consecutive days. All of the patients had a standard home exercise program. The addition of PEMF to ice therapy produced better overall treatment outcomes than ice alone, or PEMF alone in pain reduction and improvement of ulnar nerve entrapment.

Another study focused on a much broader test group that included not only fracture patients, but patients suffering with infections, osteomyelitis, sprains, strains, and other musculoskeletal conditions. Researchers conducting this study found that PEMF treatment was successful in nearly 80 percent of patients.

Intensity of the PEMF: One of the primary goals of using PEMF therapy in the setting of fractures is to decrease inflammation and pain while at the same time increasing new bone formation, whether or not around implanted hardware. The goal for intensity at the bone is 15 gauss. See Appendix A for the necessary magnetic field intensity. Clearly, smaller joints, such the hands, feet, and shoulders, would need less magnetic field intensity. 200-1000 gauss would work. Larger bones and around joints may require higher intensities, a minimum of 2000 gauss. Hip joints and pelvis involve a bigger area and are deeper into the body. Spinal fractures also are deeper and need higher intensity. To penetrate four to six inches into the body, a PEMF of 2000-4000 gauss would be best. High-intensity PEMF applicators are not contraindicated with implanted hardware. Caution should be used by gradually increasing the magnetic field to tolerance using the "low and slow" approach. If there is sufficient irritation in the area of the implant, maximum intensity may not be able to be achieved, especially at the earliest stages of PEMF stimulation. As healing occurs and inflammation decreases, intensity may be able to be gradually increased.

Applicators: For most fractures, a local PEMF applicator of the right intensity is all that is needed. If there is osteoporosis, many areas of the body with arthritis, diabetes, or other health conditions needing it, a whole-body PEMF system of at least 4000 gauss, preferably a "magnetic sandwich" type would be best. (See **Osteopenia/Osteoporosis** in Chapter 10.) If a lower-intensity PEMF system is used, extended treatment times may be needed and therefore a portable, battery-operated system may be best to allow more freedom of activity.

Treatment Time: For lower-intensity PEMFs, extended treatment times may be needed, even as much as up to six hours per day, especially with fresh fractures. It would be easier to determine the treatment time if there are significant symptoms. As symptoms improve, treatment time may be gradually reduced. It's possible to do around three hours twice a day instead of six hours all at once. For high-intensity PEMFs, treatment time should be between one to two hours twice a day initially, followed by regular use for an hour twice a day, depending on tolerance. For long-term management, 30 minutes twice a day would probably suffice, depending on symptoms and tolerance. Ultimately, the amount of PEMF stimulation will be determined by clinical and/or imaging evaluations, which may indicate that more extended treatment time is needed. In research for nonunion fractures, using medium-intensity PEMF devices, four to 12 hours per day of treatment was needed to achieve healing.

Supplements. Bone can't be built without adequate nutrients to support bone development. At a minimum these would include vitamin D3 5000 IU per day, a general bone-building formula, DHEA 25 mg per day, Ultra K2, Osteo-sil, Fructoborate 6 mg. and curcumin 3000 mg/day.

(See also **Bone Healing and Repair** in Chapter 10.)

Nerve Compression (Sciatica) and Whiplash

Whiplash is a neck injury due to forceful, rapid, back-and-forth movement of the neck, like the cracking of a whip. Whiplash is commonly caused by rear-end car accidents. It can involve the muscles and ligaments of the neck or if significant enough, nerve damage or damage to the discs in the neck. There is stretching and sometimes tearing of some muscles, tendons, and ligaments.

In a study of 92 patients with whiplash, pain was measured on a ten-point scale. The before/after treatment result averages were as follows: Head pain pre-treatment 4.6/post-treatment 2.1 with PEMF treatment compared with 4.2/3.5 in controls. Neck pain, 6.3/1.9 with PEMF as opposed to controls 5.3/4.6. For pain in the shoulder and arm, 2.4/0.8 with PEMF compared to controls 2.8/2.2.

Lumbar disc prolapse with radiculopathy (nerve compression, commonly known as sciatica) is particularly disabling. Radiculopathy causes damage to the nerves coming from the lower spine that can be permanent if not treated successfully and early.

Two randomized studies looked at people with either nerve compression or whiplash. PEMFs were used twice a day for two weeks. For nerve compression, 100 patients with lumbar radiculopathy pain received PEMF treatment while controls received standard medication. The PEMF group had low-intensity PEMF therapy twice a day for two weeks. The average time to pain relief and painless walking was eight days in the PEMF group and 12 days in control groups.

In the people with whiplash, PEMFs resulted in a 50 percent reduction in head pain, a 70 percent reduction in neck pain, and a 67 percent reduction in shoulder and arm pain. The results would be expected to be even better with higher-intensity PEMFs over a longer period.

In another randomized controlled clinical trial,40 patients with lumbar disc prolapse were randomly assigned to either a PEMF group or a control group. PEMF produced better results on the Oswestry Low Back Disability index in terms of personal care, lifting, walking, sitting, standing, sleeping, social life, and employment, as well as evidence of improvement of nerve damage and nerve root compression.

Intensity of the PEMF: 100 – 7000 gauss. Lower-intensity PEMFs can be applied locally for aching muscles or ligament strains. For local muscles, use portable, battery-operated devices. Higher-intensity systems (4000-7000 gauss) will produce better/faster results with less treatment time needed.

Applicators: Small portable local applicators. High-intensity local applicators for deeper/faster treatment and to target the brain to generate alertness and deal with any concussions. High-intensity regional applicators for treatment of larger areas, if the back is involved.

Treatment Time: For basic health maintenance, 30 – 60 minutes twice a day. For treatment of specific issues or areas of the body, typically a minimum of 30 – 60 minutes once or twice a day. Recommendations for very short treatment times, such as eight minutes, with very-low-intensity PEMF systems will produce very unreliable and limited results.

Supplements. Probiotics 20-50 billion CFUs/D, omega-3 fish oil 3-5 g per day, branched chain amino acids, protein powder 21 g per serving, CoQ 10 100-300 mg/D, curcumin 1000-3000 mg/D, L-arginine, L-carnitine 4 g/D during periods of strenuous exercise, L taurine 100-500 mg/D, magnesium citrate 500 mg/D.

Neuropathies

Peripheral neuropathy causes serious, chronic pain, most commonly in the hands and feet, decreasing independence and quality of life if left untreated. Symptoms can vary, depending on the stage of nerve involvement and can include numbness, tingling, paresthesias, weakness, or burning pain.

Because the causes of neuropathy vary significantly among individuals, identifying the most effective treatment to address the underlying causes of the neuropathy can be exceptionally difficult. Causes of neuropathy include diabetes, shingles, alcoholism, ARDS, renal failure, autoimmune diseases, toxins, medications, viral infections, vitamin deficiencies, malabsorption, food allergy, MSG, poor diet, and others.

Ultimately, treatment should be directed at the cause, if it can be determined. Since a great part of the time, it can't be determined, treatment is directed at the affected nerves and symptoms. During this trial-and-error process of finding the most effective therapy, the person continues to suffer from severe nerve pain, loss of mobility, and other debilitating symptoms.

A number of studies have researched the effect of PEMFs on people with peripheral neuropathy. When treatments lasted longer than a few weeks, the results were similarly positive across all studies.

Research on neuropathic pain using low-power, low-frequency PEMF of 600 and 800 Hz, for 30 patients, between the ages of 40 and 68 years of age with diabetic neuropathic pain stages N1a, N1b, N2a, were randomly allocated to three groups of ten each. They found significant reduction in pain and statistically significant improvement in distal latency and nerve conduction velocity in both experimental treatment groups. Using this particular protocol, low-frequency PEMF was seen to reduce neuropathic pain and slow the progression of neuropathy, even when applied for only a short span of time.

In another study, PEMFs used for at least 12 minutes every day in the treatment of patients with intense symptoms of diabetic neuropathy experienced improvement in pain, as well as reduced paresthesia and vibration sensation, with increased muscular strength in 85 percent of patients compared to controls.

Carpal tunnel syndrome is another form of neuropathy. This type of chronic neuropathic pain affects the median nerve at the wrist. In a randomized, double-blind, placebo-controlled trial, people with severe, treatment-resistant carpal tunnel syndrome received ten months of active PEMF therapy. By the end of ten months, they experienced big improvements in their pain and other symptoms, as well as improvements in nerve conduction tests. They also reported subjective improvement on examination (40 percent), and reduction in pain scores (50 percent) and global symptoms (70 percent).

Several other studies have confirmed these outcomes when PEMFs are used to treat neuropathies. Results were more conflicting in short-term studies lasting just a few weeks or less. Some shorter studies showed improvement in pain and functioning; others showed no significant difference between the test group and the control group. Most people with peripheral neuropathy need longer-term PEMF treatment to receive the best improvements in pain. Of all the neuropathies, diabetic neuropathy and carpel tunnel syndrome appear to respond the best. Other forms of neuropathy, especially the idiopathic forms or forms of unknown cause, are the most difficult and challenging to treat, whether PEMFs are used or not.

Intensity of the PEMF: 1000 – 7000 gauss in a local, regional, or whole-body, preferably a "magnetic sandwich" system. Less than high-intensity PEMF systems may be less likely to produce sufficient change quickly. Mid- to high-intensity local applicators may be used at the source of the symptoms of the neuropathy, especially if applied early in the course of the condition. If numbness has been present and paresthesias begin to occur, this is a good sign that the nerves are waking up. However, this process can be very slow.

Applicators: Local, regional, and/or whole-body. Local high-intensity treatments would be applied to the primary symptom target of treatment. Stacked 100-1000 gauss applicators could be tried locally. A medium--intensity applicator can be applied to the site(s) of the symptoms. For high-intensity applicators, placements would depend on the type used: local applicators include a loop, butterfly, paddle, or pad. They would be used locally or occasionally applied to the lumbar spine in the case of lower extremity neuropathy or to the neck for upper extremity and to the brain for facial or neck neuropathies. For trigeminal neuralgia, the loop coil may be placed over the side of the head. If flexible, it may be conformed into an elliptical form and placed over the top of the head or the back of the head and each side. The butterfly coil would be placed over the top of the head with a wing on each side or over the back of the head and each side. The paddle coil can be placed on the side of the head and moved from one side to the other in successive treatments. If the system allows two local applicators to be used as a "magnetic sandwich" then place them on either side of the head. Whole-body PEMF therapy is recommended to maintain immune and tissue health, for stress reduction, and to balance the autonomic nervous system.

Treatment Time: 30-60 minutes twice a day, using the "low and slow" approach. Add more treatment time as needed. With significant improvement of symptoms, reduce treatment time for maintenance. It is important not to stop treatments suddenly to avoid the risk of significant rebound. Treatments are likely to be needed several months after symptoms have been eliminated. Brain remodeling may take months to years.

Supplements: Thiamine for thiamine deficiency 10-30 mg/D, magnesium citrate, 500 mg/D, P5 P100 mg/D, B12 5000 mcg/D, methylfolate5 mg/D, niacin50 mg 3x/D, pantothenic acid 20-100 mg/D, B complex, acetyl l-carnitine 150 mg/kilogram/D, mixed tocopherols 800-1600 IU/D, alpha lipoic acid 1200-2400 mg twice a day, L glutamine1-6 grams/D, Co.Q10 200 mg/D.

(Since centralization is often also associated with neuropathies, also see **Anxiety** in Chapter 10.)

Complex Regional Pain Syndrome (CRPS)

CRPS, also known as reflex sympathetic dystrophy, or RSD, is one of the most severe, extremely painful, and disabling forms of neuropathy. It is a chronic condition typically resulting from a traumatic insult. Conventional medical treatment outcomes for CRPS patients are generally poor and unsatisfactory.

There are two subtypes of CRPS based on whether or not there was a previous nerve injury. The most common form is CRPS I, with no obvious previous nerve injury. CRPS II, previously known as causalgia, has a known major nerve injury.

CRPS is considered an elaborate combination of different factors that begin at the time of initial injury, including nervous system sensitization, autonomic dysfunction, persistent regional inflammatory changes, and a lack of dermatomal distribution. Allodynia, hyperalgesia, skin temperature changes, and edema are also common. CRPS is more common in females and people with upper-extremity injury. There may also be some genetic predisposition and psychological factors that may influence its development and progression.

CRPS most commonly develops after fractures of the upper extremities, especially around the elbow, and injuries of the ankle. Concurrent musculoskeletal disease, such as rheumatoid arthritis, enhances CRPS risk. Distal injuries are more susceptible. High energy injuries, severe fractures, and prolonged general anesthesia time during repair also increase risk. Therefore, fractures treated surgically are more susceptible.

After an inciting or traumatic event, certain changes happen in the nervous system, including increased pain sensitivity and the release of pro-inflammatory molecules (cytokines). These lead to lowering of the pain threshold and the experience of excess pain (hyperalgesia) for the level of stimulus. The sympathetic and peripheral pain sensory systems begin to cross-react over time because of persistent pain signals. Peripheral pain sensors become over-sensitive to the stress hormone adrenaline. Some peripheral nerve fibers even begin to degenerate, but A-delta (Aδ) fibers which carry cold, pressure, and acute pain signals are spared. This causes an imbalance of nerve signaling, increasing Aδ pain signal activity and enhancing pain.

Sensitization of the central nervous systems (CNS) is also fundamental to the development of CRPS. This sensitization is mediated by neuropeptides, decreasing the threshold for response to mechanical and temperature stimuli. Chronically, structural CNS changes may take place. For example, the affected limbs of CRPS patients have a smaller area of representation in the somatosensory cortex of the brain than unaffected limbs. This may lead to increasing CNS symptoms as the condition continues, including movement dysfunction, neglect and impaired recognition of the limb, decreased range of motion and dystonia with flexion of fingers, toes, and wrists in some.

There is autonomic dysfunction, with warm limbs becoming cold, by progressively going from decreased sympathetic sensitivity to increased sympathetic sensitivity. This leads to excessive constriction of blood vessels and sweating, leading to the cold, clammy extremities seen in the chronic phase of CRPS. In this phase, sympathetic nervous system stress responses become exaggerated.

Immune changes are also involved with the release of pro-inflammatory molecules that lead to sensitization to noxious stimuli. In the earlier phases there is also mast cell accumulation, which, among other changes, causes increased tissue permeability and blood vessel dilatation and leakage, leading to edema and increased warmth. Later on, there is prolonged inflammation and delayed tissue repair. Auto-antibodies form against the autonomic nervous system, potentiating inflammation and exacerbating symptoms. Studies have shown that up to 70 percent of CRPS patients have anti-autonomic nerve immunoglobulin G antibodies in their serum.

From a psychological perspective, people with PTSD have a significantly increased likelihood of CRPS. In many with CRPS, PTSD began before the onset of CRPS. Psychological stress influences disease progression. Those with higher levels of anxiety, perception of disability, and pain-related fear have a worsened disease course, due to increases in anxiety-associated norepinephrine release. Catastrophizing (thinking something catastrophic is about to happen), an exaggerated negative emotional response to irritating but not painful stimuli, may also have a significant impact in the development of CRPS. This state leads to increased pro-inflammatory cytokine activity in response to painful stimuli, and the level of catastrophizing has been correlated with future pain scores. Catastrophizing also may alter brain grey matter volume in pediatric individuals, possibly affecting chronic muscle and movement function and pain development.

Current conventional treatment for CRPS is mainly symptomatic, combined with physical/occupational therapies, psychological therapy, neuropathic pain medications, anti-inflammatories, and interventional pain management procedures. Medication trials for CRPS are limited. Neuromodulation has only recently been started. The evidence for effectiveness of all these therapies is weak and their side effects are significant.

Most of the aspects of CRPS described above are similar to and would be expected to respond to the actions of PEMFs. These include reducing inflammation, improving circulation, balancing autonomic function, stimulating tissue repair, balancing immune function, helping with stress, and decreasing centralization. Therefore, PEMFs have significant potential in helping with CRPS. PEMF treatment would be focused on the local area of trauma initiating CRPS, the tissues with decreased physical health changes, stress reduction, the spinal cord area corresponding to areas with the most reactivity (neck for upper extremities, sacral for lower extremities), and the brain to impact centralization.

rTMS use for CRPS has been studied and found to significantly improve pain over time when applied over the primary motor cortex, just above the ears. The treatment inhibits the conduction of pain signals to the brain. Since people with chronic pain have decreased blood flow, rTMS increases brain blood flow. rTMS also has a pain-killing effect by acting on the opioid and endocannabinoid receptors in the brain, the areas targeted by the use of opioid drugs and cannabis or CBD. This research suggests that longer-term therapy, most likely several months, is needed to achieve and retain sufficient benefits. It is not yet known if, when therapy is stopped after sufficient improvement in symptoms is obtained, or to what extent CRPS might come back.

In one study, ten 30-minute PEMF sessions at 50 Hz, followed by a further ten sessions at 100 Hz plus physiotherapy and medication reduced CRPS edema and pain in ten days.

I personally treated a patient with this disorder using a 27.12 MHz PEMF signal. My patient was a nurse who was almost completely disabled in her left upper extremity. She used her PEMF device for approximately an hour a day. Within about one month, she experienced a 70 percent recovery, and within two months, she had essentially regained normal function with no sensitivity to touch or changes in skin temperature. She maintained her recovery with continued treatments in the home setting.

Intensity of the PEMF: 4000 – 7000 gauss in a whole-body, preferably "magnetic sandwich," system. Less than high-intensity PEMF systems may be less likely to produce sufficient change quickly. Mid- to high-intensity local applicators may be used at the source of the injury, especially when applied early in the course of the condition.

Applicators: Local, regional, and/or whole-body. Local high-intensity treatments would be applied to the brain as the primary target of treatment. For brain stimulation, portable small, battery-operated panels can be applied as a "magnetic sandwich" to the parietal cortex on both sides of the head slightly above and slightly in back of the top of the ear. Stacked 100-1000 gauss applicators could be tried locally to the area of original injury. A medium-intensity applicator can be applied to the side of the head and if necessary, alternated between the two sides of the head. For high-intensity applicators, placements would depend on the type used: local applicators include a loop, butterfly, paddle, or pad. A rigid loop coil may be placed over the side of the head. A flexible loop coil may be conformed into an elliptical form and placed over the top of the head or the back of the head and each side. The butterfly coil would be placed over the top of the head with a wing on each side or over the back of the head and each side. The paddle coil can be placed on the side of the head and moved from one side to the other in successive treatments. If the system allows 2 local applicators to be used as a "magnetic sandwich" then place them on either side of the head at the same time. Whole-body PEMF therapy is recommended to maintain immune and tissue health, for stress reduction and to balance the autonomic nervous system.

Treatment Time: 30-60 twice a day, using the "low and slow" approach. Add more treatment time as needed. With significant improvement of symptoms reduce treatment time for maintenance. It is important not to stop treatments suddenly for the risk of significant rebound. Treatments are likely to be needed several months after symptoms have been eliminated. Brain remodeling may take months to years.

Supplements: Supplements to be considered include: CBD, Palmitoylethanolamide (PEA), 5HTP, St. John's wort, SAMe, Panax ginseng, St. John's wort, melatonin, Chlorella pyrenoidosa, L-carnitine, alpha-lipoic acid, magnesium, mucuna pruriens, and/or red clover, all at higher or as-tolerated doses.

(Since PTSD is often in the picture, also see **Anxiety** in Chapter 10.)

Fibromyalgia (FM)

Fibromyalgia (FM) is a pain disorder of unknown cause with amplified pain and psychological distress. It has a diverse set of disturbances, mainly involving autonomic, neuroendocrine, and neuropsychologic systems, alongside symptoms such as sleep disturbance, fatigue, pain, daily function impairment, and often stress. FM is at its core a central nervous system disorder, since individuals with FM have abnormalities within central brain structures that normally deal with pain sensations and/or altered central nervous system processing of pain signals, leading to a hypersensitivity to pain or centralization of pain. In FM, people do not process the body's natural pain-relieving neurochemicals (such as enkephalin or endorphin) efficiently, which may be due to a dysfunction in their natural painkilling mechanisms. Environmental magnetic fields (EMFs) (vs PEMFs) may also be a contributing factor, aggravating an already overly sensitive brain.

Current treatments for FM leave a lot to be desired, leading to the risks of addiction, significant side effects, difficulty withdrawing from medication, and incomplete benefits. The goal of PEMF therapy is primarily oriented toward the brain. Local pain areas may be treated as well, particularly if there were local injuries. PEMFs may also be needed for any other health conditions that may be present as well. PEMFs have been found to be very safe and allow self-treatment in the home setting. Many people start out getting PEMF treatments in a professional setting, with some degree of benefit, eventually realizing that ongoing daily home treatment produces much better results. Counseling, physical therapy, massage and other therapies should still be considered in a complementary fashion.

A fibromyalgia study involving 56 women with FM, ages 18 to 60, randomly assigned them to low-intensity PEMF or sham therapy, 30 minutes per session, twice a day for three weeks. They were tested for general FM status, pain, depression, and general function. After active treatment ended at four weeks, they had significant improvements in test scores, which were maintained at the twelve-week evaluations. The sham group showed general health improvement at four weeks. However, there was no improvement in pain or FM symptoms, and there was some regression by twelve weeks in the general health gains made earlier.

PEMF or sham exposure treatments were provided in another study and levels of pain and anxiety were evaluated. The study was double blind, randomized, and placebo-controlled with a 30-minute magnetic field exposure, at an intensity of about 400 microT (4 gauss), < 3 kHz. There was significant benefit in reduction of pain for the FM patients with PEMF therapy.

In a double-blind, sham-controlled clinical trial involving women ages 22 to 50 years old, the active stimulation group received therapy with an 8 Hz square wave PEMF of 43 nT (0.00043 gauss) using an EEG cap with 33 small PEMF coils. Treatment sessions were provided once a week, lasting 20 minutes each time, for eight weeks. Outcome measures included blood serotonin levels, pain thresholds, activities of daily living, perceived chronic pain, and sleep quality. Improvement in pain thresholds was noted after the first stimulation session; however, improvement in other measures occurred only after the sixth week. The perceived pain after eight sessions was 39 percent less, compared with 8 percent less in the sham group. This study makes it clear that even low-intensity PEMF stimulation may offer a safe and at least somewhat effective treatment for chronic pain and other fibromyalgia symptoms.

In a broad review of the use of rTMS to the brain in fibromyalgia, rTMS was found to reduce pain by 71 percent, depression by 54 percent, fatigue by 50 percent, and tender point pain by 43 percent, while improving general health by 63 percent.

Treatment of fibromyalgia can be complicated by the degree of sensitivity of the nervous system. Following a "low and slow" protocol is necessary (see Appendix B). The most benefit to the brain in reducing nervous system hypersensitivity will come from using higher-intensity PEMFs. The goal of the "low and slow" protocol will be to reach the maximum intensity for the maximum time. Because of the hypersensitivity of the nervous system, this process may need to be very slow. While high-intensity PEMFs would eventually provide the best tissue healing benefits, and should be the goal, some people will need to use a PEMF system starting with intensities that are quite low. Low-intensity PEMFs are likely to provide symptom relief but not major changes to the brain needed for sustained long-term results.

My experience has been that even very-low-intensity, whole-body PEMF devices are not tolerated by some people with fibromyalgia. This may be especially true for PEMF systems that have multiple frequencies. Pulse therapy systems seem to be less aggravating than frequency-based systems. For that reason, either portable medium-intensity or low-intensity systems with smaller pads may need to be used to start with. The portable medium-intensity systems often have the choice of multiple programs that can be useful for helping with the anxiety and sleep issues frequently seen in fibromyalgia, as well as allowing treatment of the brain.

Even low-intensity, whole-body PEMF systems with multiple frequencies can be aggravating because so many sensory nerves in the skin are being activated at the same time. A way to decrease this possible reaction with a whole-body PEMF system is to use a smaller-area regional pad over the lower extremities to first, gradually advancing the intensities and the treatment time. Once this is tolerated a local pad may be able to be moved to the abdomen or chest. The belly, called the second brain by some, in particular has a vast number of neurons that can flood the brain with sensory input when stimulated, including the parasympathetic-relaxing vagal nerve. This risk is less for the chest, which has fewer neurons than the belly, but still a possible risk, so stimulation of the chest may be a better next option than the belly, even if there are functional bowel issues that could be helped by the PEMF.

Once these local treatments are tolerated, whole-body treatment may be attempted by following a "low and slow" protocol. This protocol should advance faster once treatments have been done for a while to other parts of the body first. Unless the whole-body, low-intensity PEMF is able to produce dramatic improvements in symptoms, at some point the decision will need to be made whether to "graduate" to a high-intensity system. It may be best to select a high-intensity system that has a reasonable range of intensity settings.

Since the goal ultimately is to treat the brain with higher-intensity PEMFs, it may be better to start off with a higher-intensity system at the lowest intensities. A possible strategy with a higher-intensity system to get even lower-intensity exposure, is to move the applicator farther from the body. This will lower the magnetic field entering the body. Some trial and error will need to be followed to find the right distance and an intensity that would work without aggravation. By already owning a higher-intensity system, the "low and slow" process may be followed gradually until the highest intensities are able to be tolerated.

One other possibility in selecting a flexible PEMF system would be to choose a medium-intensity whole-body system that allows the ability to more precisely tune frequencies, intensities, and time. This is often done with a computer accessory. This type of system would allow more precise control in the lower ranges of intensities and time. One system that I've used, the Parmeds Super, has a lower-intensity whole-body pad and smaller applicator of about 1000 gauss. This may be the only system needed, potentially helping with multiple issues. After using one of the systems for a while with some degree of success, there may still be some need left for higher-intensity equipment, whether whole-body or local/regional.

With high levels of sensitivity of the nervous system, having adequate hydration and using trace minerals and electrolytes may be especially helpful to reduce the risk of aggravation. Managing other contributing factors such as toxicities, food allergies, infections, and nutrition are also very important for success. Supplements are likely to be very important as well.

Intensity of the PEMF: The ultimate goal is to get to the highest intensities to be able to stimulate the whole brain to get adequate pain, mood, stress, depression, fatigue, and anxiety benefit. Those with the highest degrees of severity and multitude of symptoms should start with either medium-intensity, local PEMF or low- to medium-intensity, whole-body PEMF. Use a "low and slow" protocol, advancing very gradually as tolerated. If a high-intensity system is used from the start, whether a local or whole-body system, start with the lowest intensity, advancing very gradually with treatment time.

Applicators: Initially local or regional applicators may be best. The main objective is to treat the brain with high-intensity local PEMF applicators. Once tolerated, whole-body treatment may be started. When switching from local to whole-body systems, the "low and slow" process may need to be reinitiated and gradually advanced until the maximum intensity and at least 30-60 minutes per treatment session are tolerated.

Treatment Time: Treatment time to start with may need to be below the normal settings of the system. For the first few treatments it may need to be no more than five minutes at a time for one to two sessions per day. As treatment time is progressed gradually in five-minute increments, as tolerated, the ultimate goal would be to tolerate about 60 minutes per day. Most of the time, treatment would be twice a day. How long treatments need to be continued will be highly individual. Treating the brain and nervous system is a very slow process, especially when the condition has been present for a considerable time and is fairly severe. Patience and the control of anxiety is important for success.

Supplements: Supplements to be considered include: CBD, palmitoylethanolamide (PEA), 5HTP, St. John's wort, SAMe, panax ginseng, St. John's wort, melatonin, chlorella pyrenoidosa, L-carnitine, alpha-lipoic acid, magnesium, mucuna pruriens, and/or red clover.

Headache and Migraine

PEMFs have been found to be very helpful for relieving headache. One study was done in people who failed treatment with acupuncture and medications. PEMF for 15 days reduced migraine, tension, and cervical (neck) headaches, with the results lasting for up to one month after treatment. The study participants had at least a 50 percent reduction in frequency or intensity of the headaches and needed fewer painkillers. PEMF treatment was most effective for tension headaches, with 88 percent of sufferers reporting excellent or good results.

Migraine is a disorder with recurrent moderate to severe headaches. Typically, the headaches involve half of the head, are pulsating, and last from two to seventy-two hours. There may also be an aura, nausea, vomiting, and sensitivity to light, sound, or smell. It is thought to be due to in part to vasoconstriction followed by reactive vasodilatation. The aura may be due to vasoconstriction. The other symptoms are when the blood vessels become overly dilated to produce the headaches. Worldwide, approximately 15 percent of people are affected by migraine headaches.

Migraines are believed to be due to environmental and genetic factors. They involve the nerves and blood vessels of the brain. Medications are only partially successful and can have significant side effects. At this point, there is no cure for migraines. Alternative approaches to management are clearly needed. PEMF self-treatment could easily fill this gap. Food sensitivities and allergies are very common triggers of migraines and contribute significantly to the inflammation. Triggers need to be identified and eliminated as much as possible, for there to be a chance of controlling the migraines.

More recently, neurogenic inflammation is considered a probable cause of migraines. Neurogenic inflammation is initiated by activation of the peripheral nervous system rather than immunological causes. The neuronal activity leads to the release of chemicals at inflammation away from the sites of the original stimulus. Nerve cells that affect the coverings of the brain, the meninges, become overly sensitive and react to chronic stress, diet, hormonal fluctuations, and other brain activity. This neuronal over-activation leads to the inflammation. The headaches may be periodic, for example with menstrual periods, occasional or even chronic daily. Migraines may be mixed with tension headaches, sometimes causing confusion as to the cause.

As with other types of headache, PEMFs have been shown to be an effective treatment for relieving and preventing migraine. The goal of PEMFs is to help with the pain, decrease the inflammation, and reduce the sensitivity of the nerves controlling the blood vessels. The target of treatment is the brain. This is done best by using PEMFs on a regular basis even when there is no headache, as a preventative and to decrease chronic inflammation. PEMFs may be best used when combined with medication, particularly anti-inflammatories, and especially at the threat of or onset of a headache. Once a headache becomes very established, it may be very difficult for PEMFs to affect it, except maybe to shorten its course.

A migraine study with an unusual design showed that applied PEMF treatments to the area of the femoral artery in the inner upper thigh for at least two weeks were an effective short-term therapy for migraine. Short courses of therapy produced a 73 percent reduction in pain, whereas a longer course of therapy provided 90 percent relief. Longer-term treatment leads to greater reduction of migraine headache activity. One month after a treatment course, 73 percent of patients reported decreased headache activity versus 50 percent for sham treatment. Another two weeks of treatment after the one-month follow-up resulted in an additional 88 percent decrease in migraine activity.

Chronic migraine also responds to PEMFs. Medium-intensity PEMFs applied on days people were migraine-free resulted in significant decreases in the number of attacks and the length of the episodes. One sufferer was even symptom-free for one year after treatment. PEMFs were not as effective during attacks, so the study authors concluded that these PEMFs would be very effective preventive treatment for migraine.

Another study found that medium-intensity PEMFs applied to the head daily for 10 to 15 minutes for 30 days reduced the frequency and intensity of migraine attacks by 66 percent, compared to 23 percent in the placebo group.

In the aforementioned study of 90 patients with headaches resistant to medication or acupuncture, excellent or good results were reported for PEMF in 60 percent of classic migraine cases and 68 percent for cervical migraines.

Another study involved 82 patients with a variety of headaches, including migraines, tension headaches, migraines and tension headaches in combination, and cluster headaches, as well as weather-related and post-traumatic head pain. Patients were evaluated in a double-blind, placebo-controlled study with four weeks of PEMF, 16 Hz at 5 mT (50 gauss). Of those receiving active treatment, 76 percent experienced evident or definite relief of symptoms. Only two participants had worsening of symptoms.

In another study, a series of 20 PEMF treatments were given to 50 migraine patients, all of whom received PEMF at 10 Hz for 15 minutes a day. Reduced frequency and intensity of attacks was experienced by 60 percent of patients, along with a reduced use of medication over a three- to four-month period. In a second study, a case series, 50 to 60 percent of participants reported a favorable effect with

PEMF therapy. A third study of PEMF at 9.6 mT (96 gauss) and 12 Hz applied to the head for one hour was also found to alleviate migraines.

A study with single-pulse TMS was carried out in 117 individuals with four or more hours of headache of four headaches per month. The treatment protocol consisted of both preventive treatment (4 pulses twice daily) and acute treatment (3 pulses at 15-minute intervals repeated up to 3-times for each attack). The patient placed the portables TMS device cradle on the back of the head and pressed a button to deliver the sTMS pulse. The primary effectiveness endpoint (PEE), mean reduction of headache days compared to baseline, was measured over a 28-day period ending at 12 weeks. The mean reduction of headache days from baseline was 30 percent (baseline 9 days). The top three adverse events were lightheadedness (5 percent), tingling (4 percent), and tinnitus (4 percent). It's quite likely the results would have been even better with a more aggressive protocol, using more pulses per treatment session, or for prevention and treatment.

Intensity of the PEMF: The intensity of the PEMF tolerated will depend on the sensitivity of the brain. Usually, when someone is in the acute throes of a severely developing headache, higher-intensity PEMFs can be somewhat aggravating. Higher-intensity PEMFs have been found to work best, however, because they not only provide the best general stimulation deep into the brain but also act best in reducing inflammation deep in the brain. A PEMF system of at least 4000 gauss is recommended.

Applicators: A local high-intensity PEMF applicator would be the best, with a butterfly coil likely being optimal. This would be placed with each wing of the butterfly on either side of the head with the connecting part over the top. Another alternative is to place the butterfly coil over the back of the neck with the wings coming around to the sides of the neck and head. A loop coil may be conformed to be elliptical, like a dumbbell shape, and wrapped from the back of the head around to the sides of the head.

Treatment Time: For preventive purposes, daily treatment to the back of the neck or head for at least 30 minutes is recommended. Continue until the headaches stop or are dramatically reduced in frequency and severity. Once treatment is stopped, there is a strong possibility of headaches returning if the inflammation has not been completely eliminated. So, there may be many periods of trial and error with stopping and starting until control is achieved. How long it takes to obtain complete control will vary with each individual and will also relate to the degree to which the person has eliminated headache/migraine triggers.

Supplements: Some supplements to consider include: magnesium 100 – 300 mg twice a day for prevention, riboflavin 15 – 400 mg per day, methyl folate 5 mg per day, L-tryptophan, melatonin 1-3 mg per day, niacin 300 – 500 mg chewed slightly and dissolved in the mouth, and/or alpha lipoic acid 600 mg per day.

Gastric Ulcer Pains

Resolution of gastric ulcers requires clinical skill, given that they can be caused by *H. pylori* infection and/or stress. Treatment of duodenal ulcers with a 50 Hz, 20 to 25 mT (200 to 250 gauss) PEMF was 1) applied for one minute to acupuncture points specific to gastrointestinal function, compared to 2) the combination of medication plus PEMF acupuncture point stimulation, and 3) standard anti-ulcer medication. Time to pain relief, reduction of dyspeptic symptoms, and ulcer healing were compared.

Pain and dyspepsia were best controlled in the sole PEMF therapy group in ~3 days, whereas combining PEMF and drug therapy resulted in pain control in ~9 days. Ulcer healing with PEMF alone took 18 days, with PEMF and medication, 19 days, and with medication only, ~27 days. Compared with other studies in which medication plus active therapy was more effective, in this study adding medication appeared to delay improvement. In addition, other research has shown that gastric acid values improve to reduce the risk of ulcers from excess acid production.

Intensity of the PEMF: Local application of 100 – 1000 gauss minimum. Higher intensities will help as well if a system is handy, but higher intensities are not needed.

Applicators: Local or regional. Small portable battery-operated PEMF applicators can be placed over the surface of the upper abdomen in the upper half of the area between the lower end of the breastbone and the belly button. Either two applicators can be used, one above the other in the same area, or two small applicators may be stacked one on top of the other over the painful area. A pad applicator may be used as well covering the whole area. With a high-intensity

PEMF system, use a local applicator, either a butterfly coil, a paddle, or loop. Since stress is a major contributor to stomach issues, local applicators may be used to the brain in addition, preferably using 7 Hz or 10 Hz frequencies. Often, treatment of the upper abdomen over the solar plexus, with any PEMF, helps reduce stress anyway by activating the vagal nerves in the abdomen.

Treatment Time: 15 – 60 minutes at a time as needed or, for more chronic problems, twice a day until the pain and discomfort have been resolved.

Supplements: DGL chewable tablets, chew two tablets two hours after each meal and bedtime. Apple cider vinegar to help digestion of food if symptoms tolerate, 2 tablespoons and 4 ounces of water with each meal. If not tolerated do DGL for several days and try again. GI Revive or other similar gastric support supplement. For GERD: calcium carbonate (Tums EX), chew two tablets as needed, beta-carotene 25 mg/D, sodium alginate one hour after meals and bedtime.

PEMF Therapy and Chronic "Pain Brain"

The perception of pain comes from the signals that are sent from the source of the pain to the brain. All pain sends these signals to the brain, whether it's acute or chronic. When you have an injury that causes acute pain, such as stubbing your toe, your brain receives the signal sent up the spinal cord and you feel the sharp pain but, as the source of that pain heals, the pain signal disappears. The brain doesn't hold on to the memory of that pain, and the pain subsides.

However, if the source of pain lingers, the pain signals are sent continuously. The brain retains the memory of pain so that even when no physical source for the pain exists, pain is still perceived. The brain can then become the chronic source of the pain (termed centralization or, colloquially, "chronic pain brain"). In this situation, treating the brain is the most appropriate approach. In fact, many chronic pain conditions centralize quickly. The brain may perpetuate the pain signal even though the initial pain stimulus is now relatively weak, or may even be gone. Therefore, dual approaches, treating the localized source (the foot, in the example of a foot injury, if pain is still felt there) and the brain, may produce the best and fastest results. In these situations, PEMF systems are recommended that allow for whole-body and localized treatment simultaneously. Treatment should address the injured area and the spinal cord at the same time or in the same treatment session. The spinal cord may need to be treated since this is from where the pain signal is sent to the brain. There can be complicated reverberating circuits in the spinal cord as well.

In other cases, pain may be conducted downstream. A hip problem can cause knee pain, for instance. For this reason, it is ideal to treat the source of the pain, not the region to which the pain is referred. Further, identifying the cause, not just the referred location, is critical to achieving appropriate and enduring relief. In sum, the most effective chronic pain management involves treating the source of the pain and also applying PEMF treatments to the brain or along the spine. This combination allows for management of the cause of the pain and at the same time controls the pain signaling to the brain where the pain is ultimately recognized and where it may continue to reverberate.

Your mental state is critical when considering chronic pain because of the connection to the limbic area of your brain and the emotions which live there. Perception of pain varies widely depending on your mental state, as evidenced by examples like athletes injured while competing who don't feel the pain until the end of the game, or how a mother's kiss reduces pain of an injury better than a pain-reliever.

Clearly, pain can't be explained solely by the flow of nerve signals or an irregular response in the spinal cord. But most of the current research on pain and pain management focuses on these physical issues, ignoring the brain connection.

The Cortical-Limbic System Connection: Research is slowly changing our ability to understand the brain through the use of imaging tools like enhanced MRI and positron emission tomography (PET) scans. That has given us information about the interactions between the exchange of pain signals in different areas of the brain.

Pain signals travelling throughout your brain can involve or cause up to 10 percent of your brain to react. That means that 8 to 10 billion neurons (brain cells) are activated with each pain signal. Less than 100 cells in the brain are specific to pain. But all these other cells are turned on as the pain signal travels throughout the brain. Most of that nerve activity stimulated by the pain signal travels to two regions in your brain: the limbic system and the prefrontal cortex.

The limbic system is where emotions live, especially fear and sadness. The limbic system is also responsible for memory of past events. The prefrontal cortex is responsible for decision-making and short-term memory.

When a constant stream of pain signals fire in the brain, even if the pain is minimal, the whole cortical-limbic system is activated. This means that even small amounts of chronic pain can cause mental and emotional "suffering" that far exceeds the expected level of pain. Even when the source of the pain is completely healed, the brain structures affected by these continuous sensory signals remain activated, even without feeling pain, but still causing chronic suffering.

This is compounded when sensations in the body not related to pain stimulate the brain circuits of previous pain memories, causing a perception of pain or discomfort that has no identifiable source. Brain imaging research on chronic pain patients reveals a lack of a cluster of brain neurons specifically devoted to the perception of pain. These chronic pain patients did, however, have increased activity in the cortical-limbic system, which helps us understand that chronic pain is a result of a combination of unique brain states that I call the chronic "pain brain."

All of this reinforces the idea that targeting this cortical-limbic system in the brain is vitally important in the treatment of chronic pain.

How PEMF Therapy Can Help the Chronic Pain Brain: PEMF therapy is a convenient, easy-to-use therapy that can help chronic pain because of its ability to target the pain response centers in the brain to help regulate brain function. Research has shown that PEMFs can safely be used across the brain with effective results. PEMFs help reduce inflammation and overactive brain functioning through both repairing tissue and by adjusting brain frequency functions (entrainment).

Because PEMF devices can be used at home for hours at a time, even overnight, they also help with poor sleep caused by chronic pain or other body sensations, while simultaneously helping to heal the inflamed tissues causing the pain signals to be released for the same nerves that are used for pain signals. Even itching uses the same nerve pathways. PEMF therapy also helps erase the pain signals that result from old memories of pain.

While PEMF systems ranging from very-high-intensity to lower-intensity have all been found to be safe in treating the brain, I prefer more frequent use of lower-intensity, battery-operated, portable units that allow extended use throughout the day, and that also offer the option of selecting multiple brain-wave-tunable frequencies (entrainment). Extended use is often important early in the treatment process as the brain is being "re-educated" to reduce activation of the pain circuitry. Portable, battery-operated PEMF devices are convenient, can be used almost anywhere, four hours a day as needed, and can be highly effective for managing chronic pain and changing the chronic pain brain. Healing of centralized pain does not typically occur overnight, however. More powerful PEMFs may be necessary, since weaker PEMF systems usually take significantly longer to provide benefit, particularly when the source of the pain is located deeper in the body.

Intensity of the PEMF: The ultimate goal is to get to the highest intensities to be able to stimulate the whole brain to get adequate pain, mood, stress, depression, and anxiety benefit. Those with the highest degrees of severity and multitude of symptoms should start with either medium-intensity local PEMF or low- to medium-intensity, whole-body PEMF. Use a "low and slow" protocol, advancing very gradually as tolerated. If a high-intensity system is used from the start, whether a local or whole-body system, start with the lowest intensity, advancing very gradually with treatment time.

Applicators: Initially local or regional applicators may be best. The main objective is to treat the brain with high-intensity local PEMF applicators. Once tolerated, whole-body treatment may be started. When switching from local to whole-body systems the "low and slow" process may need to be reinitiated and gradually advanced until the maximum intensity and at least 30 to 60 minutes per treatment session are tolerated.

Treatment Time: Treatment time to start with may need to be below the normal settings of the PEMF system. The first few treatments may need to be no more than five minutes at a time, once or twice per day. As treatment time is progressed gradually in five-minute increments, as tolerated, the ultimate goal would be to tolerate about 60 minutes per day. Most of the time treatment would be twice a day. How long treatments need to be continued will be highly individual. Treating the brain and nervous system is a very slow process, especially when the condition has been present for a considerable time and is fairly severe. Patience and the control of anxiety is important for success.

Supplements: Supplements to be considered include: CBD 50 – 100 mg 1-3X/D, palmitoylethanolamide (PEA) 600-1200 mg 2-3X/D, 5HTP 50–100 mg two times/D and increase to the appropriate dose over a two-week period, St. John's Wort 300 mg 300 3X/D up to total of 1,300mg per day, SAMe 400 – 1200 mg/D, panax ginseng 200 to 400 mg/D, L-carnitine 1000 mg 2X/D, alpha-lipoic acid 1200 mg/D, magnesium citrate 500 mg/D, mucuna pruriens 5 g/D, or red clover 40-80 mg/day.

PEMFS and Muscle Soreness After Exercise

Delayed onset muscle soreness (DOMS) is a common, painful condition that arises from exercise-induced muscle damage after unaccustomed physical activities, including intentional exercise. DOMS can happen after yard work, snow shoveling, strenuous physical work, muscle strengthening, and gym workouts. Whiplash from a motor vehicle accident can be very similar. Various treatments have been used to reduce this, including ice packs, persistent pressure, electrical stimulation, stretching, massage, and medications. In a review of 35 studies, massage proved only slightly effective in the relief of symptoms and signs of muscle damage caused by exercise. Therefore, its benefit was too small to be practical. There is also a lack of evidence to support the use of cryotherapy, stretching, and low-intensity exercise, but there is research to support using PEMF therapy to help support muscle soreness.

One randomized, double-blind, placebo-controlled study was conducted to examine the effects of a 7000 gauss PEMF, applied for 15 minutes daily for three days, to the biceps muscle. Thirty healthy volunteers had repeated isokinetic exercise of the biceps at low and fast speeds. PEMF was applied after the exercise and objective and subjective measurements were made of muscle function and symptoms. Overall, PEMF stimulation was more effective than sham in reducing symptoms, including perceived soreness, and in improving electrical function tests of the muscles. Muscle strength (peak torque) recovered to pre-exercise levels earlier than the sham group. Other research has shown that PEMFs increase peak torque to high levels with less discomfort than electrical stimulation.

In the above study a relatively high-intensity PEMF signal was used to obtain the benefits seen. I've had personal experience using lower-intensity PEMFs after yard work right after exercise that would normally induce muscle soreness, but before the muscle soreness began. I've also had benefits when I did the therapy the morning after, when the muscle soreness was already established. In the above study, a small PEMF applicator was applied to the muscle that was exercised.

In the case of yard work or other exercises involving many muscles, a larger PEMF pad should be used or a higher-intensity, whole-body PEMF system. It may also be possible to prevent muscle soreness by using a portable PEMF system over specific muscles while exercising or immediately afterwards. In addition, PEMFs applied to muscles before exercise will increase ATP production and circulation to the muscles to potentially increase the peak torque of the muscle, allow the muscles to work longer, and reduce the likelihood of development of post-exercise soreness.

Intensity of the PEMF. The ultimate goal is to get to the highest intensities to be able to stimulate the whole brain to get adequate pain, mood, stress, depression, and anxiety benefit. Those with the highest degrees of severity and multitude of symptoms, start with either medium-intensity local PEMF or low- to medium-intensity whole-body PEMF. Use a "low and slow" protocol, advancing very gradually as tolerated. If a high-intensity system is used from the start, whether a local or whole-body system, start with the lowest intensity, advancing very gradually with treatment time.

Applicators: Initially, local or regional applicators may be best. The main objective is to treat with high-intensity local PEMF applicators. Once tolerated, whole-body treatment may be started. When switching from local to whole-body systems the "low and slow" process may need to be reinitiated and gradually advanced until the maximum intensity and at least 30-60 minutes per treatment session are tolerated.

Treatment Time: Treatment time to start with may need to be below the normal settings of the system. For the first few treatments it may need to be no more than five minutes at a time, once or twice per day. As treatment time is progressed gradually in five-minute increments, as tolerated, the ultimate goal would be to tolerate about 60 minutes per day. Most of the time, treatment would be twice a day. How long treatments need to be continued will be highly individual. Treating the brain and nervous system is a very slow process, especially when the condition has been present for a considerable time and is fairly severe. Patience and the control of anxiety is important for success.

Supplements: Supplements to be considered include: CBD 50 – 100 mg 1-3X/D, palmitoylethanolamide (PEA) 600-1200 mg 2-3X/D, 5HTP 50–100 mg two times/D and increase to the appropriate dose over a two-week period, St. John's Wort 300 mg 300 3X/D up to total of 1,300mg per day, SAMe 400 – 1200 mg/D, panax ginseng 200 to 400 mg/D, L-carnitine 1000 mg 2X/D, alpha-lipoic acid 1200 mg/D, magnesium citrate 500 mg/D, mucuna pruriens 5 g/D, or red clover 40-80 mg/day.

Clinical Relevance

Across four decades of research on magnetic fields, hundreds of studies have found benefit from PEMF therapy for pain, while a limited number that found benefit equal to placebo. None of the research to date has found that PEMFs cause harm. In this chapter, I've shared the primary pain conditions for which research has documented that PEMFs provide clear benefit, with a range of parameters in terms of frequency, intensity, and duration of treatment.

There are numerous PEMF devices available to the clinician, with a range of functional capabilities and limitations. The choice of a device should be based on the conditions to be treated and the relative strength called for to reach the target tissue or organ, as indicated by research data and clinical studies. Clinical PEMF therapy is highly relevant to pain conditions treated in the fields of chiropractic, physical therapy, acupuncture, biofeedback, naturopathy, and psychology, as well as orthopedics, physical medicine, pain medicine, neurology, neurosurgery, psychiatry, and the growing fields of integrative and functional medicine.

Our ability to relieve pain is variable and unpredictable. It depends on the source of the pain (which is many times different than the location of the pain), and whether the pain is acute or chronic. Pain mechanisms are complex and have local tissue and central nervous system aspects. Because of all these variables, pain management should be tailored to each person individually. The most effective pain management strategies require multiple concurrent approaches, especially for chronic pain. Rarely will a single approach solve the problem.

Having practiced medicine for more than 50 years, I've become very familiar with the different patterns of pain. Chronic pain (especially from arthritis, lumbar stenosis, injury, failed surgeries, etc.) is not expected to be fully cured because the underlying chronic problem doesn't go away. Because of my years of experience, I resolve to find better, more helpful healing solutions that will work to resolve the underlying causes while at the same time providing safe, effective pain relief.

I frequently recommend PEMF therapies for people in chronic pain (usually before anything else) so that they can avoid complications and side effects, and because PEMFs usually provide a reliable degree of pain relief, especially through convenient and regular treatments done at home. In my experience, almost everyone benefits from PEMF therapy and very frequently they can avoid procedures and decrease or avoid the use of medications. I usually recommend relatively high-intensity systems to combat pain, as research indicates intensity is the most important component to consider when working with PEMFs for pain management. PEMF stimulation (especially with high intensities) quiets down nerves and facilitates recovery from injury and inflammation. Even patients suffering from stubborn or systemic sources of pain have found pain relief using magnetic therapies.

Treatment Expectations

Chronic and higher levels of pain alter EEG signals. An improvement in pain will reverse these EEG changes. Even if the goal of the treatment is simply to reduce the pain level without an expectation for reducing or eliminating the cause, research shows that applying PEMFs to the brain can cause a significant decrease in pain-related changes in an EEG.

Some patients get complete pain relief after only a few PEMF treatments. Sometimes it can take up to three hours after treatment to achieve maximum pain relief. In rare cases, short courses of treatment can produce complete or partial pain relief for upwards of four months after treatment. Most people experience pain relief lasting for between eight and 72 hours. This suggests that PEMFs stimulate increased energy in the tissues, which allows the body to fulfill its healing process. Treatments should be continued until the pain is under control, and ideally should continue beyond pain relief to ensure the injury has fully healed.

Unfortunately, the longer a person waits to start treatment with PEMFs, the more challenging it is to remove the cause, which is the primary objective of using PEMF therapies. When we use PEMF therapies we are attempting to heal the tissues that are the source of the pain signal. How long it takes to achieve this depends on the tissue and the level of damage. This is the most important aspect of use of PEMFs, that is, healing the tissue, not just "numbing and dumbing" the perception of pain.

It is also important to understand expectations in pain management. Even in the best hands, pain reduction follows a spectrum from complete elimination very rapidly to gradual reduction over extended periods of time, as the body heals itself. In many patients, even a 25-30 percent reduction in pain is gratifying. We can frequently achieve even higher levels of pain reduction.

PEMF therapy does more than relieve symptoms. PEMFs also address the underlying causes of pain, including inflammation which is almost always a significant factor in the cause of pain. Giving attention to what's causing the pain is essential in finding sustainable solutions, and potentially healing the dysfunction.

Because of their many mechanisms of action, pulsed electromagnetic fields support the body and the use of PEMFs alongside other therapies can promote faster healing and relief. In that sense, PEMF therapies are an "Earth-based" therapy. For more information on PEMF therapy for pain reduction, or to discuss which PEMF machine might be right for you, call my office to speak to a member of my team.

In the next chapter, you will learn how and why PEMFs are effective for treating many other common health conditions.

PEMF Therapy for Common Health Conditions

PEMF therapy has been shown through hundreds, if not thousands, of studies to be a beneficial treatment for most common health conditions. My book, *Power Tools for Health*, describes some selected studies to support the use of PEMFs for many common health conditions. This chapter provides specific guidelines on how to think about the treatment of each condition using PEMFs, considering the magnetic field intensity to be used for the best results, and whether treatment should be applied more to a local/regional area or to the whole body, or both.

By local, I mean treating the hand, elbow, shoulder, heart, brain, knee, foot, etc. By regional, I mean the ability to treat the chest, abdomen, the whole lower back, thighs, lower legs, pelvis, etc. For our purposes here, I have combined local and regional. Whole-body PEMFs can be further differentiated into a single large pad or mat or large dual applicator system that allows two applicators to be run simultaneously. Some PEMF systems allow combinations of applicators, two large, a large and a small, or two small applicators.

None of these recommendations are absolute; they are general guidelines. Ultimately, your body will tell you what is needed to get the best results. A good part of the time, if you already own a PEMF system, it may be higher or lower in intensity than recommended. If so, you will likely need to attempt to use it to its best advantage. If the PEMF system that's already being used is not doing what is hoped for, then you may want to consider adding a PEMF system that is more likely to help.

Also, if you suffer from multiple conditions needing treatment, my general recommendation is to pick one or two to start with and then treat other conditions or areas of your body after you achieve some benefits or results from treating the first conditions. Keep in mind that brief treatments, for example, 5 minutes here and 5 minutes there, will not produce the deepest, most consistent and lasting changes. Intense treatments are often needed at the beginning of treatment, and gradually tapered to less PEMF intensity and treatment time as results are achieved. Eventually, as significant benefits are seen, it may be possible to treat multiple areas for short periods.

Relative to how a treatment time should be, the body and the problem/s being treated will determine that. Anybody saying that all you need is 8 or 12 minutes is ignoring physiology and science. The treatment time needed will depend on the health problems being addressed, and the PEMF system being used. Adjustments to the treatment times will need to be made that consider all these factors. It is also not uncommon for a local treatment to produce whole-body benefits and vice versa. However, in general treating the problem area or the source of your problem will produce the best and fastest results, even though there are benefits in another part of your body. For example, applying a PEMF for arthritis of the knee, may benefit anxiety, back pain, bladder issues, etc., because decreasing pain decreases anxiety. PEMF treatment of the knee will not only reduce inflammation and pain locally, but will also improve circulation, increase brain neurotransmitters, and affect acupuncture points and meridians in the area that affect other parts of the body. In addition, nerves often cover multiple areas of the body, so treatment of one spot can lead to other benefits in the distribution of local nerves or cross over in the spine to help other nerves or parts of the body. This is similar to the concept of referred pain. For example, numbing the pain in the part of the body called McBurney's point in the lower abdomen, which is the referred pain area of an inflamed appendix, will also decrease the pain in the appendix area.

I frequently advise that the many physiologic actions of PEMFs are not really specifically controllable by PEMF treatment. We may hope that specific responses are seen, such as pain reduction, improved circulation, reduced inflammation, etc., but they are all happening at the same time to varying degrees, depending on the state of the body and the ability of the body to respond. The body will decide in what order effects happen and physical changes are seen. This is one of the reasons I like PEMF therapy so much. The body has the wisdom to restore itself in its own time and fashion, when given a boost from PEMF therapy.

Going "Low and Slow"

Going "low and slow" means starting treatments with low intensities and the shortest treatment time, then moving up the different treatment time and intensity options gradually. The reason for doing this is to test the tissue/body to determine how receptive it is to PEMF stimulation. By itself, this is a form of diagnostic test. Some clinicians use a very-high-intensity magnetic field and place it on different parts of the body for a few seconds each, effectively scanning the body. This will tell the clinician which parts of the body are especially sensitive and need dedicated attention to heal.

Usually, a reaction over the reactive parts of the body indicates they have significant inflammation or damage. Healthy tissues largely ignore the magnetic field. Damaged or inflamed tissues will react by having pain where there was none or a sudden increase in pain. Pain is not the only possible reaction. Everybody and every body part is unique and will express its potential discomfort with the magnetic field stimulation in its own way. For example, the brain may show dizziness, the lower back may have pain or maybe even a desire to empty the bladder. These reactions are unpredictable and unique to every individual and circumstance, and are caused by a sudden change in the body or body part's usual state, even if that state is by itself abnormal.

We can have similar reactions to music, whether slow-paced, staccato, metal music, high-volume, etc. We can also have exaggerated reactions to cold or heat. For the brain, our brain's state at the time of the stimulus will determine how we react to it and whether we are "resonant" with it or not. We can be irritated or calmed by the stimulation.

Considering the brain's reactions, it is the pulsation rate of movement of the PEMF passing through the brain plus its intensity that will determine how our brain cells react. The PEMFs are essentially waves of energy passing through the brain, like waves of water passing through a pond, or like the wind passing through the trees. A breeze disturbs the leaves minimally. A strong wind creates much more reaction from the leaves and branches. However, the wind does not stay in the tree; it moves completely through and keeps on going, just as PEMFs do in the brain.

Reactions can happen with many tissues or organs in the body. The body has varying degrees of tolerability for PEMFs. Most often, this depends on the intensity of the magnetic field being applied, but occasionally it depends on the frequencies of the pulsations. It is less about the specific frequency than it is about the stimulation effects of repetitive pulses to the organ or tissue. For example, some people may react to faster pulses of lower intensities. Others may react only to slower pulses of higher intensities.

As a result of the various aspects of stimulation, the baseline status of the tissues of the body will reveal whether the PEMFs passing through it are tolerated, essentially ignored, or causing reactions. There will always be reactions, ranging from minimal to strong. An irritated, sensitive tissue or an anxious, fired-up brain will react much more strongly to a weak signal than a calm brain, nervous system, or tissue. It is because we rarely really know the state of different tissues of the body that I recommend a "low and slow" stimulation protocol.

Very healthy people in great shape may not need to go "low and slow." They may start off with one lower-intensity level, jump to a middle-intensity level and then on the third try go to the highest-intensity level. After that they may never need to go any lower or slower. I'm not an advocate of anybody going to the highest intensities right away, however.

Besides intensity, the other important treatment parameter is the total treatment time. My experience, after working with magnetic fields for 30 years, has been that intensity is more important than treatment time. Sometimes a problem is related more to the amount of the body area being stimulated at the same time. I have not infrequently seen people using very-low-intensity magnetic fields with whole-body therapy having significant reactions. They may have no or milder reactions with a small body pad. This is because of the sheer number of acupuncture points and meridians, cells, and sensory nerves being stimulated at the same time with the whole-body pads, despite the PEMFs being low-intensity. Even the same signal, at a higher intensity stimulating a smaller area, may not produce the same reaction. Unfortunately, it is hard to predict who will react how. The more excitable, that is, "hotter," the brain or nervous system is, the more sensitive these individuals will be to almost any stimulation. The more sensory nerves and other cell types that are being stimulated at the same time, especially by multiple frequencies, the more "flooded" the brain becomes with sensory input.

A "low and slow" protocol will depend on the health condition of the person being stimulated, the PEMF system being used, and the person's psychological or emotional sensitivity level. The most sensitive people will need to use an extremely "low and slow" protocol. How long it takes to reach the desired, optimal levels of stimulation is unpredictable. While the optimal level of stimulation may well be the maximum treatment time and the maximum intensity, this may not be possible for everybody. In those circumstances, individuals will have to find their maximum level of tolerance and continue to do treatment with the PEMF knowing that it is still going to produce deeper cellular benefit even though they are not at the maximum and may not be feeling significant progress.

Even though my experience has been that intensity is more important than treatment time, at some points in the progression of the "low and slow" protocol, intensity may not be able to be advanced, but treatment time may. To understand this better, the analogy I use is athletic training. It is a stop-start or stair-step process: train to the level tolerated, stop if it can't be handled, move back to the previous level tolerated, do that for a while, then try to advance again. How fast this "training process" will be depends on the shape the body's in at the time. As PEMFs produce healing in the body, this "training process" will be able to advance. The goal would be to advance to the optimal level desired, after which the amount of training would be adjusted based on time available and treatment goals.

Some of this PEMF "training process" will also depend on the organ and the tissue being treated. Stimulation is not uniform or equal throughout the whole body because of the configuration of the applicators used. Whole-body stimulation produces different results than local treatments. Generally, whole-body stimulation is at lower levels of intensity than treatments with local applicators, because of the design of the applicators. Local applicators would be a better indicator of the state of health of the local area being treated.

In Appendix B, I provide a variety of "low and slow" protocols. Any one of these may be followed as they are, or the protocol may have to be adjusted based on personal experience and reactions. To adjust the protocol, with each treatment session you would either do:

- much slower progressions of intensity while maintaining treatment time steady, or
- maintain intensity while gradually increasing treatment time, or
- gradually advance treatment time and intensity with each treatment session, or
- various combinations of these.

Most Health Conditions Didn't Happen Overnight

Most of the time, PEMF therapy is used for chronic problems that have become significant enough for a person to decide that a more aggressive, alternative, safer, and more effective approach needs to be taken than has previously been tried. Optimally, PEMF therapy should be started very early in the process of a chronic problem developing. The sooner the right PEMFs are used for a problem, the better and sooner the results will be. Improvement also depends on the severity of the problem and the tissue involved. The more severe and damaged the tissue is, the longer it takes to repair. Some tissues take longer to repair than others, if ever. As a result, it's critical to have the right PEMF system, have clear and appropriate expectations for treatment, and to let the body do the repair it needs to do. PEMFs don't do the healing. They stimulate the healing. The body does its own healing. PEMFs don't raise the dead. Dead tissue is still dead tissue. A scar is still a scar. A scar is transformed or bridged dead tissue. PEMFs may make the scar prettier, but that's all. Bottom line, the body has to be allowed to do the job it can do.

Treating Multiple Areas of the Body

Most people who seek PEMF therapy have multiple health issues. For example, they have multiple areas of the body with arthritis or aches and pains. It is natural to want to be able to eliminate all pains at the same time with the same effort. What many people do is spend a few minutes treating each area. This is not likely to produce much benefit. Any given area may need considerable time, maybe even for 30 minutes to 60 minutes at a time for weeks to months to reach a sufficient level of healing, especially when the problem is more severe.

I recommend that one or two priority areas be selected for intense treatment to begin with. As these areas improve, they may need a small amount of time to be maintained, often at a higher level of intensity, while new, lower-priority areas may begin to get treated more intensely, similarly to the first set of priority areas. High-intensity, whole-body PEMF therapy, especially with the "magnetic sandwich" approach, is more likely to help multiple areas simultaneously.

If multiple areas of the body are largely unique, for example, arthritis of the knee from an old injury, degenerative disc disease of the back, shoulder pain from rotator cuff issues, neuropathy of the feet from diabetes, etc., they can be treated according to the approach mentioned above. However, if there are multiple problems in the body that are due to a single, probable cause, such as autoimmune disease from rheumatoid arthritis, lupus, Lyme disease, diabetes, etc., then a whole-body approach will produce better results than treating individual areas where pain is being experienced. While whole-body treatment is being used, individual areas may still get individual treatment for better pain relief. The goal of the whole-body treatment is to deal with the cause and not just use a local, symptomatic approach.

The Need for Daily PEMF Treatment

I frequently consult with people who have been getting periodic PEMF treatments in a professional setting. If this is solving the problem, that is worthwhile. However, if after a few treatments in a professional setting, the problem shows that it needs continuing treatment, daily home treatments become necessary. Most chronic problems need daily treatment until the problem has begun to heal itself, after which daily treatment may not be needed for maintenance. Usually, though, at the beginning stages of using PEMF therapy most people need daily treatment to begin to get control of the issues.

Some problems, such as bone-on-bone arthritis, chronic degenerative disc disease, spinal stenosis, chronic tendinitis, MS, Parkinson's disease, and many more are truly chronic and may never be able to be fully healed. That means that intense PEMF treatments will begin to improve the problems and then need to continue to be maintained with a lower level of daily treatment. When intensive therapy has made a big difference, treatments are typically cut back. If they are cut back and some of the problem begins to return, this is an indicator that healing has not been completed. This process of stopping and starting may need to be done several times to confirm that continued therapy is necessary.

This stopping and cutting back approach can be especially helpful with pain issues. When PEMFs help pain but the pain returns in three hours, then perhaps treatment should be started again to achieve longer periods of relief. If a treatment helps the pain and the pain doesn't come back for two or three days, then treatment may be able to be shifted to every other day. Pain that comes back is a clear indication that the tissue has not healed. Again, the goal of PEMF therapy is not only to remove the pain. The goal is to heal the tissue completely so that the pain doesn't come back.

Twice-a-Day Treatments: I usually recommend twice-a-day treatments. Every treatment initiates a healing sequence of events in the tissues. Most of the time, these healing events do not last all day. They taper off as the day goes on. That means they need to be repeated periodically. In some cases, they need to be repeated more often than twice a day, and that will need to be individually determined.

The other reason to do twice-a-day treatments is that every treatment produces multiple benefits in the body beyond the tissue being treated, especially with whole-body PEMF therapy. As a result, I say that a morning treatment "shakes off the cobwebs" from the night before. The second treatment, usually in the evening, "shakes off the stress" in the body that is natural and which progressively builds up as we go through our daily activities. Clearly some people need the nighttime treatment more than others depending on how "stressful" their day has been. Just normal daily living causes "stress" to the body even though it is not perceived as stressful. This normal daily "stress" is a necessary physiologic (versus mental) adaptation response but, unfortunately, also adds to our aging process. The second PEMF treatment of the day is a physically de-stressing treatment, even though it may not be a mentally, psychologically, or emotionally de-stressing treatment. These latter types of stress also contribute to the total stress load. PEMFs can help with these types of stress as well.

Types of PEMF Devices to Use by Intensity and Area of Treatment

In the following table, the ranges of magnetic field therapy (low, medium, or high) are somewhat arbitrary and based more on available equipment. The table lists the conditions, the strength group of the magnetic field in gauss that should be considered, whether treatment should be local and/or whole-body, and the areas that should be treated. The strength groups are low, medium, and high. For our purposes, the intensities are: 0.1 – 10 gauss for low intensity; 10 – 500 gauss for medium intensity; 500 – >1000 gauss for high intensity. Some would argue that high intensity would be anything over 1000 gauss. A large percent of PEMF systems studied in research do not reach magnetic field intensities greater than 100 gauss. Very few PEMF systems studied in research do not reach magnetic field intensities greater than 5 gauss (500 microTesla). Very few whole-body systems reach above 5 gauss, especially those combined with crystals and other stimulating components.

Low-intensity PEMFs tend to be whole-body systems. Most local therapy systems fall into the class of medium- or high-intensity. Local therapy devices basically treat a small area, depending on the size of the applicators. Magnetic fields typically extend beyond the edges of the PEMF applicators and vary with the system. These local PEMF devices and/or applicators can certainly be moved around to treat multiple individual areas. Because of the intensity and the natural drop-off in the magnetic field, even a local applicator may need to be moved around a specific spot to be most effective. For example, treating arthritis of the knee, depending on how badly the knee is affected, may require a local applicator to be placed on one side of the knee for a while, followed by another part of the knee, etc., to treat the whole knee. If that is the case, it may be more efficient to use a medium- to high-intensity device to get better, faster results.

And "x" in the table indicates what intensity may be best for treating a given condition and where to apply the applicator for that condition. In addition to suggesting local versus whole-body and intensity, I discuss other considerations for treatment approaches in a bit more depth as I go through each condition separately later in this chapter.

Type of PEMF System and Intensity by Condition

	Local			Whole body			
	Intensity - in gauss			Intensity - in gauss			
	low	medium	high	low	medium	high	
Condition	0.1–10	10–100	100–>1000	0.1–10	10–100	100–>1000	**Area/s to be treated**
Addiction		x	x			x	brain
Adhesions, abdominal			x				belly
Alkaline Balance, Systemic			x		x	x	kidneys/full body
Alzheimer's disease			x				brain
Anxiety, Panic, and PTSD Disorders		x	x			x	brain/solar plexus
Arthritis (Osteoarthritis)		x	x		x	x	affected joints
Athletic performance		x	x		x	x	affected areas + whole body
Autoimmune	x	x	x	x	x	x	affected areas + whole body

	Local			Whole body			
	Intensity - in gauss			Intensity - in gauss			
	low	medium	high	low	medium	high	
Condition	0.1–10	10–100	100–>1000	0.1–10	10–100	100–>1000	Area/s to be treated
Back pain		x	x		x	x	back
Bladder Conditions		x	x				bladder
Bone Healing and Repair		x	x		x	x	affected bones
Breast implants		x	x				breasts
Bruising		x	x				bruised area/s
Burns		x	x		x	x	affected areas + whole body
Cancer		x	x		x	x	organs; whole-body for leukemia/lymphoma
Cancer, bone cancer/mets			x		x	x	areas with cancer/mets
Cancer, brain radiation therapy			x				brain
Cancer, breast		x	x		x	x	breasts and whole body
Cancer, chemotherapy				x	x	x	whole body, brain and/or abdomen
Cancer, head, neck and oropharyngeal		x	x				head and neck area
Cancer, liver			x		x	x	liver area

Condition	Local Intensity - in gauss			Whole body Intensity - in gauss			Area/s to be treated
	low 0.1–10	medium 10–100	high 100– >1000	low 0.1–10	medium 10–100	high 100– >1000	
Cancer, lung		x	x		x	x	lung/s
Cancer, pancreatic			x		x	x	pancreas/ whole body
Cancer, stage IV			x		x	x	areas with cancer/mets
Carpal tunnel syndrome		x	x				wrist
Cataracts	x	x					eye/s
Chronic Fatigue Syndrome (CFS)			x	x	x	x	brain/ full-body
Complex regional pain syndrome (CRPS)			x		x	x	brain/ full-body
Concussion and traumatic brain injury (TBI)			x				brain
Dental Issues		x	x				local dental area
Depression		x	x				brain
Diabetes		x	x	x	x	x	whole-body and local if needed
Ear problems		x	x				ear/s
Eczema and dermatitis		x	x	x	x	x	affected areas
Ehlers Danlos Syndromes		x	x		x	x	brain/ full-body

	Local Intensity - in gauss			Whole body Intensity - in gauss			
	low	medium	high	low	medium	high	
Condition	0.1–10	10–100	100–>1000	0.1–10	10–100	100–>1000	Area/s to be treated
Endometriosis			x		x	x	pelvis/lower abdomen
Enuresis, nocturnal		x	x				bladder and brain
Epilepsy			x				brain
Erectile dysfunction			x				genital area/pelvis
Eye conditions	x	x					eye/s
Fibromyalgia		x	x	x	x	x	brain
Fungal skin infections		x	x	x	x	x	affected areas
Gall Bladder Disorders		x	x				gall bladder area
Glaucoma	x	x					eye/s
Heart Conditions		x	x				heart
Hepatitis, Viral		x	x				liver area
Interstitial cystitis/bladder pain syndrome (IC/BPS)			x				bladder/ pelvis
Intestinal Function		x	x				abdomen
Joint replacements and implanted prosthetics			x				affected joints
Kidney disease			x				kidney areas

	Local			Whole body			
	Intensity - in gauss			Intensity - in gauss			
	low	medium	high	low	medium	high	
Condition	0.1–10	10–100	100–>1000	0.1–10	10–100	100–>1000	**Area/s to be treated**
Lyme disease			x	x	x	x	whole-body and local if needed
Memory loss		x	x				brain
Migraine			x				brain
Multiple sclerosis			x		x	x	brain
Obesity		x	x		x	x	whole body, brain and local if needed
Osteopenia and osteoporosis						x	whole body
Pain management		x	x	x	x	x	local and brain
Pancreatic Conditions		x	x		x	x	upper abdomen
Paraplegia and spinal cord injury		x	x		x	x	whole body, spinal cord and local if needed
Parkinson's disease		x	x		x	x	brain
Premenstrual syndrome (PMS)		x	x		x	x	lower abdomen; back if needed
Prostate hyperplasia - benign prostate hyperplasia (BPH)			x				bladder, sacrum

	Local			Whole body			
	Intensity - in gauss			Intensity - in gauss			
	low	medium	high	low	medium	high	
Condition	0.1–10	10–100	100–>1000	0.1–10	10–100	100–>1000	**Area/s to be treated**
Scleroderma or progressive systemic sclerosis (PSS)		x	x		x	x	affected areas
Shingles		x	x				affected areas
Sickle cell disease		x	x		x	x	whole-body and local as needed
Sleep		x	x		x	x	brain
Smoking cessation		x	x				brain
Stem cell therapy		x	x		x	x	whole-body and local as needed
Stomach problems		x	x				stomach area
Stroke			x				brain
Tendinitis/ tendinosis		x	x				local area/s
Testosterone		x	x				testes and brain if needed
Tinnitus			x				brain
Tremor		x	x				brain
Vascular disease		x	x		x	x	whole-body and local as needed
Wounds		x	x				affected areas

PEMF Treatment Recommendations

Each of the following conditions begins with short overview of the condition itself, followed by the general goals of PEMFs for treating it. Specific recommendations are provided for PEMF intensity, applicators to use, suggested treatment times, and potential supplements that can also be helpful.

All of these recommendations have to be individualized based on your individual circumstances. These are suggestions and guidelines and are not rigid. These recommendations are based on an evaluation of a large body of scientific PEMF evidence, my 50 years of broad clinical experience, including 16 years of holistic medicine experience and 30 years of experience working with PEMFs. You already have a PEMF system which may or may not fit the recommendations I share below. Whatever you have may be tried, and your results will need to be considered. All PEMFs provide some degree of benefit albeit not necessarily optimal. Even less-optimal local or whole-body therapy may produce some systemic benefits. Remember, your goal is to achieve healing, not just putting a Band-Aid on a problem by simply feeling better. If healing is not able to be satisfactorily accomplished, a problem is likely to continue and even worsen. I often told my patients "pay now or pay later, but, if you pay later, you might not like the interest."

Supplements and Nutrition: PEMFs stimulate the body to produce more energy in order to function, repair, and heal itself as optimally as possible. The success of PEMF actions depends on the state the body is in at the time PEMF therapy is begun. A healthy diet that provides the body with a sufficient amount of proteins, fats, carbohydrates, water, vitamins, minerals, enzymes, and other nutrients is essential for maintaining the body's state. Appropriate nutritional and herbal supplements can also be very helpful. PEMFs add the stimulus to activate all these elements.

It is beyond the scope of this book to provide comprehensive instruction about nutrition, supplements, and herbs. However, for each condition, I make some basic supplement recommendations. These are suggestions and it is not always practical or reasonable to take all of them. It's also not possible to provide dosing information, because individual circumstances and many other factors, including co-morbidities and your general state of health, need to be considered. Other supplements and nutritional advice may be needed, as well. As a result,

I recommend consulting with a professional skilled in nutrition, supplements, and herbs to guide you on the individualized, unique combination of nutrition, supplements and/or herbs that you should follow.

I use a shorthand for the times per day supplements could be used. For example, three times per day would be 3X/D and 500 mg 2 to 3 times per day would be 500 mg 2-3X/D. When supplements are taken multiple times a day, they would normally be spread out throughout the day. For example, 2 times per day would normally be in the morning and at dinnertime or bedtime, depending on the supplements. For 3 times per day, supplements could be taken morning, dinnertime, and bedtime. The timing of the supplements will depend on the supplements themselves and instructions given on the supplement containers unless a nutritionist or other professional advises otherwise. Many of the supplement recommendations are taken from the authoritative book *Nutritional Medicine* by Alan Gaby (Concord, NH: Fritz Perlberg; 2017.)

Note: For certain of the conditions below, I suggest the use of a "magnetic sandwich" approach to applying PEMF applicators. For more information about this approach, see Appendix C.

Addiction

Addiction is often associated with anxiety and depression. Treatment of addiction is primarily focused on the brain, and can be done locally with a sufficient intensity magnetic field. If lower intensity is used, treatment times may need to be considerably longer, possibly even several hours a day. Trial and error becomes important. It may be valuable to do treatments every hour, with breaks of half an hour to an hour in between, especially when dealing with cravings and withdrawal symptoms.

When cravings occur, therapy may be applied at the onset and continued until the cravings have reduced to a level of comfort or disappeared. Cravings often occur when the addictive substances are being withdrawn or tapered. With significant improvement in cravings and withdrawal symptoms, treatment times may be able to be reduced and spread out over longer periods of time between treatments. Much current research is done using high-intensity PEMFs applied directly to the brain. Often high-intensity treatment times can be significantly shorter. The body's response to PEMF therapy will determine how much treatment time is needed. With higher intensities the going low and slow approach is important.

Addictions occur to many different substances, including among others: alcohol, opioids, cocaine, benzodiazepines, barbiturates, tobacco, sugar, salt, and caffeine. There are also many types of behavioral addictions. While psychospiritual and psychological approaches to dealing with addictions are important, they do not always account for the biochemical aspects of addiction. A person's urge to use a particular drug or continue a particular behavior may be as strong biochemically as the need to take sugar for hypoglycemia, water for thirst, or food for hunger. In this case, counseling by itself may not be enough to prevent relapse. Strengthening the body and brain can be the difference between successful abstinence and chronic relapses.

PEMFs help to "strengthen" the body and brain, helping to decrease the risk of addiction, lower the use of the drugs or substances involved during addiction, and help with the withdrawal symptoms when stopping the use of a substance. In the case of withdrawal from benzodiazepines and alcohol, there is a risk of seizures and delirium tremens (DTs). PEMFs may help to reduce these risks.

PEMF therapy may need to be continued for months, even years, depending on the presence of addiction triggers. Long-term treatment is also important for shifting and maintaining brain physiology and even brain structures, so that the predisposition to addiction may be able to be helped as well.

While intensity is very important, the frequencies of the PEMF system are also important. With high-intensity systems, lower pulse rates are better. With frequency-based systems, the best frequencies are likely to be alpha, theta- and gamma. Beta may be able to be used to generate alertness but this should be watched for the possibility of increasing anxiety. Adequate rest, nutrition, and hydration are also critical to achieve and maintain benefits.

Intensity of the PEMF: 100-7000 gauss. Applications would be to the brain.

Applicators: Portable- battery-operated PEMF applicators placed over the sides of the head or two applicators stacked on the left forehead during the day at 7 Hz, 10 Hz or 40 Hz. Trial and error will determine which frequencies work best. For sleep, use one or two applicators under the pillow through the night at 3 Hz or 7 Hz. Local high-intensity PEMFs may also be applied to the sides of the head or over the left forehead as well.

Treatment Time: Portable, battery-operated PEMFs can be applied for hours at a time during the day, as needed. During nighttime, they will be used throughout the whole night. High-intensity treatments would be between 30 to 60 minutes at a time, 2-3 X/day, as needed. More treatments may be needed during the early stages of withdrawal and decreased as symptoms begin to resolve. Maintenance treatment with 30 minutes twice a day may be needed for months, and especially when episodes of urge to use again occur.

Supplements: Niacin 500 mg/D time release or 500 mg niacinamide 2-3x/D, glutamine 1 or more gm/D, magnesium 500 mg 1-2X/D, P5 P 100 mg/D, B12 sublingual 3000 – 5000 μg/D, thiamine 100 mg/D, zinc 25 mg/D + copper 1-4 mg/D (if no cirrhosis), L taurine 1000 mg 3X/D, evening primrose oil 4 g/D, acetyl l-carnitine 2000 mg/D (in 2-3 divided doses), L tyrosine one – 3 g/D, melatonin sustained-release 3–12 mg at bedtime, or L-tryptophan 50 mg/Kg body weight/day.

Adhesions, Abdominal (Including Pelvis)

Peritoneal adhesions are abnormal fibrous connections between peritoneal surfaces in the abdomino-pelvic region of the body, resulting from incomplete peritoneal repair. Peritoneal healing is a complex process involving control of bleeding, inflammation, new blood vessel formation, development of granulation tissue, extracellular matrix (ECM) deposition, and tissue remodeling. Surgery-related tissue trauma, ischemia, infection, inflammation, and foreign body reaction all complicate peritoneal healing. Postoperative peritoneal adhesions (PPA) are inevitable with any abdomino-pelvic surgery. PPAs occur in 95 percent of surgeries.

Adhesions can develop anywhere in the abdomen and pelvis. Most the time they are due to prior surgery, but they can also happen from inflammation or infections. Pelvic adhesions can happen due to endometriosis and infections in the fallopian tubes which extend into the abdomen and pelvis. Usually, they develop silently. Common symptoms are frequent or persistent abdominal cramps. In worst case scenarios, they can lead to bowel obstruction. Unfortunately, surgery to break down adhesions, called lysis of adhesions, can provide temporary relief but lead to further adhesion development because any invasion of the abdomen can create adhesions, even with the small puncture wound during laparoscopy.

A person's body size will dictate the intensity of the magnetic field used to abdomino-pelvic treat adhesions. Because of the need for adequate depth of penetration, considering the inverse square law, a minimum of 500 gauss is recommended for small, thin bellies. To decrease inflammation in the belly, and using about 4-6 inches as the distance from the skin on the front of the abdomen to the back through which the PEMF needs to penetrate, the optimal magnetic field would be between ~1800-3800 gauss. Therapy to the whole belly is needed; 30 minutes a day may suffice.

Ideally, anybody having abdominal surgery should have PEMF therapy as soon as possible following surgery. This is most likely to happen in somebody who already has a PEMF system. Adhesions begin to form the first day following surgery, the extent of which depends on the body's aggressiveness in repair. Symptoms can show up months to years later.

It is unknown for how long PEMF therapy would be needed to prevent adhesion development. But even one to two weeks of PEMF therapy may be helpful. Needless to say, anybody using whole-body PEMF therapy for any other purposes or for health maintenance would still get a benefit in preventing adhesion development or reducing existing adhesions. Once adhesions have formed, it is unknown how long treatment needs to be continued, because they may be fairly thick and dense. In this situation, regular daily use may be advisable, especially to prevent further bowel obstructions. If adhesions cause recurrent abdominal cramps or any bowel obstructions, PEMF therapy should be started as soon as feasible.

In the case of chronic inflammatory bowel disease and endometriosis, continuous PEMF therapy daily would also be helpful, not only for the underlying condition, but also to manage and prevent adhesion development. Again, in these situations PEMF therapy may be needed for 30 to 60 minutes twice a day for the underlying conditions.

Intensity of the PEMF: 2000-7000 gauss.

Applicators: A regional applicator covering the whole belly, or at least from the bellybutton to the pubic bone.

Treatment time: 30 – 60 minutes twice a day, for active treatment, when there are symptoms and after abdominal or pelvic surgery; 30 minutes a day for preventive maintenance.

Supplements: Serrapeptase, nattokinase and/or lumbrokinase, inflamase, bromelain 200-400 mg three times a day, curcumin 1000 – 3000 mg 1-2X/D, garlic, zinc 25 mg/D + copper 1-4 mg/D, MSM 3000-9000 mg/D. Many of these supplements may decrease clotting, resulting in bruising or bleeding. Consult with your nutritionist or doctor.

Alkaline Balance, Systemic

There is a significant interest in alkaline diets. Having too much acidity in the body creates many metabolic and functional issues. Alkaline balance does not mean that the body should be alkaline, rather that it should not be acidic. Greater, out-of-normal pH changes in the body, whether acidic *or* alkaline, require the kidneys to work harder to maintain a neutral systemic pH. A chronic, mild, acidic state, often caused by a more acidic diet is best dealt with by changing the diet. It is beyond the scope of this book to talk about diets for this situation.

Systemic acid-base (alkaline) balance is very dependent on kidney function, in more significantly acidic pH states, PEMFs may be able to help somewhat with kidney function. It may be inadequate without the underlying cause of the acidic state being addressed as a priority. In the case of even mild kidney failure, PEMFs may be able to help the kidneys to perform their pH-balancing duties more efficiently. For this purpose, a local PEMF could be helpful applied on the back over the kidneys. Because of the depth of the kidneys in the body, the ideal magnetic field intensity would be close to 2000 gauss.

Systemic inflammation increases the acid pH burden in the whole body, due to an accumulation of local tissue acidity. Whole-body PEMF therapy could be useful in this situation. A medium- to high-intensity PEMF system would be best for this purpose.

Intensity of the PEMF: 1000-4000 gauss to be able to penetrate into the kidneys and general vascular system.

Applicators: Regional over the kidneys, or whole-body, preferably a "magnetic sandwich" type system.

Treatment time: 30 minutes twice a day.

Supplements: The most important thing is adequate hydration. Routine use of bicarbonate or acid neutralizing tablets or drinks for the stomach are not recommended, except for occasional indigestion or heartburn since they will put a strain on the kidneys long-term. There may be other undesirable long-term effects for the body.

Alzheimer's Disease

Alzheimer's Disease (AD) is the most common form of dementia. There is no cure. Current treatments only help with the symptoms. AD worsens as it progresses, and eventually leads to death. Most often, AD is diagnosed in people over 65 years of age, although the less-prevalent early-onset Alzheimer's can occur much earlier.

The cause and progression of Alzheimer's disease are not well-understood. Research indicates that AD is associated with plaques and tangles in the brain. There are several competing other theories to explain the cause of AD: that it is caused by reduced formation of the neurotransmitter acetylcholine, the amyloid theory, the tau theory, and the idea that age-related myelin (the cover of nerve fibers) breakdown in the brain releasing iron, causing damage. Normal, natural myelin repair processes which are triggered by the iron contribute to the development of protein deposits such as beta-amyloid and tau. Also, oxidative stress and rebalancing of biometal metabolism may be significant in the formation of the disease.

People with AD exhibit a 70 percent loss of local brain cells that make norepinephrine. Norepinephrine acts as an internal anti-inflammatory agent in the microenvironment around the neurons, glial cells, and blood vessels in the brain cortex and hippocampus. It has been shown that norepinephrine stimulates mouse microglia to suppress production of cytokines, which are responsible for the breakdown of amyloid.

As I've noted many times before, PEMFs have general functions and actions relating to all cells, including brain cells. It is these general effects of PEMFs that may help people with or predisposed to AD, even though the PEMFs are not addressing AD specifically. The challenge is getting people to start therapy earlier in their disease process, and especially doing prevention in those at high risk, that is, those with strong family histories.

Various studies have explored whether PEMFs help AD from different aspects, using various PEMF devices. All showed some benefit. Inflammation is the constant factor in AD, as it is in most diseases. Therefore, if we do nothing but address chronic inflammation, we could have a substantial impact on the development and progression of AD.

PEMFs may not only address the development and progression of AD but may also help to improve brain function, increase brain energy by stimulating ATP, improve circulation and memory, help any pre-existing brain damage and help with many of the conditions that contribute to AD, including the effects of diabetes, alcohol, smoking, and brain atherosclerosis. While whole-body PEMF therapy may help many of the contributing factors to AD, the focus of treatment here will be the brain itself.

Intensity of the PEMF: 100 – 1000 gauss using gamma frequencies, 30-100 Hz, especially 40 Hz. High-intensity PEMFs between 4000 – 7000 gauss. Higher-intensity, whole-body PEMFs from 150-7000 gauss for general whole-body benefits.

Applicators: Portable, battery-operated PEMF applicators placed over the sides of the head or two applicators stacked on the left forehead during the day at 7 Hz, 10 Hz or 40 Hz. Trial and error will determine which frequencies work best. For sleep, use one or two applicators under the pillow through the night at 3 Hz or 7 Hz. Local high-intensity PEMFs may also be applied to the sides of the head or over the left forehead as well. Local applicators applied to either side of the head just above the ears, of whatever intensity, but preferably higher intensity. For high-intensity systems, use the local applicators, including loop, butterfly, paddle, or pad. The loop coil may be placed over the top or side of the head. If flexible, it may be conformed into an elliptical form and placed over the top ahead and each side or the back of the head and each side. The butterfly coil would be placed over the top of the head with a wing on each side. The paddle coil can be placed on the side of the head and moved from one side to the other. Whole-body applicators for whole-body treatment. If the system allows the "magnetic sandwich" approach, this would be the most efficient, being sure that the head is lying on the bottom coil or using a bottom whole-body pad combined with a local coil applied to the head.

Treatment Time: 30 – 60 minutes twice a day. If there is significant improvement in symptoms/memory, maintenance may be able to be reduced to

30 minutes twice a day, as long as this level of stimulation maintains the benefit. Treatment is expected to be lifelong.

Supplements: B12 5000 µg/D, P5P 100 mg/D, methylfolate 3 mg/D, niacin 50 mg 3x/D or 1.5 g/D, thiamine 100 mg/D, magnesium citrate 500 mg/D, acetyl l-carnitine 2000 mg/D, beta-carotene 50 mg/D, phosphatidylserine 300 mg/D, ginkgo biloba 120 mg/D, DHEA sulfate 10 – 25 mg/D, NADH 10 mg/D before breakfast, Inositol 3 g 2X/D, CoQ10 200 mg 2X/D, mixed tocopherols 1000 IU 2X/D, Fiji water (has high levels of silica) 1 L/D.

Anxiety, Panic, and PTSD Disorders

While these conditions can be considered primarily psychological or emotional, they can be significantly helped by brain tuning. Brain tuning using PEMFs can also support counseling efforts. Counselors using PEMFs report that using PEMFs prior to or during counseling makes the counseling more effective. The reason is that PEMFs help people to "chill out" and be more relaxed before or during counseling. Because counseling is often not covered by insurance and can be expensive in the long run, anything that can help counseling or help the individual to decrease the need for counseling is important and supportive.

Unfortunately, one of the most common approaches to dealing with chronic anxiety disorders is medication. Medications for anxiety carry significant risks of dependency and addiction. Effectiveness of medications and counseling have been found to be limited, ranging from 3 to 70 percent. Even the so-called non-addicting medications, the SSRIs, are very hard to get off once started. Also, these common anti-anxiety medications can increase the risk of dementia.

While brain chemistry is very much involved in the production of anxiety, and is the basis for the use of medications, brain chemistry can be controlled to a significant extent by tuning the brain with almost no risk. Neuroscience research, using quantitative EEG (QEEG) or brain mapping, found a number of patterns of imbalance in brainwave frequencies: deficient Alpha frequencies (8 – 13 Hz) in the frontal lobes of the brain, excessive beta frequencies (>13 Hz) in many parts of the brain, and even higher Alpha frequencies (>11.5 Hz).

The approach to treatment with PEMFs would be to use PEMF coils applied to the head (transcranial magnetic stimulation, TMS) using medium- to high-intensity devices. Devices that allow control over frequencies can be used at low to medium Alpha frequencies (8 – 10 Hz) applied to both forehead areas, or on both sides of the head just above and slightly behind the midline of the upper part of the ear. A low and slow approach may be necessary to begin with. The ultimate goal would be to get to the highest intensity tolerable. Some people use a portable PEMF system, which can be used as a spot treatment when anxiety starts or even up to hours at a time for maintenance and prevention, allowing a person to be up and about. Currently available portable systems have a maximum intensity of about 200 gauss. The higher-intensity systems require access to an electrical outlet for the equipment to operate. Both the higher-intensity and the lower-intensity systems can be combined, although not at the same time.

High-intensity PEMFs have extensive research behind them. They can be applied to the frontal lobes as well and to the sides of the head. Some experimentation may be needed to see which positioning applications work best. One treatment session could be to the forehead areas and a subsequent session could be to the sides of the head. Many PEMF applicators have "butterfly" coils, allowing one side of the butterfly to be used on each side of the head, whether placed over the top of the head or the back of the head coming to the front. But any kind of PEMF applicator applied to the forehead areas or either side of the head will still work. High-intensity, whole-body systems, if you have one, can still be effective with the smaller applicators applied to the head.

The only precaution in using higher-intensity PEMFs to the brain is the very rare risk of seizures. PEMFs can be used safely and effectively even in those individuals on seizure medications. Some research has indicated that seizures seen with high-intensity PEMFs are coincidental to the person being in a state where they would have had a seizure anyway. If there is concern about this, the use of PEMFs could be discussed with your practitioner. Also see **Epilepsy** later in this chapter.

Even with PEMF treatment, medication may still be needed, hopefully at a lower dose. Before stopping or reducing medication, consult with your practitioner. At least some counseling is likely to be needed at some point to deal with the potential foundational causes and triggers of anxiety. Behavioral therapy may help to identify, reduce, or remove reactions to triggers.

Since the gut has more neurons than the brain and also produces numerous neurotransmitters and chemicals, and the gut and solar plexus is controlled by the vagus nerve, PEMF stimulation of the solar plexus area can be helpful for the treatment of anxiety, as well, and especially for PTSD. Research has shown that

PTSD can be helped significantly by vagal stimulation. PEMF stimulation of the solar plexus may help any gastric issues associated with anxiety, panic, and PTSD.

The vagus nerve can also be stimulated at the top of the neck, using a single coil at the base of the skull just below the ear, or with a high-intensity system with the butterfly coil placed on the back of the neck across both sides of the neck at the base of the skull. It may be possible to combine brain stimulation and vagal nerve stimulation in the same treatment session. Some individual trial and error may be needed to determine whether neck stimulation would be as good as solar plexus stimulation, or a combination of both.

Intensity of the PEMF: 100-7000 gauss.

Applicators: Portable battery-operated PEMF applicators placed over the sides of the head or two applicators stacked on the left forehead during the day at 7 Hz or 10 Hz. Trial and error will determine which frequencies work best. For sleep, use one or two applicators under the pillow through the night at 3 Hz or 7 Hz. Local high-intensity PEMFs may also be applied to the sides of the head or over the left forehead as well. Local applicators applied to either side of the head just above the ears, of whatever intensity, but preferably higher intensity. For high-intensity systems, use the local applicators, including loop, butterfly, paddle, or pad. The loop coil may be placed over the top or side of the head. If flexible, it may be conformed into an elliptical form and placed over the top ahead and each side or the back of the head and each side. The butterfly coil would be placed over the top of the head with a wing on each side. The paddle coil can be placed on the side of the head and moved from one side to the other. Whole-body applicators can be used for whole-body treatment. If the system allows the "magnetic sandwich" approach, this would be the most efficient, being sure that the head is lying on the bottom coil or using a bottom whole-body pad combined with a local coil applied to the head.

Treatment Time: Since even high-intensity PEMFs have been found to be very safe when applied to the brain, the amount of treatment time needed for results will be highly individual and may even be used for hours a day, based on tolerance and results.

Portable battery-operated PEMF applicators at the highest intensities may be tolerated for hours at a time to control anxiety symptoms throughout the day.

See **Sleep** for further directions for use at night. The portable PEMF systems can be combined with higher-intensity systems, you just wouldn't use them both together at the same time. For higher-intensity systems, do 30 – 60 minutes twice a day. If there is significant improvement in symptoms, maintenance may be able to be reduced to 30 minutes twice a day, as long as this level of stimulation maintains the benefit. Treatment is expected to be lifelong.

Supplements: Minimize caffeine and eliminate aspartame. Niacinamide 2500 mg/D in divided doses, magnesium citrate 500 mg 1- 2X/D, B12 sublingual 1000 – 5000 µg/D, methyl folate 1-7 mg/D, P5P 100 mg/D, B complex, omega-3 fish oil 3 g/D, L-tryptophan one – 3000 mg/D taken two – three divided doses (avoid if taking SSRIs), DHEA 50 mg/D. Theanine, CBD, chamomile, and other relaxing herbs may also be tried.

Arthritis (Osteoarthritis)

It typically takes years for osteoarthritis (OA) to develop. Symptoms of an evolving arthritic process can start as long as two to five years after an injury to the joint, while, without any obvious injuries, it can take as much as 20 years between the beginning of the first flare and the total destruction of the cartilage. There are many factors that go into determining this timeline. Changes in the fundamental structures of the joint tissues (the "extracellular matrix") and the presence of inflammation play a key role in OA, causing an imbalance between tissue growth and tissue breakdown, favoring breakdown. Connective tissue cells also play a role in OA because they secrete a wide range of inflammatory molecules.

Research is done on OA in guinea pigs, which develop arthritis very quickly, often with fairly severe arthritis at about two years of age, and have evidence of arthritis beginning between three to six months of age. OA development in Guinea pigs is very similar to humans. This research shows that the fundamental underlying process of progression of arthritis can be slowed or stopped, even in the presence of fairly severe arthritis (OA) with PEMF treatment. Results include cartilage becoming significantly thicker, much less cartilage damage and degeneration, and exaggerated bone thickness under the joint capsule is less. PEMF treatments counteracted OA progression, maintained cartilage structure, and increased proteoglycan content, cell appearance and general cell integrity. Even in animals at later stages of OA, PEMFs were still effective at counteracting progression especially cartilage breakdown. Humans have a much slower metabolism and similar results are possible but would require much longer PEMF exposure, at much earlier stages. At the very least this research shows that healing arthritis with PEMFs is biologically feasible.

The above research shows that the best treatment approach is to prevent progression of the OA process at the earliest stages. The later the stage and the more severe the problem, the more challenging it is to treat OA no matter what you do, short of joint replacement. PEMF stimulation is most effective for treating pain and improving function in OA, with the benefits being most obvious at about eight weeks following treatment, and with virtually no toxicity or side effects. Continuing PEMF treatment will provide benefits over the lifespan of the person. It is not likely that OA will be reversed, except maybe in its mildest forms, however. PEMFs also have the potential to stimulate regeneration of cartilage in those individuals with a sufficient amount of cartilage left in the joint from which new cartilage cells can grow.

PEMF stimulation increases cell growth and extracellular matrix (ECM) production. ECM molecules include collagen II, glycosaminoglycans (GAGs), and proteoglycans (PGs), IL-1b and IGF-1. PEMFs inhibit inflammation-producing prostaglandin E2 (PG-E2), helping to reduce inflammation, and increase joint capsule cells. Breakdown of the joint capsule by the presence of inflammation and a reduction in support molecules is critically important in the development of OA. In addition, local joint tissue stem cells and collagen synthesis increase with PEMFs. Increased proteoglycans provide more lubrication to joints. Stem cells help to repair and regenerate tissues. PEMFs can be used in conjunction with platelet rich plasma (PRP) and stem cell therapies to greatly improve the value of these therapies.

The main goal in PEMF therapies is to decrease inflammation. The secondary aspects of PEMF stimulation will happen in any event once the destructive actions of inflammation are controlled. PEMFs also have a secondary simultaneous value in reducing pain. The PEMF signal chosen will depend mostly on the depth of penetration and the area of treatment needed. An additional consideration is the ease of application. The goal is to deliver the optimal magnetic field intensity of 15 gauss throughout the joint for as long a period of treatment as needed. This will be highly individual, depending on the amount of pain and dysfunction.

Somebody who has "bone-on-bone" arthritis will need much more intense treatment, with the primary goal being to improve pain and dysfunction.

It is commonly thought among doctors that the only clear reasons to do joint replacement are if the pain is intolerable and there are severe limitations in function. The decisions hinge around quality-of-life considerations. PEMF therapy is unlikely to reverse a "bone-on-bone" situation.

Hyaluronic acid injections into a joint may have some value, but may become unnecessary with intensive PEMF therapy. The benefits from these injections often do not last very long. The basic function is to provide more cushioning to the joint, until the injection becomes absorbed.

A lack of cartilage is often regarded as the main problem with OA. However, the ligaments tendons and muscles that support the joint are also important. Muscle strengthening exercises and physical therapy may still be very useful to slow progression. Low-level laser is often used with additional benefit. But PEMFs have the greater advantage of working much deeper in joints, especially the larger joints.

Treatment times per day spent doing PEMF stimulation will depend on the severity of the OA and the intensity of the PEMF signal. For mild cases of OA, the least treatment time may be suitable. Next would be moderate, and the most time needed would be for those with severe OA. Ultimately, it comes down to how much treatment time one cares to spend to achieve acceptable results. Some degree of reduction in pain and improvement in function may be acceptable to some individuals, for example even 10 to 20 percent. For others, the goal is complete pain reduction and elimination of dysfunction. Individuals' use of the PEMF system and their own emotional and physical circumstances will determine to how much stimulation time they will be willing to commit. Since the PEMF signals normally do not create significant risk, it's hard to overdo PEMF treatment, except potentially in the use of very-high-intensity magnetic fields.

Joints may be classified by depth and volume. The most superficial joints (type 1) are the hands, feet, wrists, elbows, sacroiliacs and TMJs. Next (type 2) would be shoulders, neck, knees, and ankles. The joints that are the deepest and with the greatest volume (type 3) include the hips and thoracic and lumbar spine. Though the spine may involve only one level, it is much more common for there to be multiple levels. Even if there is only one level there is a reasonable probability that it would spread to other levels over time, given the mechanics of the spine and the underlying health condition of the body. In addition, most often, people will have joints in multiple areas of the body that are simultaneously involved and, in addition, possibly multiple health conditions. In this situation, for treatment efficiency, both in treating multiple areas and considering total treatment time, a whole-body PEMF system is likely best.

Intensity of the PEMF: See the table below for the recommended intensities for the different joint types.

Intensity Needed to Treat Different Joint Types

Joint type*	Intensity		
	Low	**Medium**	**High**
1	X	X	
2		X	X
3		X	X
Multiple areas			X

*Type 1. hands, feet, wrists, elbows, sacroiliacs and TMJs
*Type 2. shoulders, neck, knees, and ankles
*Type 3. hips and thoracic and lumbar spine

Applicators: Most times the right intensity (from the Table above) using a local PEMF device will work the best. A high-intensity, whole-body PEMF system should be considered for multiple areas farther apart, such as the knees, back, and the neck in the same person. If there are multiple levels involved in the spine, a PEMF system with a large enough applicator would be better. If multiple members of a family need PEMF therapy, then a higher-intensity, whole-body PEMF system would be most efficient for everyone. A high-intensity PEMF system can also be used even for type 1 joints, even though that intensity may not be necessary.

Treatment Time: This will be highly individually variable. In more severe situations, longer treatment time will be the rule, especially when first starting treatment, using the "low and slow" principle. Typical treatment times would be between 30 to 60 minutes, once or twice a day. Whether to use twice a day is based on individual needs and results after a few treatments. If adequate results are not seen with 30 minutes twice a day, then longer treatment times may be necessary. Most often, treatments done for one to two months with treatment times longer than 30 minutes twice a day could be scaled back to just 30 minutes twice a day. At some point, it may even be possible to cut back to about 15 minutes twice a day, depending on the intensity of the PEMF system and the treatment results.

Often when treatment is cut back, symptoms may reappear, telling you that more treatment time is needed. This process of stopping, scaling up and scaling back is likely to be repeated many times before some stability is reached. Recall that it's unlikely that the arthritis process will be reversed except maybe in the mildest forms. However, enough symptom improvement may be achieved that it could be weeks or months before symptoms return. When symptoms return, you're being told by the body that you're not done yet. Patience is very important for managing arthritis. Usually, it takes years to decades for arthritis to develop, so it can't be expected that it could normally be reversed rapidly, even with the most diligent PEMF treatment.

Supplements: Anti-inflammatory supplements could significantly complement the value of the PEMF therapy. Niacinamide 500 mg 3-6X/D, glucosamine sulfate 1500 mg/D, chondroitin sulfate 800 – 1200 mg/D, SAMe 400 – 1200 mg/D, CBD 25-100 mg 1-3X/D, palmitoylethanolamide (PEA) 600-1200 mg 2-3X/D, curcumin 1000-3000 mg 2X/D, MSM 3000-9000 mg/D, omega-3 fish oil 3000 mg/D, hyaluronic acid oral 200-1000 mg/D, bromelain 200-400 mg three times a day. Serrapeptase, nattokinase and/or lumbrokinase, inflamase, or collagen can be added, as well.

Autoimmune Disease

Autoimmune disease occurs because the body's immune system attacks the body's own healthy tissue. This happens because the tissues are not recognized by the body as "self." Whatever is not seen by the immune system as "self" is considered a threat and needs to be removed. Parts of the body subjected to high stress are more prone to immune reactions because of the damage to the tissue. One of the most common causes of immune reactions are infections of any kind. People may have genetic predispositions to overreaction of the immune system. Generally speaking, most therapies are aimed at reducing the amount of inflammatory response caused by an autoimmune reaction.

The most common autoimmune diseases are rheumatoid arthritis, thyroiditis, celiac disease, diabetes type I, vitiligo, rheumatic fever, pernicious anemia, lupus, alopecia, blood disorders, and many more. It's rare that an autoimmune condition can be reversed. Most therapies are aimed at controlling the degree of autoimmune activity. The combination of at least three autoimmune diseases in the same person has been defined as multiple autoimmune syndrome (MAS). About 25 percent of people with autoimmune disease will develop additional autoimmune diseases. MAS is being identified more frequently, and somewhat simplistically, given the level of knowledge at the moment, has been classified as three types, based on the associated conditions. These patterns are not exclusive. Of note, all autoimmune diseases taken together are the third major cause of death behind cancer and cardiovascular disease in the United States.

PEMF therapy is aimed primarily at reducing the inflammation caused by the autoimmune condition and controlling the inflammatory damage. Autoimmune disease is often associated with significant increases in stress, and PEMF therapy can help significantly with reducing the stress response. Even though autoimmune diseases are given disease labels because of the part of the body they attack, they are actually a whole-body problem. Treating the organ attacked can help that particular organ but it does little to protect other parts of the body from similar attack.

PEMFs have many actions (see Chapter 3) which help autoimmune conditions to varying degrees. The most important is the reduction of inflammation in both the identified organ and in the body as a whole. Inflammation in the areas of the body that have not been identified as having the autoimmune condition, such as the kidneys, lungs, heart, etc., often still have significant, perhaps not obvious, inflammation. These other areas with inflammation could become targets for the immune system, hence the MAS, mentioned earlier.

My book *Power Tools for Health* discusses a number of autoimmune conditions in some detail, including arthritis, chronic fatigue syndrome, fibromyalgia, intestinal dysfunction, Lyme disease, multiple sclerosis, osteoporosis, pancreatic disease, scleroderma, and skin conditions. The optimal approach to dealing with these and many other autoimmune diseases is to do both local and whole-body PEMF treatment. There is also no evidence or experience showing that PEMFs interfere with conventional medical approaches to autoimmune diseases, or that PEMF therapy will increase the risk for an autoimmune disease.

The goal with PEMF therapy is not only to treat the identified autoimmune-affected organ, but also to treat the whole-body to reduce stress and inflammation and to prevent any additional autoimmune damage and progression of autoimmune problems. People with autoimmune conditions often have significant sensitivity to many things, including nutrition, supplements, medications, environmental stimulants, etc., and have often failed or had to stop many therapies. Therefore, the best approach to dealing with autoimmune conditions is to go "low and slow" more than usual.

If there is little history of sensitivities, then a whole-body PEMF system with significant control over intensities, treatment time, and frequencies (ITFs) is recommended. Systems that have many built-in programs do not adequately allow for control of ITFs. There are medium-intensity whole-body PEMF systems that have the option for a relatively small additional cost to allow this level of control, usually by adding a computer interface. This allows the go "low and slow" approach. The goal would be to start off with the lowest intensity and the shortest treatment times. Programs should be chosen that are the least likely to produce irritability, such as using Theta (7-10) or Alpha (8-13) frequency programs. After beginning use, the person's experience will guide whether other frequencies can be used that would not be irritating or cause aggravations. Appendix B has some tables for what this "low and slow" approach could look like, based on treatment time and intensity. Always start with the lowest intensity and the shortest treatment time. Ultimately, it has to be individualized, so these tables are just guidelines.

For those with a strong history of sensitivities and milder single organ involvement, a pulse-type, as opposed to a frequency-type, PEMF may be more tolerable. A system with many frequencies may be overstimulating to the body and it would be difficult to figure out which frequencies are overstimulating. Sometimes it's an individual frequency, sometimes it's a combination. A pulsed system is more like a metronome with a very simple pulse pattern, and is often more tolerable, even to treat a wider area and with higher intensities. Whichever system is used, a "low and slow" approach should always be employed.

The fewer treatment variables, the easier it is to control them to avoid sensitivity and still get results. The path to avoid PEMF treatment challenges and find benefits can be extremely slow and frustrating. Many people with these conditions will need naturopathic or functional/integrative/ alternative/holistic health treatments for a while to "cool things off" before starting PEMF therapy. Sometimes PEMF therapy can be combined at the same time with these other approaches. Adequate hydration and nutritional status will make PEMF therapy more effective.

Intensity of the PEMF: 100-7000 gauss. It's best to have a system with a range of magnetic field intensities with the opportunity to eventually be able to tolerate high intensity, to effectively reach deeper into the organs and soft tissues of the body, including the vascular system.

Applicators: The size of the organ(s) involved will dictate the size of the PEMF applicators. Thyroid would take a smaller applicator. Multiple joints in the body being involved would require a medium-sized applicator, such as a 6 to12 inch ring. This would require multiple coil placements to treat individual joint areas. A liver, lung or belly would require a larger applicator system. A PEMF system should be used that has multiple intensity settings, from low to medium to high. The ideal system would be whole-body and preferably a whole-body "magnetic sandwich" system since autoimmune disease is a systemic problem, even though it may manifest mostly in one organ.

Treatment Time: Treatment with PEMFs for autoimmune disease will be a lifetime process. PEMFs, like medications, usually tune down the level of inflammation and the aggressiveness of the immune response and help to control and repair tissue/organ damage. PEMFs help to moderate the effects of life events that contribute to the ups and downs of immune processes. Experience shows that PEMFs can help to decrease the severity and duration of episodes of autoimmune exacerbations and reduce organ dysfunction and damage.

Supplements: Anti-inflammatory supplements could significantly complement the value of the PEMF therapy. CBD 25-100 mg 1-3X/D, palmitoylethanolamide (PEA) 600-1200 mg 2-3X/D, curcumin 1000-3000 mg 2X/D, MSM 3000-9000 mg/D, omega-3 fish oil 3000 mg/D, hyaluronic acid oral 200-1000 mg/D, bromelain 200-400 mg three times a day. Serrapeptase, nattokinase and/or lumbrokinase, inflamase, or collagen can be added, as well. Also see the individual organ topics in this chapter.

Back Pain (see Chapter 9)

Bladder Conditions

The most common bladder conditions that can benefit from PEMF therapy include urinary incontinence, overactive bladder, enuresis, interstitial cystitis, prostate hyperplasia/benign prostatic hypertrophy (BPH), bladder cancer, and recurrent bladder and urethral infections. Stress or overflow incontinence involves the stretching and weakening of pelvic muscles that support the bladder. PEMFs have been developed and FDA-approved to stimulate and strengthen pelvic muscles. These are done in professional settings and, like other muscle strengthening activity, need to be repeated regularly to maintain the muscle toning improvements. Interstitial cystitis and prostate hyperplasia/BPH will be addressed in separate topics below.

Urinary urge incontinence, overactive bladder and enuresis overlap in their physical processes. BPH shares mechanisms with overactive bladder as well. The common themes with these conditions include the involvement of the bladder, the spinal cord, and the brain. The bladder has increased irritability and sensitivity to stretching of the bladder wall and muscle. As a result, even small increases in bladder volume send signals to the spinal cord, and then to the brain, to activate the urge to urinate. After some time, the bladder wall muscle, which is not stressed enough, begins to shrink, becoming even more sensitive to stretching. This sets up a vicious cycle.

Medical treatments for these conditions are only somewhat effective and do not prevent progression of the problem. PEMF treatment addresses several elements of the problem, which is why it may be even more effective than conventional treatments, which really only address the functional element of the urinary tract. The combination of PEMF therapy with conventional therapies may even be more effective. Once PEMF therapy has been started, at some point medications may be reduced or stopped.

The goal of PEMF therapy is to address the three components: the bladder, spinal cord, and the brain. PEMF therapy decreases the sensitivity of the bladder muscle, reduces inflammation in the bladder tissue, and helps the spinal cord and brain to be less sensitive to the exaggerated signals throughout this urination system. In some cases, it is necessary to treat the whole pelvic area and possibly the abdomen due to "crosstalk" between the intestinal tract activity and the urinary tract. The common mediator in this vicious cycle is the spinal cord and brain. Stress can play a significant role in exaggerating the whole problem. My recommendation is to start PEMF stimulation with the bladder and see if that solves the problem. If not, then the next step would be to treat the sacrum, where the nerves from the spinal cord enter the pelvic area to control bladder function. The final step would be to add treatment to the brain, both to decrease brains stress reaction and also to desensitize the brain to the signals coming from the spinal cord and bladder.

However, there is no reason that someone would decide to simply treat all three components from the get-go anyway. In other words, the process could work in reverse, that is, with this more aggressive approach results may happen faster and be more sustainable thereafter, decreasing treatment to the brain, followed by decreasing treatment to the spinal cord and finally treatment to the bladder alone. How long the bladder alone would be treated will be highly individual. The body will tell you what you should be doing. This is because each body is unique and will react uniquely to PEMF treatments. So, each person will have to in a sense create their own unique treatment protocol.

The PEMF device needed will have to deliver sufficient intensity of the PEMF through the whole volume of the bladder, including when the bladder is distended. Treating the distended bladder is important to decrease the sensitivity of the bladder muscles to stretching when being filled. This does not mean that the treatment should only be done when the bladder is distended, but it does mean that the bladder should be treated as well when it is distended (full) and when not distended.

Overactive bladder issues tend to be more common in women entering perimenopause and often continue into menopause. Part of this is related to the reduction of hormones in this part of a woman's life. Men experience andropause, which is a reduction in hormones in their bodies as they age. Frequent urination issues go along with prostate enlargement. Bladder focused treatments can still be helpful for enlarged prostate but a prostate PEMF protocol may need to be added. See the prostate hyperplasia topic.

Intensity of the PEMF: Full distention of the bladder measures about 15 cm (~6 inches) from front to back. Then, one has to add the distance from the skin over the lower abdomen to the front part of the bladder wall. Based on the goal of delivering about 15 gauss throughout the bladder to reduce inflammation, at least a 4000 gauss magnetic field would be required. This level of intensity would be sufficient as well for treating the sacral nerves and the brain.

Applicators: Local/regional PEMF applicators will work best. Even better would be a "magnetic sandwich" approach, that is, applying an applicator to the front of the abdomen above the pubic bone and one over the sacrum. This would accomplish the goal of getting both the bladder and the sacral nerves stimulated. The other alternative setup would be to treat over the bladder and the brain at the same time. This type of double stimulation would make treatment times more efficient.

Treatment Time: Each area should be stimulated for about 30 minutes twice a day. Once significant improvement in symptoms is seen, maintenance could be accomplished by 15 minutes twice a day. The body will tell you how much treatment time is needed and how often, once an initial course of treatment at the 30-minute level is done for at least a month. It may take weeks to months of twice-a-day treatments to determine whether this level of treatment time needs to be continued. If symptoms return any time treatments are cut back, this tells you that more treatment time is needed. Your body will tell you what your maintenance program needs to be to maintain the benefit. There is a chance that treatments will need to be continued indefinitely.

Supplements: A partial list to improve bladder function includes: Bladderwrack, Gosha-jinki-gan, Horsetail, and/or Saw palmetto. There are others possible nutrients for bladder function. As a result, I recommend consulting with a professional skilled in nutrition and supplements to give guidance on nutrition and the supplements that could be used. The PEMFs are expected to work synergistically with any supplements.

Bone Healing and Repair

PEMF therapy is useful in the treatment of acute injuries like breaks or fractures (whether fresh, delayed, stress, or nonunion fractures), incorporation of bone grafts, bone infections (osteomyelitis), radiation damage to the bone (radionecrosis), death of bone (osteonecrosis), avascular necrosis, bone surgery (osteotomy), and for the prevention and treatment of more chronic bone conditions, including osteoporosis and osteopenia. Osteopenia and osteoporosis are often associated with chronic inflammation, whether steroids are used or not. Osteolysis often occurs next to a prosthesis that causes either an immunological response or changes in the bone's structural load. Osteolysis may also be caused by pathologies like bone tumors, cysts, or chronic inflammation. Radionecrosis happens due to radiation damage. Osteonecrosis results from the loss of blood supply to the bone; one of the most common sites is in the hip (femoral osteonecrosis), also called avascular necrosis. Without blood, the bone tissue dies and the bone collapses.

As with most other conditions for which PEMFs are used, removing the underlying cause is critical to being able to have successful results with PEMF therapy. But, even when the underlying causes are removed, left on its own, the bone damage will take a long time to heal properly. Even normal fractures take a long time to heal to a point where the fracture site is no longer vulnerable to failure. When failure of the fracture site happens, typically after three-six months, this could be called the delayed union or nonunion. It can take several years to get complete healing of the bone even though the bone may be usable after 12 to 16 weeks. Frequently, these days, fractures receive plates or screws, called internal fixation. Plates and screws, like prostheses, create inflammation in the bone, which has to be dealt with. This is usually why these plates and screws are removed so they do not create long-term problems for the bone, including osteomyelitis.

Research using an 18 gauss magnetic field found that the daily hours per day of magnetic field use had significant effects on the length of time to healing of nonunion fractures. At less than <= 3 hours fractures healed at 188 days, three to six hours healed 29 days earlier, six to nine hours healed 41 days earlier and at >9 hours per day they healed 76 days earlier, taking about 112 days. The more hours per day the bones were treated, the faster heating occurred. Still, healing took between two to three months' time. Increasing the average daily dose of PEMF treatment from one hour to 10 hours reduced the time required to heal by 45 to 50 percent in those with scaphoid, tibia, and tibia/fibula nonunions for nine months or more. For those with nine-month nonunion tibia and tibia/fibula fractures the reduction in healing time was 60 percent.

Magnetic field intensity may not always correlate with healing time; the study above show that the hours of treatment time clearly made a big difference in healing times. Higher-intensity PEMFs may accelerate the time to healing and the total treatment time may be able to be reduced significantly.

Many of the causes of bone problems are not as simple as a basic fracture. They may be more similar in some ways to nonunion fractures, having been there relatively chronically. This may normally take longer to heal than a simple fracture.

Intensity of the PEMF: There is no specific magnetic field intensity needed for bone repair and regeneration. Inflammation is a common factor for most of the causes of PEMFs, including osteoporosis. The effects of PEMFs on inflammation will be used as the guide to determine the magnetic field intensity needed for a given bone site. See Appendix A for details. PEMF therapy is usually provided locally using medium- to high-intensity PEMFs. Intensity recommended should be >200 gauss, even up to or beyond 4000 gauss. It is not recommended to use intensities high enough to cause muscle contractions in the area of the fracture or bone lesion. Muscle contractions around the bone lesion or fracture site will disturb the healing of the bone.

Applicators: Local, medium- to high-intensity applicators. A single loop applicator with an internal circumference large enough to allow the applicator to be placed around the bone site may work best. Another good option to increase the magnetic field around the bone lesion would be to use a butterfly coil, being similar to a "magnetic sandwich." For individual vertebral lesions, a paddle or butterfly coil may work best. For vertebral issues involving multiple levels, an elliptical loop coil or half-body pad may cover the whole area.

Treatment Time: Based on the above study, the treatment time recommended is no less than three hours per day, especially at the beginning of a course of treatment. It's possible that with a higher-intensity PEMF system such as 1000-4000 gauss, the treatment time may be able to be reduced to 90 minutes per day using 30-minute sessions three times per day. It will have to be an individual decision on what time can be committed to treatment. It's highly probable, especially with higher-intensity PEMFs, that treatment time could be 5-6 hours per day, to achieve more rapid healing. Treatment would be continued until full bone healing has been achieved, based on imaging results.

Supplements: Bone can't be built without adequate nutrients to support bone development. At a minimum these would include vitamin D3 5000 IU per day, a general bone building formula, DHEA 25 mg per day, Ultra K2 15 mg/D, 1 Osteo-sil/D, Fructoborate 6 mg/D and curcumin 3000 mg/day.

Breast Implants

Breast implants and breast reconstruction with implants are very common. Unfortunately, problems with implants are very common as well; 27 percent of women report implant rupture and an additional 10 percent report implant (capsular) contracture. Contracture is associated with stiffening of scar tissue around the implant that then can lead to pain and very hard areas of the breasts. The most common issues are breast pain, sensitivity, asymmetry, infection, and swelling. Scar tissue formation around the implant is expected and serves to keep the implant in place. Unfortunately, scar tissue production can be unpredictable and exaggerated and may also result in immune responses, especially with silicone implants. Implant contracture can range from mild to severe. About 75 percent of contractions happen within two years, but can also happen years later. Implant rupture is the most common cause of late-onset contraction. Infection as a result of biofilm development is a common cause of excessive scar formation.

PEMFs have been found to help with infections and reduce the aggressiveness of scar formation. PEMF therapy can be used through the whole spectrum of implants, from before implants are placed, following implant placement, during the whole time implants are in place, and with the development of symptoms or implant problems. PEMFs do not harm the implants themselves. They are also safe after reconstructive surgery and implant placement. The goal of PEMF therapy is to reduce inflammation, which then serves to help with pain and excessive scar formation.

Intensity of the PEMF: Medium- to high-intensity PEMFs would be needed for local application. Most implants are now placed underneath the chest muscles, placing them deeper into the body, thus the need for higher intensity, typically between 500 to 6,000 gauss. 2000 gauss would be needed at four inches beyond the skin, through the thickest part of the breasts and implant, combined. If the back of the implant is eight inches from the skin, the intensity would need to be about 6000 gauss. It is not recommended to use a PEMF system at intensity levels that cause muscle contractions of the chest wall or pectoral muscles.

Applicators: Local applicators are all that are needed. Using a whole-body pad and lying on the back would not typically produce enough magnetic field intensity to be sufficient on the surface of the chest. A loop coil, butterfly coil opened out, or half body pad placed on the front of the chest would serve best. It is not recommended to use a coil that generates heat.

Treatment Time: Treatment time should be about 15 minutes to 30 minutes twice a day, for one to two months, once symptoms are improved, followed by 15 minutes twice a day for maintenance.

Supplements: The most important supplements are those that help with inflammation, especially, curcumin, Boswellia and hyaluronic acid. It's hard to recommend specific supplements and nutrition because they need to be individualized. I recommend consulting with a professional skilled in nutrition and supplements to give guidance on the supplements that should be used. It is rare that surgeons would provide this guidance.

Bruising

Bruising frequently happens after a blunt injury, contusion, or around wound, surgical or traumatic injuries. It can be made significantly worse when somebody is on anticoagulants. Bruising happens because blood seeps into tissue around the injury accompanied by swelling. Since the blood does not belong in the tissue, it sets up an inflammatory reaction until it is gradually absorbed by the body. My earliest experiences with magnetic fields showed me their amazing value in removing bruising, often as early as 24 hours following the injury. Bruising and swelling improve rapidly following the use of PEMFs, depending on the extent of the bruising and swelling.

Intensity of the PEMF: Most bruising is relatively shallow, occurring in the skin and muscles. A local medium- to high-intensity PEMF would work best, from 200-1000 gauss. It's possible that the higher-intensity systems will produce better and faster results.

Applicators: The size of the applicators would be determined by the size of the bruise. Most often small, local applicators with a diameter between two to 10 inches are enough. Small, portable PEMF devices may be adequate.

Treatment Time: I recommend aggressive treatment time to get the best results. With small, portable PEMF devices treatment time can be continuous for hours, even overnight, if available, until the bruising and swelling have subsided. Devices supplied by conventional electrical outlets should be considered for several hours, until there's clear evidence of the bruising improving. Treatment may be repeated multiple times during the day and/or over several days. Unless the bruising is severe and extensive, results should be seen rapidly within 24 to 48 hours.

Supplements: The most important supplements are those that help with inflammation caused by the injury and the blood leaking into the tissues, especially curcumin, Boswellia, and hyaluronic acid.

Burns

A burn is damage to your body's tissues caused by heat, chemicals, electricity, sunlight, or radiation. Scalds from hot liquids and steam, building fires, and flammable liquids and gases are the most common causes of burns. Another kind is an inhalation injury, caused by breathing smoke. There are three types of burns:

First-degree burns damage only the outer layer of skin.

Second-degree burns damage the outer layer and the layer underneath.

Third-degree burns damage or destroy the deepest layer of skin and the tissues underneath.

Burns can cause swelling, blistering, scarring and, in serious cases, shock, and even death. They also can lead to infections because they damage your skin's protective barrier. Treatment for burns depends on the cause of the burn, how deep it is, and how much of the body it covers. Antibiotic creams can prevent or treat infections. For more serious burns, treatment may be needed to clean the wound, replace the skin, and making sure the patient has enough fluids and nutrition.

A wound is a disturbance of the integrity of the epidermal and/or deeper tissue. The wound induces a net flow of ionic current through the injured cells and fluid exudate, which form a low electrical resistance pathway around the perimeter of the wound. Flow of this ionic current between normal and injured tissue plays an important role in stimulating tissue membrane repair processes essential to restore the tissue to normal function. The biological activity of a cell can be affected by weak, externally applied PEMFs. See **Wound** for more discussion about the use of PEMFs to help repair wounds.

PEMFs can accelerate healing of soft tissue wounds. Healing of wounds in general requires that the supply of nutrients and oxygen be optimized, which allows tissues surrounding the wound to grow. Another goal of skin wound repair is to restore the physical and chemical barrier functions. The most important principle of wound management is to provide a natural physiological environment that will restore the physical and barrier functions of the skin.

The goal of PEMF therapy is to accelerate healing of the burned skin and surrounding tissues. PEMFs do this by increasing circulation, reducing edema, stimulating RNA and DNA for repair, increasing growth factors and stem cells, and decreasing inflammation, among their other actions.

Intensity of the PEMF: 100 – 1000 gauss.

Applicators: Local, regional, or whole-body. Applicators would be applied to local burn areas. Regional applicators would be applied to larger areas of burns. Whole-body applicators may be used in general for general health support and to simultaneously help with healing local or regional burn areas.

Treatment Time: 30 – 60 minutes twice a day. In the early stages of burn treatment 15 – 30 minute treatment times multiple times a day may be needed to gain the most control over swelling, pain, and inflammation. Once the more urgent state is addressed, treatment may be decreased somewhat per day and used until full burn wound healing has been completed.

Supplements: Collagen, vitamin C 2000-5000 mg twice a day, mixed tocopherols, zinc citrate 25 mg twice a day combined with 2-4 mg/D copper; magnesium citrate 500 mg/D, vitamin A 25,000 IU/D, mixed tocopherols 400 IU/D, B12 5000 IU/D sublingual, P5P 100 mg/D, pantothenic acid 20-200 mg/D, citrus flavonoids 500-1000 mg 2-3 times/D, biotin 600 µg/D, hyaluronic acid oral 200-1000 mg/D.

Cancer

Developing PEMF treatment recommendations for cancer is complicated by the fact that there are many types of cancers, potentially in all areas of the body, and the conventional medical system treatments are many and varied, as well. In addition, cancer can be local, regional, and systemic. There is the primary cancer and metastatic cancer, with variable degrees and locations of metastatic activity. There are different degrees of severity, and aggressiveness, complicated by the underlying health status and age of the individual. Some people even have multiple cancers. Cancers have a myriad of presentations with many different body systems involved. Cancers also have highly variable degrees of response to various therapies. Different tissues have different response rates to PEMFs. So, ultimately, PEMF treatment recommendations have to be highly individualized. A major goal of PEMF therapy is to help with the primary cancer as well as working to prevent spread or metastases.

The PEMF treatment recommendations below are highly generalized and only suggestive at best. While most people who look at PEMF therapy as an adjunctive or alternative approach for the specific cancer in the specific location, our goal should be not only focused on the short term but also the long-term needs. The reality is that people often look for PEMF therapy after they have gone through multiple rounds of conventional approaches and have moved into a state of dire need. This limits the potential value of PEMF therapy. There are also people with cancer who look to alternative approaches as a priority and avoid conventional therapies. Neither of these positions can be disputed. It's always a matter of personal choice. No therapeutic approach is guaranteed to be completely successful, as success depends on the definition and goals of the individual. Most, but not all, of the time my experience has been that PEMF therapy provides some amount of value to people who have chosen this therapy as part of their healing journey. Sometimes it provides a great deal of value. Tailoring the right PEMF system to the individual's situation and clearly defining expectations is very important to good results.

Intensity of the PEMF: Most of the time the PEMFs will need to be medium or high intensity, either local, regional, or whole-body. High-intensity, whole-body "magnetic sandwich" will normally achieve the best results most efficiently, both short-term and long-term. Local, superficial, and deeper cancers can be managed well with local medium- to higher-intensity PEMF therapies. These would be most helpful for short-term needs, and may be all that is necessary for some cancers, depending on the nature of the cancer. Primary cancers involving a larger organ, such as a lung, liver, bowel, or bladder, can be considered regional in their activity and will typically need a higher-intensity magnetic field, unless the cancer is very superficial and close to the applied magnetic field.

Applicators: For the PEMF device chosen, the applicators available will determine the type of magnetic field it will produce. For local cancers, the recommended magnetic field applicator intensity should be able to produce no less than 500 gauss, as long as the cancer at its farthest distance from the applicator is less than two inches. Usually, regional cancers involving a larger area are deeper in the body. Even though a cancer may appear to be less than an inch in diameter on imaging studies, that does not mean that its "sphere of activity" is less than an inch. It is almost always better to think deeper and wider than what the imaging shows. For regional cancers, the minimum magnetic field for a wider applicator would likely need to be between 4000-7000 gauss. High-intensity, whole-body, "magnetic sandwich" systems essentially remove all the guesswork and can be used for most aspects of cancer, including metastatic spread and long-term whole-body needs.

Treatment Time: Always use the "low and slow" approach. The minimum treatment time should be no less than 30 minutes twice a day, to the primary cancer site. For multiple areas needing treatment, each significant area may need 30 minutes at a time. Using whole-body "magnetic sandwich" PEMF allows for multiple areas to be treated simultaneously for 30 minutes twice a day. However, even with these whole-body treatments, local or regional areas may need additional stimulation. Combined treatments may need to be done for several hours a day. How many times a day to repeat the treatment will depend on the cancer in the person. The minimum should be twice a day. In some cases, especially with cancer pain, the treatments may need to be many times a day for optimal results.

Supplements: I always emphasize the need for good nutrition and appropriate supplements in the setting of cancer. There is enough scientific evidence to emphasize this need. It's hard to recommend specific supplements and nutrition because they have to be individualized. I recommend consulting with a professional skilled in nutrition and supplements to give guidance on the supplements that should be used. There are many practitioners who specialize in helping with cancer. It is rare that oncologists would provide this guidance.

Cancer Bone/Metastases

There are primary bone cancers and secondary bone cancers. Primary bone cancers include multiple myeloma (the most common), osteosarcoma, chondrosarcoma, and Ewing's sarcoma. Secondary bone cancers are those that are metastasized from primary cancers in other areas of the body. In both situations, the most common symptom is pain as a result of destruction of the bone and the nerves in the affected area. Fractures happen more easily in the affected bones and may involve collapse of the vertebrae.

The goal of PEMF therapy is to not only treat the underlying involved bone area or areas but also to help the rest of the body deal with the cancer. (See **Cancer** above.) The earlier in the process that PEMF is started when cancer invades bone, the better and faster the results. Most of the time medical treatments may involve pain medications, radiation, and medication to stimulate bone growth. PEMF therapy works well alongside other treatments. My experience over the years has shown that PEMFs can make a significant reduction in bone pain. PEMF therapy has been FDA-approved for decades for the treatment of nonhealing fractures, which is what bone metastases really do. Therefore, PEMF therapy may not only help with the underlying cancer bone pain, but also help to stimulate new bone formation and reduce progressive destruction of the bone.

Intensity of the PEMF: Medium- to high-intensity PEMFs are needed for specific local application at the primary cancer or metastatic sites. The lower the intensity of the magnetic field the more treatment time is needed. I usually recommend medium- to high-intensity fields, depending on where the cancer is, with higher-intensity fields being preferred at an intensity of at least 4000 gauss.

Applicators: The goal of therapy is not only to target the area of the bone with the cancer but also to help the whole body. When the whole-body is treated, the body is healthier in general and has more physical healing and immune resources available to target the sites of the cancer itself, and will not need as much for any of its other needs. A high-intensity, whole-body PEMF system is recommended, preferably a whole-body "magnetic sandwich," dual-applicator system. The dual-applicator system provides whole-body treatment for general health as well as an applicator available for the local cancer site. This type of dual system also makes treatment times more efficient, so that less treatment time would be necessary, as when individual applicators are used.

Treatment Time: 60 minutes two to three times a day, especially at the beginning, using a "low and slow" approach. Once the pain is controlled, treatment time may be able to be reduced. I recommend a minimum of 30 minutes twice a day for ongoing treatments. Repeat evaluations, including imaging studies and blood markers, and the status of symptoms and function, following the initiation of PEMF therapy will help to guide how to adjust the protocol. Treatment would be lifelong.

Supplements: New bone can't be built without adequate nutrients to support bone development. At a minimum these would include vitamin D3 5000 IU per day, a general bone building formula, DHEA 25 mg per day, Ultra K2, Osteo-sil, Fructoborate 6 mg. and curcumin 3000 mg/day. Also, the cancer needs to be addressed with targeted supplements. I recommend consulting with a professional specializing or skilled in nutrition and supplements for cancer to give guidance on the supplements that should be used.

Cancer, Brain Radiation Therapy

Brain radiation therapy is most commonly used for metastatic brain cancers and also for acoustic neuromas and trigeminal neuralgia. But the radiation used to destroy cancer cells can also hurt normal cells in the area radiated. Side effects vary from person to person, depending on how much of the brain is being radiated, and are caused by the cumulative effect of radiation on the cells. This means they develop over time and most patients do not experience any side effects until a few weeks into their treatment. Side effects may be unpleasant and perhaps temporary, disappearing bit by bit after therapy is complete. Acute (short term) side effects include some of the most common side effects of radiation therapy for brain tumors:

- Fatigue is very common with radiation treatment and tends to begin a few weeks into therapy. Fatigue typically resolves slowly over the weeks and months following treatment.
- Hair loss may occur where you received radiation. Hair typically starts to regrow a month or so after treatment. However, your hair might not grow back exactly as it was before treatment and for some, the hair loss becomes permanent.
- Muffled hearing during treatment. This typically resolves in 2-4 weeks after finishing treatment.

- Skin irritation in the treatment area. It may include being red, irritated, dry, or sensitive, looking like a sunburn.
- Short-term memory loss and difficulty thinking can occur, especially with whole-brain radiation, but may also happen with local radiation depending on the area of the brain being treated.
- Brain tissue swelling can develop during treatment, resulting in a headache or pressure feeling. If this happens medications may be needed to decrease swelling.
- Side effects of radiosurgery are usually related to sending high doses of radiation to particular areas of the skull. For instance, if you are treated for an acoustic neuroma (a tumor involving the nerve that controls hearing), you might lose some hearing. Treatment for trigeminal neuralgia can lead to tingling or numbness of the face.

The side effects mentioned above tend to occur during treatment, up until a few months after treatment. Long-term effects can happen months to many years after cancer treatment and the risks vary depending on the areas included in the field of radiation and the radiation techniques used.

Long-term side effects after a few months following treatment, even up to years in some cases, include:

- Low risk of a second cancer in or near the radiation field from exposure of healthy tissue to radiation.
- Radiation necrosis of the tissue at the site of the tumor. Surgery may be needed to remove the necrotic tissue.
- Damage to healthy brain tissue can cause headaches, seizures, or even death.
- Harm to the pituitary gland and other areas of the brain which can affect hormone levels in the body, including thyroid and sex hormones, future fertility issues for women, and cause sexuality concerns for men.

It may not be possible to use PEMF therapy during the course of radiation. PEMFs may be used to treat the brain and head prior to radiation if there is adequate time. The intent is to try to get the tissues around the head and the brain as healthy as possible, even to the extent of reducing swelling around the tumor, prior to the radiation. There is a risk that magnetic fields may protect the tissues being radiated from the effects of radiation. The goal of radiation is to eliminate or significantly reduce the tumor. There is no point doing radiation if this cannot be achieved due to protection provided by the PEMF therapy.

It may be best to wait one or two weeks following radiation therapy before PEMF therapy is started. PEMF therapy can be done to the whole head or, in the case of very focused radiation therapy, to the area of the radiation field. On the other hand, because radiation cannot be completely isolated and laser focused, whole head stimulation of with PEMFs may be very reasonable. The goal of PEMF therapy is to reduce the amount of collateral inflammation in the head and brain caused by the radiation. There is no significant research to guide what the likely benefits would be in this specific setting. We are extrapolating from the general knowledge about what PEMFs would do with all tissues, including the brain. Since PEMFs increase ATP in tissues, they may help significantly with brain fog, fatigue, memory, swelling, circulation, hair loss, and hearing issues. If there were seizures before the radiation started, PEMFs may help to decrease inflammation related to the seizures, since radiation may not eliminate seizures entirely. By improving the health of the brain in general, it's possible that recurrences of cancer may also decrease. There is no guarantee with radiation therapy that it would reduce or eliminate the tumor completely, in which case it could potentially regrow. Adding PEMF therapy after radiation may decrease this risk of regrowth.

Intensity of the PEMF: Since whole brain/head PEMF therapy will be needed, and one of the goals of the therapies is to reduce inflammation, the PEMF magnetic field needs to penetrate the entire head with at least 15 gauss per the intensities in Appendix A. The average human head measures 6-7 inches in width and 8-9 inches in length. This means that a PEMF intensity of about 7000 gauss is needed or a minimum of 4000 gauss. If a 4000 gauss magnetic field is used, treatment would need to be done to the front and the back of the head. Treatment should follow the "low and slow" approach. Generally, PEMFs can be used with other medications as needed. If anti-seizure medications are being used, it's important to watch for side effects; the dose of these medications may need to be reduced. This may be true for other medications, as well.

Applicators: The best applicators will likely be a butterfly type coil or a loop coil placed on the top of the head. In the case of the butterfly coil, one loop (wing) of the butterfly coil would be on each side of the head, with the center of the butterfly at the top of the head. The loop coil would also be placed at the top of the head, like a halo. If the loop coil placed on top of the head is too large, one end of it can be squeezed together to make it a better fit. A paddle applicator is not as helpful, although it could be tried at the side of the head. This would require the paddle to be placed on each side of the head for a balanced treatment. It's also possible with a "magnetic sandwich" to use two applicators at the same time on each side of the head. Since many of these brain cancers are spread from other parts of the body, making this a stage IV cancer, high-intensity, whole-body PEMF is recommended separately, followed by a session with a lower whole-body pad combined with a loop applicator applied to the head.

Treatment Time: Using the "low and slow" approach is very important for this type of treatment. Both time and intensity need to be gradually ramped up based on the body's ability to tolerate the treatments. The goal would be to reach a minimum of 30 minutes twice a day, depending on symptoms, ability to tolerate the PEMF treatments, and other practical health and function constraints. PEMF therapy may likely need to be continued indefinitely to get as much recovery from the radiation damage as possible.

Supplements: PLEASE NOTE. Radiation oncologists frequently advise against nutritional supplements while ongoing radiation therapy. Consult with your radiation oncologist about the use of supplements during radiation. Experts believe that there is no harm in doing supplements after radiation is completed. Vitamin C 2000 as 4000 mg/D combined with 300-600 mg of grapeseed extract, mixed tocopherols 500 IU/D, zinc 50 mg 3X/D + copper 1-4 mg/D (not if there is cirrhosis), selenium 200 – 250 µg/D, glutamine 30 g/D, P5 P 100 mg/D, B12 sublingual 1000-5000 micrograms/D, thiamine 400 mg/D, methylfolate three – 5 mg/D, beta-carotene 75 mg/D, evening Primrose oil (GLA) two – 4 g per day, alpha lipoic acid 1200 mg 2X/D, and probiotics.

Cancer, Breast

PEMF therapy for breast cancer can be considered for prevention, during treatments, following treatments and long term.

Relative to prevention, inflammation in the breast over long periods of time is a highly likely stimulant to the development of breast cancer, although not necessarily in all cases. A strong family history of breast cancer, positive BRCA genes, significant chronic fibrocystic disease of the breasts, trauma or other significant insults to the breasts, breast implants, and significant obesity are all risk factors for breast cancer. Even cancer.gov writes, "Chronic inflammation may be caused by infections that don't go away, abnormal immune reactions to normal tissues, or conditions such as obesity. Over time, chronic inflammation can cause DNA damage and lead to cancer." Any woman with any of these contributing factors should consider routine PEMF therapy for prevention, not only to the breast, but also for the whole body.

Typical breast cancer treatments include lumpectomy, mastectomy, chemotherapy, radiation, and longer-term hormone suppression therapy. Lymph node sampling creates its own issues with lymphedema. PEMF therapy has a significant role for anybody recovering from surgery, accelerating healing times and reducing the risk of complications. PEMF therapy has been found to often dramatically increase the effectiveness of the chemotherapy in reducing side effects, especially neuropathy. PEMFs can be used before and after radiation therapy to reduce the collateral damage from the radiation to healthy tissues, including the heart, which is often in the path of the radiation field in the left chest. Routine use of PEMFs following these more aggressive procedures will also help reduce the risk of recurrences. While recurrence is more often in the same breast as the breast cancer, it also tends to recur more often than elsewhere in the opposite breast.

Another important aspect of using PEMFs is a long-term benefit to reduce the risk of metastases. Nearly 35 percent of women diagnosed with early-stage breast cancer will develop metastatic disease within 10 years. One breast cancer researcher from Northwest University in Chicago reports that 40 to 60 percent of women at the time of initial diagnosis will have breast cancer stem cells in the bones. This is one of the reasons that bone metastases are common 10 or more years after initial treatment. Inflammation in the body is likely to be one of the more significant factors contributing to the breast cancer stem cells becoming activated in the bones. This information suggests that women having their initial diagnosis of breast cancer should strongly consider whole-body PEMF therapy for the rest of their life following initial diagnosis and treatment. The purpose of the

PEMF therapy in this setting is to continually work on reducing inflammation in the body, especially in the bones. Daily whole-body PEMF therapy will help to restore health for other health problems as well.

Intensity of the PEMF: Therapy can be local, regional, or whole-body. The intensities in general should be medium to high. Local therapy would be to the breast itself. Regional therapy would be to regional metastases, such as to the liver, the lungs, vertebrae, and other regional bone metastases. The preferred and recommended treatment would be whole-body, for the reasons mentioned in the previous paragraph. Given the investment required for adequate intensity magnetic fields, for local or regional use, it would be most cost-effective to proceed from the start to have a higher-intensity, whole-body PEMF, particularly the "magnetic sandwich" approach. Since many women with breast cancer develop breast cancer post-menopause, they may also have osteopenia or osteoporosis, and therefore require higher-intensity whole-body PEMFs anyway. Having the right PEMF system from the start will provide many multiple benefits beyond the breast cancer. The minimum intensity magnetic field for local treatment is 1000 gauss. For regional or whole-body purposes, a minimum of 4000 gauss would be better, given the depth into the body that the magnetic fields have to reach. A 6000+ gauss allowing the "magnetic sandwich" approach would be the optimal intensity needed.

Applicators: To treat the breast or breasts only, a local, small, magnetic pad PEMF system is needed. For regional therapy, a half-body pad of sufficient intensity, for example, 4000 gauss could work. A PEMF whole-body system is the most recommended, allowing the "magnetic sandwich" treatment approach for optimal lifetime results.

Treatment Time: PEMF treatment around the time of procedures (chemotherapy and/or radiation) may need to be more intense. Typically, up to 60 minutes twice a day may be needed for the first few weeks or months after the end of conventional breast cancer treatments. After healing and recovery, PEMF therapy is geared to lifetime health maintenance and the typical recommendation is whole-body PEMF stimulation twice a day in the morning and evening for 30 minutes. More time may be added if other needs arise.

Supplements: I always emphasize the need for good nutrition and appropriate supplements in the setting of cancer. There is enough scientific evidence to emphasize this need. It's hard to recommend specific supplements and nutrition because they have to be individualized. I recommend consulting with a professional skilled in cancer nutrition and supplements to give guidance on the supplements that should be used, and there are many practitioners who specialize in helping with cancer. It is rare that oncologists would provide this guidance.

Cancer, Chemotherapy Complications

Chemo drugs kill fast-growing cells, such as cancer cells. But because these drugs affect the entire body, they affect normal, healthy cells that are fast-growing, too. Damage to cells causes side effects. The severity of side effects varies significantly from person to person and from chemo agent to chemo agent. Side effects are a very common aspect of cancer therapy.

Normal cells most likely to be damaged by chemo are:

- Blood-forming cells in the bone marrow
- Hair follicles
- Cells in the mouth, digestive tract, and reproductive system
- Some chemo drugs can damage cells in the heart, kidneys, bladder, lungs, and nervous system.

Doctors try to give chemo at levels high enough to treat cancer, while keeping side effects at a minimum.

Common chemotherapy side effects include:

- Fatigue
- Hair loss
- Easy bruising and bleeding
- Infection
- Anemia (low red blood cell counts)
- Nausea and vomiting
- Appetite changes
- Constipation
- Diarrhea

- Mouth, tongue, and throat problems such as sores and pain with swallowing
- Peripheral neuropathy or other nerve problems, such as numbness, tingling, and pain
- Skin and nail changes such as dry skin and color change
- Urine and bladder changes and kidney problems
- Weight changes
- Chemo brain, which can affect concentration and focus
- Mood changes
- Changes in libido and sexual function
- Fertility problems.

Some side effects of chemotherapy may not happen for several weeks to months after the chemo is completed. Use of PEMFs during chemotherapy may not only help chemo work better but may also help to reduce the side effects. Waiting to start PEMF therapy after symptoms have begun may not work as well as using it throughout the course of chemotherapy, or starting PEMF therapy afterwards.

While PEMF therapy may be targeted to specific problem areas with side effects, whole-body PEMF therapy will produce the best and most efficient results. Additional focused PEMF therapy could be applied locally for problems such as urine, bladder, and kidney issues, nausea, fatigue, and peripheral neuropathy. See **Cancer** above for general help applying PEMFs in the setting of cancer.

Intensity of the PEMF: Most efficient treatment would be using high-intensity, whole-body PEMFs with significant control of intensity. Whole-body treatment will help in the control of the cancer and healing of tissues damaged by the treatments. Treatment of local problems would require magnetic field intensities based on the depth of penetration needed to reduce inflammation. See Appendix A.

Applicators: Whole-body, magnetic field "sandwich" is the most efficient way to deal with problems in multiple areas the body. Additional local or regional treatment can be applied for problems not responding to whole-body treatment. Frequency-based, medium- to high-intensity local PEMFs may be needed for brain entrainment purposes to reduce fatigue, brain fog, and neuropathy. Nausea may require both brain and abdominal treatments. PEMF therapy should be able to be used together with other therapies to reduce symptoms. Most other therapies that control symptoms do not help with healing, which is why combinations of PEMF therapy and medications can be expected to be more effective.

Treatment time: Because of the toxicities associated with chemotherapy, the "low and slow" approach is critical. Individuals in this situation often lack motivation to do treatment and may require their support system to help out with encouragement and applicator placements. The goal would be to reach the maximum intensity and up to an hour of total treatment at a time, two to three times per day. The success in managing symptoms, especially for how often they recur, will determine how long and how often treatments need to be done. Any treatments used for chemo side effects should help with the underlying cancer process, as well.

Supplements: I always emphasize the need for good nutrition and appropriate supplements in the setting of cancer and chemotherapy. There is enough scientific evidence to emphasize this need. It's hard to recommend specific supplements and nutrition because they have to be individualized. There are specialized sets of supplements for many of the individual side effects encountered. I recommend consulting with a professional skilled in cancer nutrition and supplements to give guidance on the supplements that should be used, and there are many practitioners who specialize in helping with cancer. It is rare that oncologists would provide this guidance.

Cancer, Head, Neck, and Oropharyngeal

See **Cancer** above. PEMFs may be helpful to the primary cancer itself, but may be especially helpful following chemo, before and after surgery and/or radiation. The incidence of distant metastases in head and neck squamous cell carcinoma (SCC) is relatively small in comparison to other cancers. Metastases occur most often in the lungs.

Intensity of the PEMF: High-intensity PEMFs are necessary for the head and neck area to be able to reach all the tissues equally throughout the whole neck area, especially to be able to benefit lymph nodes.

Applicators: Local applicators would do best, particularly the butterfly coil or loop coil folded into an ellipse or oval around the neck. Metastases can be treated with higher-intensity regional applicators or whole-body PEMF therapy.

Treatment Time: Between 30 – 60 minutes twice a day in the first stages of treatment. As significant improvement is seen, treatments may be cut back to 30 minutes twice a day indefinitely for health maintenance.

Supplements. See supplement recommendations in **Cancer** above.

Cancer, Liver

See **Cancer** above. Liver cancer can occur as a primary condition or a secondary condition from liver metastases. Regardless of whether it is primary or secondary, liver cancer should be treated generally as well as specifically. PEMFs are not expected to cure or kill the cancer. Occasionally, liver cancer may be seen to shrink.

Primary liver cancer can metastasize most commonly to the lungs and bones. As with all other cancers, high-intensity whole-body PEMF therapy is recommended, preferably at the earliest stages before obvious metastases have developed. Combination therapies will usually provide the best results. PEMFs can be used in combination with chemotherapy, surgery, or embolization procedures and before and after radiation.

Intensity of the PEMF: Follow the intensity recommendations in Appendix A. Since the liver is a large organ, a magnetic field intensity of a minimum of 4000 gauss is recommended.

Applicators: A regional applicator may be used but a whole-body, high-intensity PEMF system is recommended. A regional applicator would include a half-body pad or an elliptical coil applied over the liver on the front of the lower chest and upper abdomen. Whole-body PEMF therapy should be done using a "magnetic sandwich" approach or, if using a single pad, with the bottom of the two pads and loop coil, apply the pad below the body as well as the loop coil on the front of the body.

Treatment Time: A "low and slow" approach should be used. The goal is to reach maximum intensity for an hour twice a day. Once significant results are achieved, treatment may be able to be reduced to 30 minutes twice a day while monitoring test results. It is likely that treatment will be required for months followed by a maintenance protocol.

Supplements. Liver and antiviral supplements should be combined. At a minimum, liver supplements can include milk thistle, alpha lipoic acid, and acetyl cystine, acetyl l-carnitine, zinc, selenium, tocotrienols, licorice root and vitamin C. There are many more possible anti-cancer supplements. As a result, I recommend consulting with a professional skilled in nutrition and supplements to give guidance on nutrition and the supplements that could be used. A nutritionist specializing or skilled in working with cancer would be best. The PEMFs are expected to work synergistically with any supplements, as well as decreasing inflammation in the liver and improving liver function.

Cancer, Lung

See **Cancer** above. There are many forms of both primary and secondary lung cancer, with primary starting in the lung itself and secondary from metastases from other cancers elsewhere in the body. The two major forms of primary lung cancer are non-small cell and small cell. The overall five-year survival rate for all stages is 14-17 percent for non-small-cell lung cancer and 6 percent for small-cell lung cancer.

Inflammation is a very important contributor to the development of lung cancer. The inflammatory components include a buildup of inflammatory white blood cells, promoting tumor progression by releasing a variety of cytokines, chemokines, and cell-toxic mediators. Inflammation also affects many aspects of the cancer process, including the proliferation and survival of cancer cells, angiogenesis, tumor metastasis, and tumor response to chemotherapy and hormones.

One of the most important causes of inflammation in the lung is smoking. Other contributing factors include air pollution, autoimmune disease, radon, and recurrent infections. Cancers like low-oxygen environments, so they are more commonly seen in people with chronic obstructive pulmonary disease (COPD), who have lower than normal oxygen levels in their lungs.

Research has been limited on the use of PEMFs for lung cancer but one study showed significant impact on cancer cells. Lung cancer tumor tissue obtained during surgery from twenty patients was evaluated for biochemical and physical changes using deep electron microscopy. All had PEMFs preoperatively to reduce tumor resistance to standard therapy. PEMFs caused cellular changes to the cancer cells, showing a marked anti-tumor effect. Changes were best after 20 to 30 treatment sessions. Highly differentiated (mature) adenocarcinomas were the most sensitive to the PEMFs.

The goal of PEMF therapy is to help to heal inflammation in the lung, which not only contributes to the development of the cancer, but also causes it to continue to grow and spread. In addition, PEMF therapy increases blood supply and oxygen exchange in the lungs, making the environment less hospitable to the cancer.

With metastatic cancer, the other parts of the body from which the metastases spread need PEMF therapy as well. Whole-body, high-intensity PEMF therapy is the best and the most efficient use of treatment time. Individuals with cancer would be best served by considering long-term needs, for whatever health issues may unexpectedly arise. So, the investment in a more efficient PEMF treatment system should be evaluated and considered. The cost, not just in dollars but also in health, of not considering future needs can be considerable and regrettable. PEMFs can be used along with surgery, chemotherapy, and before and after any radiation therapy, as well as other medications.

Intensity of the PEMF: Because of the size of the lungs, high-intensity PEMFs are needed. The average diameter of the chest from the front to the back is about 6-9 inches, depending on which part of the chest is measured. That means that a magnetic field intensity of between 4000-7000 gauss is necessary to provide at least 15 gauss of magnetic field intensity from the front to the back of the chest.

Applicators: Appropriate intensity regional applicators may be used. They would have to be applied to the side and back of the left chest, and the front and the back of the right chest to deliver the needed magnetic field intensity. If the lung cancer is secondary to cancer elsewhere in the body, the other parts of the body would need to be treated as well. A more efficient alternative would be to use a dual pad, whole-body, "magnetic sandwich" PEMF system. The whole-body system would also be helpful to maintain the general health of the body and work to prevent and deal with metastatic disease.

Treatment Time: Using the "low and slow" approach, the recommend treatment time goal is 60 minutes twice a day. Improvements in lab work, symptoms, and imaging studies may allow treatment time to be decreased to about 30 minutes twice a day, indefinitely.

Supplements: See supplement recommendations in **Cancer** above.

Cancer, Pancreatic

The causes of or risks for pancreatic cancer include chronic pancreatitis, age, heredity (family cancer syndrome and BRCA2 gene), smoking, heavy alcohol use, excessive processed and red meat, other history of cancer, abdominal obesity, sedentary lifestyle, diabetes and chronic hepatitis. People often have several of these risk factors. Over 80 percent of cases occur between the ages of 60 and 80.

Pancreatic cancer can spread into other parts of the belly and the liver, and also to the lungs, bone, brain, and other organs. Because pancreatic cancer disseminates early and progresses locally rapidly more than 3/4 of patients diagnosed with it cannot be offered curative treatment.

By the time somebody is diagnosed with pancreatic cancer, PEMF treatment, to have some value to either improve symptoms and perhaps to delay progression and dissemination, needs to be done aggressively and early. The temptation may be to simply do local high-intensity treatments to the pancreas area, but because of the rapid dissemination, a high-intensity whole-body "magnetic sandwich" system should be strongly considered and used aggressively.

Intensity of the PEMF: 4000-7000 gauss is recommended. Lower-intensity systems may provide some general benefit for symptom relief and somewhat improve vitality, but the risk may be too high to bother.

Applicators: If the decision is made to do local treatment, a regional applicator over the whole upper abdomen would be better than a smaller local device just to treat the pancreas itself. Again, by the time the cancer is discovered it will have started causing problems in the whole upper abdomen, not just the pancreas itself. The best system is likely to be a high-intensity "magnetic sandwich" PEMF system. Every treatment session could include treatment with the two whole-body pads first, followed by laying on the lower whole-body pad combined with a loop coil to the upper abdomen.

Treatment Time: A" low and slow" approach may be needed depending on the general status of the person. It may need to be advanced faster than used with other conditions, in order to be more aggressive. The minimum recommended treatment time is 60 minutes two to three times per day.

Supplements. See supplement recommendations in **Cancer** above and **Pancreatitis**.

Cancer, Stage IV

The same issues that apply to stage IV cancer apply to cancer in general. (See **Cancer,** above). The difference is that in stage IV, the cancer has now spread to another organ or multiple organs in the body from its original source. It may range from being mild to severe. There may be other significant health issues at the same time. Treatments for stage IV cancer are complicated and often challenging to deal with, and may include chemotherapy, immune modifying agents, surgery, and/or radiation. Life expectancy with stage IV cancer depends on many factors, as well. Five-year survival rates vary by cancer and range from 5.5 to 72 percent for the top 12 most common cancers, and vary by cancer type, grade, genetics, and many other traits.

The goal of PEMF therapy in the setting of stage IV cancer is to increase general health, reduce symptoms from the cancer or treatments, help the body to control the cancer at its current level or better, facilitate the effectiveness of any other standard or experimental conventional medical system treatments being used, help any other alternative approaches to be more effective, and/or reduce inflammation in the body that may make cancer growth more likely. Since often, especially for solid organ cancers, cancer stem cells are already in many places of the body, the aim of PEMF therapy is to reduce local factors that may cause cancer cells to take root and grow. It is not a replacement for other therapies, especially rescue therapies with imminent organ failure. My experience has been that PEMFs help to support any other approaches being taken to deal with the cancer and other health conditions.

I believe it is important to work with integrative health practitioners to obtain the optimal benefits for the circumstances. Every health discipline has something to offer; no one type of practitioner is supreme or absolute. Survival of a person, in general and with stage IV cancer in particular, I believe is ultimately spiritually determined. After 50 years of medical practice and being part of the care of hundreds of stage IV cancer patients, I'm only one of the participants helping. I bow to the Ultimate Decision-Maker. After all, "nobody gets out of here alive." Everyone leaves and shuffles off this mortal coil. We do the best we can to maintain our residence in these bodies, guided by spirit.

In my experience, combining PEMF therapies along with other integrative approaches in the stage IV cancer setting, a number of individuals with short-term survival expectations have lived four years or more. Whether the PEMFs were a major contributing factor to their extended survival, we can't say for certain. However, almost all were thankful for the benefits they received which made them feel considerably more comfortable in their journey.

It is a personal choice which path people want to take in dealing with stage IV cancer. There is no judgment. It's impossible to know which path was right or not. I respect each person's choice. If PEMFs are part of the choice to continue with various treatments, then I hope they can have an impact in helping.

Ultimately, the decision on which PEMF system to use has to be individualized. This often will require a consultation with a professional with clinical expertise with cancer, as well as in the use of PEMFs. A professional with expertise with only one particular PEMF system can still be very important and helpful, understanding the strengths and limitations of the system they are using. It may also be helpful to engage a professional who has wider knowledge of PEMFs and access to different types of PEMF systems to have flexibility in making the best recommendations. To take a quote from Dr. Abraham Maslow, "If your only tool is a hammer, you see every problem as a nail."

I believe that stage IV cancer will require at least a whole-body "magnetic sandwich" system and/or additional applicators for local use. Different PEMF systems can be configured in many ways to produce "magnetic sandwich" configurations. The better option, normally, would be to have two whole-body pads running together. This makes treatment more efficient, decreasing total treatment time. Smaller applicators may be used for specific needs, often combining a whole-body pad with a local applicator. It's even possible to combine two local applicators in two different areas or in a "magnetic sandwich" approach.

The whole-body approach is to decrease inflammation throughout the whole body, thereby decreasing the burden of the immune system with many fights in many locations. The whole-body approach with the right magnetic field intensity will also help any local needs, while at the same time being able to use a local applicator where also needed.

Intensity of the PEMF: 4000 – 7000 gauss either/or whole-body and local. The need for these intensities is to reach deep into the body wherever an anti-inflammatory and support action is needed.

Applicators: Local, whole-body, and preferably whole-body "magnetic sandwich." A local portable PEMF device may be needed for sleep or for other local treatments over extended treatment times.

Treatment Time: The "low and slow" approach will always be needed at the beginning of PEMF stimulation. I recommend 30-60 minutes twice a day at a minimum, morning and evening, combining local and whole-body treatment time as needed. Depending on the amount of pain or other health issues present, more time may be added throughout the day.

Supplements: See supplement recommendations in **Cancer** above.

Carpal Tunnel Syndrome

Carpal tunnel syndrome causes pain, numbness, and tingling in the hand and arm. The condition occurs when the median nerve to the hand is squeezed or compressed as it travels through the wrist. It tends to get worse over time, so early diagnosis and treatment are important. Early on, symptoms can often be relieved with simple measures like wearing a wrist splint or avoiding certain activities. If pressure on the median nerve continues, this can lead to nerve damage. To prevent permanent damage, surgery to take pressure off the median nerve may be needed.

The carpal tunnel is a narrow passageway in the wrist, about an inch wide. The floor and sides of the tunnel are formed by small wrist bones called carpal bones. The tunnel protects the median nerve and tendons that bend the fingers and thumb. The roof of the tunnel is a strong band of connective tissue called the transverse carpal ligament. Because these boundaries are very rigid, the carpal tunnel has little capacity to "stretch" or increase in size. The median nerve provides feeling in the thumb and index, middle, and ring fingers. The nerve also controls the muscles around the base of the thumb. The nine flexor tendons that bend the fingers and thumb also travel through the carpal tunnel.

Carpal tunnel syndrome occurs when the tunnel narrows or when tissues surrounding the flexor tendons swell, putting pressure on the median nerve. These tissues are called the synovium. Normally, the synovium lubricates the tendons, making it easier to move your fingers. Most cases of carpal tunnel syndrome are caused by a combination of factors. Studies show that women and older people are more likely to develop the condition.

Other risk factors for carpal tunnel syndrome include:

- Heredity. This is likely an important factor. The carpal tunnel may be smaller in some people or there may be anatomic differences that change the amount of space for the nerve, and these traits can run in families.
- Repetitive hand use. Repeating the same hand and wrist motions or activities over a prolonged period of time may aggravate the tendons in the wrist, causing swelling that puts pressure on the nerve.
- Hand and wrist position. Doing activities that involve extreme flexion or extension of the hand and wrist for a prolonged period of time can increase pressure on the nerve, such as happens with the wrong night-time hand position.
- Pregnancy. Hormonal changes during pregnancy can cause swelling.
- Health conditions. Diabetes, rheumatoid arthritis, and thyroid gland imbalance are conditions that are associated with carpal tunnel syndrome.

Night-time symptoms are very common. Because many people sleep with their wrists bent, symptoms may awaken you from sleep. During the day, symptoms often occur when holding something for a prolonged period of time with the wrist bent forward or backward, such as when using a phone, driving, reading a book, or typing.

Inflammation of the nerve and the other components of the tunnel and swelling are the primary factors involved. The primary goal of PEMF therapies to reduce the inflammation, decrease swelling, and help to heal the nerve and other tissues. Ongoing prevention, especially during the night, is needed with a wrist splint to keep the level of inflammation and irritation at a minimum. If working at a computer keyboard, an ergonomic mouse and proper keyboard positioning may be necessary.

Intensity of the PEMF: 100 – 1000 gauss.

Applicators: Local applicator of a whole-body system, a small system using electrical power, or a portable battery-operated system with one or two small applicators. The best results would be with two applicators stacked with appropriate orientation to increase the PEMF intensity applied over the carpal tunnel.

Treatment Time: With a battery-operated system, treatment can be hours at a time, including overnight, if needed for a more severe issue. A minimum of 30 to 60 minutes per use, at least twice a day. Because of the normal waxing and waning of symptoms, depending on activity, some amount of daily maintenance may be necessary.

Supplements: P5P 100-200 mg/D, B12 5000 µg/D, alpha lipoic acid 1200 mg 1-2X/D, Agmatine – dose per the bottle, magnesium citrate 500 mg/D, CBD oil 50-100 mg 2-3X/D (just the CBD component, not the total hemp).

Cataracts

Cataracts are a superficial condition as far as the depth in the body is concerned. As is typical for most health conditions, except for those individuals interested in health maintenance, people look for PEMF therapy when the cataract situation is relatively serious and advanced. In this setting it is very hard to determine what the value of PEMF therapy would be. At least, PEMF therapy for cataracts is very simple. People who are doing whole-body PEMF therapies for health maintenance are more likely to experience a preventative value from PEMF therapy. Cataract is defined as the loss of lens transparency because of opacification of the lens. Most cataracts are age-related in adults, with onset between age 45 to 50 years. In children, hereditary and metabolic causes are most common.

The eye lens is composed of fibers contained by a thin capsule. The lens fibers migrate from the edge toward the center. From there, the nucleus or center of the lens has older lens fibers. Newly formed lens fibers are in the outermost layers of the lens, known as the cortex. Opacity of the lens is a direct result of oxidative stress. Based on location of opacification within the lens, age-related cataracts are classified into three types: cortical, nuclear, and posterior subcapsular cataracts. The lens cells are metabolically active cells, undergoing various changes that eventually make them insoluble. These cells gradually migrate to the lens center and are progressively compressed, resulting in hardening of the center of the lens, called nuclear sclerosis. This sclerotic center makes the lens opaque to light.

The goal of PEMF therapy in the presence of cataract is much more preventative than therapeutic. The earlier in the cataract process PEMF therapy is started, the more likelihood of preventing the development of cataract. Once the cataract is dense, the only solution really is to replace the lens. I encourage people to get routine eye examinations to detect changes in the lens at the earliest stages. PEMF therapy at this point is simple and inexpensive. Besides, PEMF therapy for this use could be helpful for other problems of the body as well.

Intensity of the PEMF: The front part of the eye that includes the lens is very shallow, so the intensity the magnetic field does not need to be as high. All PEMFs help with oxidative stress and individuals who need help with cataracts often need help to other parts of the eye, such as to prevent and treat glaucoma or macular degeneration. The intensity should be between 100 and 200 gauss, at a minimum, using a portable battery-operated PEMF system. This could also be used for other needs anywhere in the body that would lend themselves this level of intensity of magnetic field.

Applicators: Small, round coil applicators will work. One or two applicators may be used at a time, placed right over the eye. Often the easiest way to apply an applicator would be over the frame of glasses. The applicators can be taped over the glasses and then just wear the glasses. If this is not tolerable or practical, the coils can be taped, using paper tape, to the temples, with the coil advanced forward with the leading edge even with the front of the eye. Another option would be to tape coils onto a mask with holes for the eyes. The image that comes to mind is the Lone Ranger mask. You may have to be inventive in finding ways to keep the coils in place for the treatments.

Treatment Time: If treatments are started very early in the course of the condition, 15 minutes per day may suffice. Otherwise, I would recommend 30 minutes twice a day, especially at the beginning, and then continuing at this level for several months to see what eye examination results show or if symptoms significantly improve.

Supplements: Since cataract formation is largely an oxidative stress problem, I recommend broad-spectrum antioxidants. Several different antioxidants may be needed. It's hard to recommend specific supplements and nutrition because they have to be individualized. I recommend consulting with a professional skilled in nutrition and supplements to give guidance on the supplements that should be used.

Chronic Fatigue Syndrome (CFS) / Myalgicencephalomyelitis (ME)

The older term used for this syndrome is CFS. The current terminology is ME. ME/CFS is defined by incapacitating fatigue of at least six months duration, neurological problems, and a constellation of symptoms that can resemble other disorders, such as mononucleosis, multiple sclerosis, fibromyalgia, AIDS-related complex, Lyme disease, post-polio syndrome, and autoimmune diseases such as lupus. Research studies suggest that CFS results from a dysfunction of the immune system, involving a disruption of fundamental mechanisms of central nervous system (CNS) function such as the sleep-wake cycle and the stress related hypothalamic-pituitary-adrenal axis. A history of viral infections is common. Psychological stress responses are part of the syndrome. It's likely that ME/CFS is caused by multiple factors acting together, which is why there is no gold standard therapy and definitive diagnostic test. The goal of PEMF therapy is to keep the whole-body healthy, since no specific cause can be targeted for elimination. As a result, daily, long-term, whole-body PEMF treatment should be considered to achieve the best and most enduring results, in addition to other treatment modalities, such as nutrition, lifestyle, and psychological support.

PEMFs often help with the neurological aspects and the pain components, improving the level of energy with activity, sleep, stress, and immune function.

Counseling is often needed. It may be very useful to do PEMF water treatment. (See **Water.**)

Intensity of the PEMF: Going "low and slow" is paramount in ME/CFS and escalation to optimal levels often may only be able to happen very slowly. While whole-body PEMF therapy is the preferred approach, the intensity of the magnetic field may be a challenge. Many people with ME/CFS have very significant sensitivities to many aspects of life, including EMFs. Though PEMFs are not EMFs in their actions in the body, PEMF systems with multiple frequencies can create a stress response in the body. To be sure that any aggravations are not caused by the PEMFs, it's important for these individuals to eliminate or reduce as much EMF exposure as possible, including Wi-Fi, smart meters, cell phones, and now especially 5G. (See Chapter 2.)

Individual frequencies or the combinations of frequencies may cause treatment challenges, so controlling the total number of treatment variables becomes very important in achieving benefit. In addition, the intensity needs to have fairly discrete control, from low to medium to high. Devices that have multiple programs with variations in frequencies and intensities would be the most challenging to see results without aggravations and PEMF therapy would be stopped before significant healing and symptom reduction benefits could be seen. Most often I recommend a PEMF system with intensities under 1000 gauss, and preferably under 500 gauss. Many individuals can't tolerate even more than one gauss. But it's possible to go up to higher intensities with the pulse-type magnetic systems, since they have fewer variables to control.

Applicators: Depending on the constellation of issues present, not only from the ME/CFS problem itself, but also from other concurrent health issues such as arthritis, perimenopause, diabetes, etc., a range of applicators may be needed, from local, to regional, to whole-body. If a whole-body system is used, appropriate local and regional applicators should be considered as well. Problems with mitochondrial function and ATP production are common in ME/CFS, making whole-body treatment especially important. Since the fatigue may be associated with various hormonal problems, including adrenal insufficiency and a central brain-related cause (hence the encephalitis part of the ME), a frequency-based local applicator to be used for the brain would be helpful. Some people need to run a PEMF system all night to help sleep. A regional applicator, such as a half-body pad may be useful for related gastrointestinal, urinary tract, and/or pulmonary issues. So, an individualized PEMF system will need to be put together that will address as many issues in the same person as possible.

Treatment Time: This will have to be highly individualized and expect a lengthy "low and slow" process. Some people have to start off with only one or two minutes of PEMF treatment at a time, with the lowest intensities. The body's responses will determine how quickly the intensity and time can be increased. We can almost say that we have arrived when the highest intensity can be used for 60 minutes at a time at least twice a day. Often these levels cannot be achieved but the PEMF therapy will still be providing significant benefits and the results will be seen over months to years. See Appendix B for examples of the low and slow process.

Supplements: I always emphasize the need for good nutrition and appropriate supplements for people with ME/CFS. It's hard to recommend specific supplements and nutrition because they have to be individualized. There are specialized sets of supplements for many of the individual symptom patterns and causes encountered. I recommend consulting with a professional skilled in nutrition and supplements to give guidance on the supplements that should be used. The PEMFs are expected to work synergistically with any supplements used. Doctors rarely make recommendations for supplements.

Complex Regional Pain Syndrome (CRPS) (See Chapter 9)

Concussion and Traumatic Brain Injury (TBI)

Concussion and TBI are notable more for the symptoms and functional issues they cause than for the type of injury and the findings on diagnostic studies. Except for the more severe types of penetrating brain injuries, the consequences of both mild TBI (concussion) and TBIs associated with loss of consciousness at the time of the trauma, the symptoms and functional problems can be very similar. Diagnostic studies, especially imaging studies, are uniformly not revealing. The ones that can be revealing are rarely used, and include SECT scanning, QEEG or MRI with DTI. PEMFs have been found in numerous research studies to be helpful for TBI, in a range of intensities from low to medium to high. The most consistent and longer-term results appeared to be best achieved with high-intensity local therapy to the brain. The treatment parameters are not yet certain and depend on the intensity the magnetic field used and the length of treatment time. While it appears that PEMFs can significantly improve function and symptoms, how long results will last is highly individual and it appears that short courses of treatment are more likely to show a loss of benefit. It's likely that better results would be seen with higher-intensity, longer-term treatments, best handled with daily treatments the home setting. At this point it is not known to what extent the brain lesions are actually healed versus having mostly a functional and symptom benefit.

Various ancillary therapies may be needed as well, including counseling, speech and language therapy, cognitive and physical rehabilitation, as well as medications as needed. PEMF therapy may be able to reduce the side effects of and dependency on medications, primarily as a symptom management tool.

Intensity of the PEMF: Medium- to high-intensity magnetic fields applied locally to the brain are recommended for the best results. Portable battery-operated PEMFs that allow selection of various frequencies can be used to address numerous symptoms often seen in these individuals, such as brain fog, anxiety, and sleep issues. These portable PEMFs can be used for more extended periods of time, such as through the night, and do not restrict activity. These are typically around 200 gauss for a single coil and 100 gauss each when two coils are used together. The portable PEMFs can be combined with high-intensity PEMFs depending on symptoms and needs. High-intensity PEMFs penetrate the brain better to achieve functional results and help with the inflammation in the brain seen with TBI.

Since whole brain/head PEMF therapy is needed, and one of the goals is to reduce inflammation, the PEMF magnetic field needs to penetrate the entire head with at least 15 gauss, per the intensities in Appendix A. The average human head measures 6-7 inches in width and 8-9 inches in length. This means that, at minimum a PEMF intensity of 4000 gauss is needed to about 7000 gauss. If a 4000 gauss magnetic field is used, treatment needs to be done to the front and the back of the head, separately or combined across the sides of the head. Treatment should follow the "low and slow" approach. Generally, PEMFs can be used with other medications as needed. If anti-seizure medications are being used, it's important to watch for side effects indicating the dose of these medications may need to be reduced. This may be true for other medications, as well.

Applicators: For the medium-intensity magnetic fields, the two small applicators should be applied to the head, alternating between the front and the back at the same time, and side to side at the same time. High-intensity PEMF systems allowing the "magnetic sandwich" approach with two separate applicators will simplify treatment times. Apply the applicators on the sides of the head at the same time, and to the front and back of the head at the same time, to see which approach produces the best results. Some PEMF systems have a butterfly coil that can be placed over the top of the head with a loop on either side of the head. If there is only one applicator, then it would be applied on each side of the head separately during the same treatment session.

Treatment Time: I did a pilot study using a medium-intensity PEMF of 100 gauss per coil using two applicators that showed significant results when the applicators were placed front and back for an hour, followed by side to side for an hour. The study went on for three months, followed by a month of evaluation without treatment. During the month off, everybody lost about half of the benefit they saw during the course of actual treatments. Based on the results with this study, it is not known whether longer-lasting results would be seen with more treatment time per day or if treatment duration with this protocol would have been better done over six months or more. The conclusion was that the treatments produced significant functional and symptom improvements. Everybody in the study developed a headache within the first couple of days that resolved after another three to four days on its own.

Higher-intensity PEMFs of 4000-7000 gauss are recommended to be applied for 30 minutes twice a day. A "low and slow" approach should be used with these higher-intensity systems; 60 minutes twice a day could be tried to see if there's a difference between 30 and 60 minute treatments. After several months, and if significant improvements are seen, treatment times may be able to be reduced down to about 15 minutes twice a day for maintenance purposes. After symptoms have steadily improved for at least a month, treatment holidays could be tried to see if symptoms recur. If they do recur, further courses of treatment should be used for a month before trying treatment holidays again.

Supplements: At the very least I recommend alpha lipoic acid, N-acetyl cysteine, vitamin B12, acetyl L-carnitine, glutathione, magnesium, CBD, curcumin and Co Q10. Because other brain-support supplements may be considered, I always emphasize the need for good nutrition and appropriate supplements in those with TBI. It's hard to recommend specific supplements and nutrition because they have to be individualized. I recommend consulting with a professional skilled in nutrition and supplements to give guidance on the supplements that should be used. PEMFs work synergistically with any supplements used. Doctors caring for TBI rarely make recommendations for supplements.

Dental Issues

Magnetic fields have been used in dentistry for prosthetics, during orthodontia, periodontal disease, dental infections and abscesses, cavitations, dry sockets, dental and jaw pain, fractures of the jaw and radionecrosis, osteomyelitis of the jaw, bruxism, temporomandibular joint disease (TMJ/TMD), and maxillary and mandibular reconstructions. Treatments are normally applied locally.

Intensity of the PEMF: Because the teeth and dental structures are superficial the intensity the magnetic field does not need to be as high. PEMFs between 100 and 1,000 gauss are normally adequate.

Applicators: Portable battery-operated PEMF devices are sufficient, allowing one or two applicators to be used at the same time. They would normally be placed next to the dental structure being treated, whether it's a tooth, abscess, jaw, or TMJ. In the case of TMJ, one applicator may be placed over each TMJ area. If many jaw structures are involved, a larger magnetic pad can be used under the jaw. This is more challenging for the upper teeth (maxilla), where the PEMFs would have to be wrapped around the maxilla or placed locally if there is a specific spot needing treatment. With higher-intensity magnetic fields, a flexible applicator can be used to target the whole dental area, placing it over the front and bending it over the sides of the jaw/lower face. Since magnetic field is the strongest at the coil, bending the coil as opposed to the whole applicator may be all that is needed.

Treatment Time: Treatment time will depend on the problem being treated and the treatment response. An active tooth abscess may require hours of treatment until a definitive procedure is performed to drain the abscess. After abscess drainage, treatments need to be continued regularly until the tissue has healed. If the pain goes away and the problem is resolved, treatment may be able to be stopped unless it recurs. With cavities, a PEMF can provide temporary relief until the cavity is properly dealt with through the placement of a filling. With orthodontics, coils may be placed over the areas of the most discomfort and continued until the discomfort is gone. The most discomfort happens after initial placement or adjustments of the orthodontic appliance(s). Bone issues can be dealt with similarly to what was discussed in **Bone Healing and Repair** above. This includes mandibular and maxillary surgical procedures.

Supplements: I always emphasize the need for good nutrition and bone healing and inflammation-reducing supplements. Specific supplements and nutrition have to be individualized. I recommend consulting with a professional skilled in nutrition and supplements to give guidance on the supplements that should be used. Doctors and dentists rarely make recommendations for supplements. Also see supplement recommendations for **Bone Healing and Repair**.

Depression

Depression is considered to be primarily a brain issue. As with most other health conditions, it has a spectrum of severity from mild to severe. A separate category of more severe depression can also be considered as treatment-resistant depression. Most depression is managed with medication, but when even this fails, it is treatment-resistant. PEMF therapy is an important alternative to helping with depression and can be used well in conjunction with other treatments. All PEMF treatments are oriented towards the brain, so they are considered local. Milder forms of depression may be readily dealt with using moderate level PEMFs. More significant depression may require higher-intensity PEMFs. The FDA has approved high-intensity PEMFs, called rTMS or *repetitive Transcranial Magnetic Stimulation*, for treatment-resistant depression. This has to be done in professional offices. Insurance coverage is usually reserved for treatment-resistant depression, not common depression. As a result, home-based PEMF therapy is a reasonable alternative for more common, not treatment-resistant, depression, and when used earlier in the course of depression it may be able to prevent progression to the treatment-resistant form.

A 1000 Hz 40 gauss PEMF has been found in research to help with acute depression. This frequency was designed into the FlexPulse™ device, and can be used alone or during the transition onto medication, primarily in mild to moderate forms of depression. This multipurpose device can also be used for accompanying brain fog, pain, and/or insomnia. Depression is frequently accompanied by anxiety. (See **Anxiety, Panic, and PTSD** above.) Successful treatment of the anxiety may determine the value for the treatment for depression, and vice versa.

With FDA-approved rTMS treatment, depressive symptoms decrease following daily rTMS treatments (5/wk) as early as two or three weeks after starting treatment. A standard acute course of 20 to 30 treatment sessions over six weeks will very likely be needed to achieve more stable results. People who fail treatments or have recurrence may need to continue weekly treatments for longer periods of time. The response rates in studies were 15 to 24 percent and remission rate of 14 to 17 percent with active rTMS. For those receiving sham treatments, the response was 15 percent, and 8 percent had relapses. People who did respond may have had benefit for three to six months. The treatment protocols were very rigorous and not equivalent to using high-intensity PEMFs available for use by consumers at home.

> **CAUTION: PEMFS SHOULD NOT BE USED FOR DEPRESSION WITHOUT ACCOMPAN-YING CARE FROM A LICENSED PROFESSIONAL. IT IS RECOMMENDED THAT THE PRO-FESSIONAL BE INFORMED THAT PEMFs ARE BEING USED CONCOMITANTLY WITH PROFESSIONAL CARE. DO NOT STOP, ALTER, OR REDUCE MEDICATIONS WITHOUT THE ADVICE OF YOUR PRESCRIBING PROFESSIONAL. FOLLOW CONTRAINDICATIONS AND CAUTIONS (SEE CHAPTERS 4,5,6 AND 11).**

Intensity of the PEMF: For milder forms of depression, a portable, battery-operated PEMF of about 100 – 200 gauss can be applied to the left forehead at about the hairline. A 1000 Hz, 40 gauss PEMF may help with milder acute depression. If a higher-intensity PEMF system is available for other reasons, it can also be used for milder forms of depression. For more moderate or more significant depression, higher-intensity PEMFs can be applied to the forehead, ranging in intensities from 1000 gauss and higher.

Applicators: Local 100-200 gauss applicators can be applied to the forehead or to the sides of the head, especially if anxiety is present. Some trial and error may be required to determine which placements provide the most benefits. Higher-intensity magnetic fields can be placed over the forehead and/or over the top of the head. The best coil would be a butterfly placed over the top of the head, one loop layered on top of the other, like a halo. A loop coil can be shaped into a smaller circumference and be placed over the top of the head. A paddle coil can be tried at the left side of the head or over the flat part of the forehead.

Treatment Time: For low-intensity portable PEMFs the recommended treatment time is between one to two hours twice a day. For high-intensity PEMF systems recommended treatment time is between 30 to 60 minutes twice a day. Once significant improvement has been achieved, maintenance therapy is recommended for three to six months.

Supplements: A number of supplements that may help with depression include St. John's wort, SAMe, 5-HTP, omega-3, saffron, and others. It's hard to recommend specific supplements and nutrition because they have to be individualized. I recommend consulting with a professional skilled in nutrition and supplements to give guidance on the supplements that should be used.

Diabetes

Diabetes is a complex condition that involves the whole body. Chronically elevated blood sugar is the primary problem with diabetes that ends up causing the myriad of problems associated with this condition. The elevated levels of glucose start combining with blood proteins through a process known as glycation. Protein glycation reactions lead to the production of advanced glycation end products (AGEs) which are thought to be the major causes of different diabetic complications. AGEs are the cause of aging and the development, or worsening, of many degenerative diseases, such as atherosclerosis, chronic kidney disease, and Alzheimer's disease. All the tissues in the body are affected by AGEs, including the skin, the eyes, the brain and nervous system, joints, and the immune system, among others. The impact of the damage of diabetes is more obvious and common in some organs than others, specifically vision, heart disease, kidney disease, wound healing, and neuropathy. These areas of damage tend to occur fairly late in the diabetic process and are common causes of death and disability.

Production of AGEs is constant as long as blood sugar is elevated. In other words, the production of damage in the body from diabetes/AGE's "never sleeps."

The earlier in the course of diabetes prevention of damage from AGEs is started the better the control of the problems caused by the AGEs.

For diabetes, daily PEMF treatments to both involved local areas and the whole-body is the goal. Whole-body treatment is the most efficient to help all the tissues of the body. If there are complications in specific organs, these can be dealt with locally, as well. Inflammation is a constant factor in diabetes. PEMF treatment will need to be lifelong, especially if there's organ damage or at least until the hemoglobin A1c is less than 5.7 on a consistent basis, at least over three to six months and remains that way.

Even an A1c under 5.7 still produces a significant amount of AGEs. A more optimal A1c level would be around 5. Unfortunately, the medical community is often satisfied with an A1c of 7. That is because they are often dealing with A1c's over 10 or 12, so a decrease to 7 feels successful. An A1c >6.4 is considered diabetes. A1c's between 5.7-6.4 are considered prediabetes. This is actually a bit of a name game. Factually, A1c's between 5.7-6.4 are mild diabetes. AGE damage is still being done between 5.7-6.4. Any spike, at any time, in blood sugar level increases production of AGEs. Occasional spikes are not our biggest concern. It is the chronic daily spiking and/or consistently elevated A1c's that create the long-term damage.

Intensity of the PEMF: Because of the amount of inflammation in the body as a result of the diabetic process, the intensity of the magnetic field is very important to be able to reach through all the tissues of the body adequately. See Appendix A for a guide to the magnetic field intensity needed to go through the whole-body and/or individual organs. If an adequate intensity whole-body PEMF system is used, there may be decreased need for local treatments, especially if treatment is started early enough before significant organ damage is apparent. Generally, PEMF intensities between 4000-7000 gauss work best and most efficiently. While lower-intensity PEMFs will provide at least some degree of limited benefit, longer twice daily treatment times may be necessary.

Applicators: Whole-body PEMF is best. Most whole-body systems provide for local applicators as well. Generally, local applicators are stronger than the whole-body pads. Relying on local applicators to treat specific organ damage, without using adequate intensity whole-body therapy at the same time to limit damage everywhere, will not be effective. It may only make sense if diabetes is controlled with an A1c consistently under 5.7, and ideally closer to 5.

Treatment Time: If there is significant damage in the body that needs to be repaired, the targeted treatment time should about one hour twice a day. Longer treatments can be used if desired. After evidence of organ damage and/or symptoms show significant improvement, treatment times may be able to be reduced to no less than 30 minutes twice a day. Because PEMF treatment is anti-aging, and because years of diabetes can have created significant damage throughout the body, lifetime treatment is recommended. This would be true for anti-aging whether there was a history of diabetes or not.

Supplements: There are at least three categories of supplements that should be considered: those targeted toward glucose control, those for inflammation, and those for specific organ needs. These are too numerous to list here. Supplements and nutrition need to be individualized. As a result, I recommend consulting with a professional skilled in diabetic nutrition and supplements to give guidance on the nutrition and supplements that should be used. Doctors rarely make recommendations for supplements. Referrals to a dietitian/nutritionist by doctors is common practice. Unfortunately, it is uncommon for dietitians to recommend supplements.

Ear Problems

There are many types of ear problems. The focus here will be on those that are associated with infection and chronic inflammation. They can be divided into external ear (ear canal) and inner ear. The inner ear is at the end of the ear tubes (eustachian). It has three main parts:

- Cochlea, the auditory area of the inner ear that changes sound waves into nerve signals.
- Semicircular canals, which sense balance and posture to assist in equilibrium.
- Vestibule, the area of the inner ear cavity that lies between the cochlea and semicircular canals, also assisting in equilibrium.

The most common ear conditions are otitis externa, otitis media, serous otitis, and labyrinthitis. Serious otitis is most frequently associated with blockage of the eustachian tubes caused by inflammation in the back of the throat, such as with a cold.

Otitis externa is an acute condition and usually treated with antibiotics. Otitis media is also usually associated with an acute infection, whether caused by viruses or bacteria. This is also usually managed appropriately with antibiotics. The trouble with these conditions begins when they become chronic, causing hearing loss and balance issues. When they become chronic, decongestants and antihistamines are frequently used and occasionally surgery has to be resorted to. PEMFs can be tried before considering surgery, even in children. They can be used to the side of either ear to treat chronic otitis externa, chronic otitis media, chronic serous otitis and labyrinthitis. The eustachian tubes can be stimulated from the top of the neck just forward from of the angle of the jaw bone.

Intensity of the PEMF: 100-1000 gauss.

Applicators: Smaller-size, local applicators are best. With loop applicators, the edge of the loop or edge should be applied just over the side of the ear. With pad applicators, it is necessary to find the edge of the magnetic coil in the pad. The edge should be positioned over the side of the ear. If two applicators are available, try to use them at the same time. If only one applicator is available then it will have to be positioned over each area to be treated for the needed time.

Treatment Time: 15-30 minutes twice a day or repeated multiple times a day as needed to each area requiring treatment. Treatment may be needed for several weeks. Separate treatment may be required to the ear and to the eustachian tubes.

Supplements: Multivitamin/mineral, xylitol 9– 10 g/D as a chewing gum or syrup primarily as a preventative for otitis media, vitamin C 1000-3000 mg 2X/D, D3 2000 – 5000 IU/D, grapeseed extract 100 mg 2X/D, quercetin 1000 mg 2X/D.

Eczema, Dermatitis, and Psoriasis

Eczema and psoriasis are autoimmune conditions. Dermatitis simply means inflammation of the skin. It may be autoimmune, and happens with eczema or psoriasis. Causes of these conditions vary depending on the type. Some types, like dyshidrotic eczema, neurodermatitis, and nummular dermatitis, may have unknown causes. Different forms include atopic, autoimmune, contact dermatitis (due to contact with an irritant such as poison ivy or detergents), seborrheic dermatitis (due to skin mites), or stasis dermatitis from venous insufficiency, among many others. Inflammation is the one denominator all of these conditions have in common. It is because of the inflammation that steroids, whether oral or creams, are frequently used. The steroid creams simply suppress inflammation but do not help to heal the underlying skin. Eczema and psoriasis are frequently due to IgG food allergies. While there are many culprits, the most common are dairy, eggs, and gluten. Removing the cause is the most important strategy for dealing with these skin conditions, but it is not always possible to identify the cause. In this case, PEMF therapies may be helpful to not only improve the inflammation but also to heal the skin, by stimulating collagen, hyaluronic acid, fibroblasts, and stem cells, reducing the damage from oxidative stress and sun exposure, and reducing aging.

Intensity of the PEMF: Direct stimulation of the skin can be done locally for specific problem areas with relatively low-intensity PEMFs and a minimum of 15 gauss. Each area of the skin needs to be dealt with separately. If lower intensities are used, multiple areas of the body will need to be treated at the same time. However, to stimulate the skin throughout the body or over larger areas at the same, a higher-intensity system will be needed, for example 4000-7000 gauss, to penetrate from one side of the body to another.

Applicators: Applicators may be local, regional, or whole-body. For extensive lesions, whole-body stimulation is the most effective. The best would be a "magnetic sandwich" system. If there have been multiple lesions in multiple areas of the body that respond and return, whole-body PEMF treatment should be strongly considered.

Treatment Time: Each area with lesions will need between 30-60 minutes twice a day early on to decrease the inflammation. Treatments need to be continued until the lesions are healed. Stopping treatments before the lesions are healed, even though symptoms are improved, will allow the lesions to return. Skin lesions tend to come and go and may rotate among different areas of the body.

Supplements: Supplements to consider include curcumin, borage or evening Primrose oil (GLA), MSM, hyaluronic acid, collagen, CBD creams or balms, probiotics, and/or omega-3 fatty acids. Psoriasis is often treated with light therapy. A study in Brazil using 45,000 units of vitamin D3 per day for 6 months, showed complete resolution in everybody, without any evidence of risk or harm. It is assumed that the light therapy is increasing vitamin D3 in the body, producing the results. Lower levels of vitamin D3 may have a little benefit.

Ehlers-Danlos Syndromes (EDS)

Ehlers-Danlos syndromes (EDS) are a group of connective tissue disorders that can be inherited and are varied both in how they affect the body and in their genetic causes. Affected individuals have joint hypermobility (joints that stretch further than normal), skin hyperextensibility (skin that can be stretched further than normal), and tissue fragility.

Ehlers-Danlos syndromes (EDS) are classified into 13 subtypes. Each EDS subtype has a set of clinical criteria that guide diagnosis. A patient's physical signs and symptoms are matched up to the major and minor criteria to identify the subtype that is the most complete fit. There is significant symptom overlap between the EDS subtypes and the other connective tissue disorders, including hypermobility spectrum disorders. A definitive diagnosis for all the EDS subtypes when the gene mutation is known requires confirmation by testing to identify the responsible variant for the gene involved in each subtype. For those who meet the minimal clinical requirements for an EDS subtype, a "provisional clinical diagnosis" of an EDS subtype can be made. Expanded molecular testing should be considered to see to which category they belong.

The prognosis depends on the type of Ehlers-Danlos syndrome and the individual. Life expectancy can be shortened for those with the Vascular Ehlers-Danlos syndrome due to the possibility of organ and vessel rupture. Life expectancy is usually not affected in the other types. There can be a wide or narrow range of severity within a family, but each person's own manifestations of EDS will be unique. While there is no cure for the Ehlers-Danlos syndromes, there is treatment for symptoms, and there are preventative measures that are helpful for most. More than 90 percent of those with classic EDS (cEDS) have a mutation in one of the genes for type V collagen. The skin is hyperextensible and abnormal scarring can range in severity. Most with cEDS have extensive atrophic scars at a number of sites. They may have easily bruised skin or spontaneous bruises. Some may have progressive cardiac-valvular problems. Vascular fragility leads to the bruising.

An important sub-type is hypermobile EDS (hEDS). A number of conditions can be part hEDS but not proven to be the result of hEDS. Some include sleep disturbance, fatigue, postural orthostatic tachycardia, functional gastrointestinal disorders, dysautonomia, anxiety, and depression. These conditions may be more debilitating than the joint symptoms and often impair daily life.

Adults diagnosed with joint hypermobility syndrome (JHS)/hEDS often experience joint pain in multiple joints, which can vary from localized to widespread pain in nature and severity. Chronic widespread pain is frequent; 50 percent of cases have predominantly neuropathic, hyperlagesic pain even in asymptomatic areas (generalized secondary hyperalgesia), evidence of a sensitized central nervous system (See **CRPS** in Chapter 9). Fatigue varies from mild to severe, which may be the most disabling complaint. Neurologically oriented symptoms (joint position sensory deficits), psychological dysfunction (anxiety, depression), and systemic complaints (organ dysfunction, dysautonomia) often show up, as well.

PEMF therapy can be very important in the management of EDS because of the impact of PEMFs on collagen, fibroblasts, soft tissue repair, joint repair, and pain management. Vascular fragility may be improved by improving the collagen content of blood vessels in helping to fortify the soft tissue of blood vessels, as well as many other soft tissues.

Since EDS is a genetic disorder involving all soft tissue, higher-intensity, whole-body "magnetic sandwich" PEMF therapy is necessary. Local therapies can be useful for local symptom management. Since atrophic skin scarring is common, a wound management approach is also taken.

The goals with using PEMFs in EDS are pain management, stimulating collagen production, helping with arthritis, reducing the progression of arthritis, helping with general musculoskeletal function, decreasing muscle spasms, and generally maintaining the health of the body. Physical therapy is very important in dealing with EDS, as well, and can be enhanced by PEMFs.

Intensity of the PEMF: 400-7000 gauss.

Applicators: Whole-body "magnetic sandwich" is the most important applicator for the long-haul treatment of this condition. Higher-intensity local applicators may be used as well for spot treatments for particularly problematic areas.

Treatment Time: 30-60 minutes two to three times/day using a "low and slow" protocol to start. Treatment will be lifelong. With significant improvement, treatment times may be reduced for maintenance, guided by symptoms and function. It is very important not to cut back significantly on treatment intensity and time because of the need for continuous stimulation of collagen throughout the body and to deal with the natural insults of daily living that are more exaggerated in EDS and accumulate and become more exaggerated over time.

Supplements. See the supplement recommendations for **fibromyalgia** and **CRPS** in Chapter 9, and for **arthritis** and **tendinitis** in this chapter.

Endometriosis

The uterus is lined with tissue (endometrium). Endometriosis is a disease in which tissue that is similar to the endometrium grows in places outside the uterus, usually in the pelvis. These patches of tissue are called "implants," "nodules," or "lesions." They are most often found:

- on or under the ovaries
- on the fallopian tubes
- behind the uterus
- on the tissues that hold the uterus in place
- on the bowels or bladder
- in rare cases, the tissue may grow on your lungs or in other parts of your body.

The cause of endometriosis is unknown. Endometriosis is most common in women in their 30s and 40s, but it can affect any female who menstruates. It occurs in six to ten percent of women. Infertility is common. About 25 to 50 percent of infertile women have endometriosis, and 30 to 50 percent of women with endometriosis are infertile.

Women are at higher risk if:

- a mother, sister, or daughter have it
- periods started before age 11

- monthly cycles are short (less than 27 days)
- menstrual cycles are heavy and last more than seven days.

They have a lower risk if:

- they have been pregnant before
- their periods started late in adolescence
- they regularly exercise more than four hours a week
- they have a low amount of body fat.

The main symptoms of endometriosis are:

- pelvic pain, which affects about 75 percent of women with endometriosis; it often happens during your period.
- infertility
- painful menstrual cramps, which may get worse over time
- pain during or after sex
- pain in the intestine or lower abdomen
- pain with bowel movements or urination, usually during periods
- heavy periods
- spotting or bleeding between periods
- digestive or gastrointestinal symptoms
- fatigue or lack of energy.

Endometriosis is most often diagnosed by laparoscopy and ultrasound or MRI. There is no cure for endometriosis. Treatments are mostly to manage the symptoms.

The most common treatment for endometriosis pain is pain relief drugs. Other treatments include hormone therapy, including birth control pills, progestin therapy, and gonadotropin-releasing hormone (GnRH) agonists, which can cause a temporary menopause, but also help control the growth of endometriosis. Studies have shown that GnRH agonists cause significant reduction in pelvic pain in women with endometriosis, however they are approved for continuous use for only up to six months due to side effects secondary to very low estrogen, like bone loss, vaginal atrophy, dryness, and hot flashes.

Surgical treatments are for severe pain, to remove the endometriosis patches or cut nerves in the pelvis that carry pain. The pain may come back within a few years after surgery. If the pain is severe, a hysterectomy may be an option and sometimes removing the ovaries and fallopian tubes. Treatments for infertility caused by endometriosis include laparoscopic surgery and in vitro fertilization.

In a study of high-intensity PEMFs (HIPEMF) applied to the pelvic area, pelvic pain was reduced by 90 percent. The authors thought the rapid pain relief produced by the device was due to as a possible neurological effect involving accelerated healing at the cellular level. Another report of HIPEMF of 18 female women with acute (n=13) and/or chronic(n=8) pelvic pain, found marked, even dramatic relief, in 15 women (83 percent) even after only a few treatments. Other research indicates that even treatment of the temporal areas of the head may help. Researchers found normal menstrual function, alleviation of pain, and decrease or disappearance of premenstrual syndrome. Improvement of ovarian function was seen in 93 percent of the patients.

The goal of PEMF therapy is to reduce pain, inflammation, stabilize ovarian function, scar and adhesion formation, improve bowel and bladder function, reduce progression, and possibly even help fertility. PEMF therapy may be best to try before considering surgical procedures and if GnRH agonists have to be stopped due to side effects or long-term use.

Intensity of the PEMF: 4000 – 7000 gauss.

Applicators: Regional applicators applied to the pelvic area. Depending on the intensity of the PEMF used, treatment may need to be done both over the pubic/lower abdomen area as well as over the sacral area.

Treatment Time: 30 – 60 minutes twice a day. Treatments likely need to be continued for months at a time. Once pain has improved, deeper pelvic lower abdominal treatment work needs to continue to more adequately resolve the endometrial implants.

Supplements: See supplement recommendations for **Bladder Conditions** and **Abdominal Adhesions.**

Enuresis, Urinary Incontinence (See Bladder).

Epilepsy

Epilepsy is one of the most widespread and devastating neurological disorders, characterized by abnormal neural activity in the brain, leading to spontaneous recurrent seizures. Seizures are classified into two groups: generalized and focal. Generalized seizures affect both sides of the brain and can be broken down into two types: absence and tonic-clonic.

Focal seizures are located in just one area of the brain, and are also called partial seizures. They can be classified into simple focal, seizures, complex focal seizures, and secondary generalized seizures. Simple focal seizures affect a small part of the brain. These seizures can cause twitching or a change in sensation, such as a strange taste or smell. Complex focal seizures can make a person with epilepsy confused or dazed. The person will be unable to respond to questions or direction for up to a few minutes. Secondary generalized seizures begin in one part of the brain, but then spread to both sides of the brain. In other words, the person first has a focal seizure, followed by a generalized seizure.

Seizures may last as long as a few minutes. They come out of the blue and can create significant risk of injury when they happen during activities, including during driving a vehicle. Sometimes they last long enough to deprive the brain of oxygen and therefore cause further brain damage or even death. It can take hours for a person to recover from a seizure.

Epilepsy can be caused by different conditions that affect a person's brain. Some known causes include stroke, brain tumor, brain infection from parasites (malaria, neurocysticercosis), viruses (influenza, dengue, Zika), bacteria, traumatic brain injury or head injury, loss of oxygen to the brain (for example, during birth), some genetic disorders (such as Down syndrome), other neurologic diseases (such as Alzheimer's disease). For two-thirds of people the cause of epilepsy is unknown.

There is new evidence that localized brain inflammation, whether immune-related or nonspecific, can cause persistent and treatment-resistant seizures. Evidence also shows that seizures can cause inflammation too, influencing the occurrence and severity of seizures, and seizure-related neuronal death.

Despite significant advances in drug development, traditional anti-epileptic drugs can't target particular groups of brain cells and epileptic neural circuitry. One-third of people with seizures continue to experience intractable seizures even on anti-epileptic drugs. If drugs don't work, surgery or vagal nerve electrical stimulation may be necessary. Surgery is invasive and its effects are irreversible and associated with many neurological deficits, such as memory, speech, movement, and visual impairments.

Vagal nerve stimulation (VNS) is also invasive lifelong. Efficacy at 18 months is 40 to 50 percent, with seizure reduction of 50 percent or more. People with posttraumatic epilepsy and tuberous sclerosis do best with VNS. Few patients achieve complete seizure freedom, and about a quarter of patients have no benefit in seizure frequency. Some have only milder and shorter seizures. Complications from VNS include postoperative hematoma, infection, vocal cord palsy, lower facial weakness, pain and sensory-related issues, aseptic reaction, cable discomfort, surgical cable break, oversized stimulator pocket, and battery displacement. Hardware-related complications include lead fracture/malfunction, spontaneous VNS turn-on, and lead disconnection. Although these complications are uncommon, they may cause major suffering and even be life-threatening. Repeated surgeries are needed for battery and lead replacements and complications also may occur with these surgeries.

Since these procedures may not be fully effective and carry significant risk, PEMF therapy should be considered first because it can be very effective and have low risk, particularly when applied in the home setting long-term. In addition, VNS is a more indirect approach and does not address the underlying causes in the brain, including inflammation. As a result, PEMF therapy may be of significant value before invasive procedures are considered or to help with the side effects of drugs.

Another approach to chronic seizures is the ketogenic diet. This has been used primarily in children who do not respond to medications. It can be 40 to 70 percent effective in reducing seizures at least 50 percent. Ten to 33 percent of epileptics who adopt a ketogenic diet become seizure-free. Occasionally, medications can be discontinued or dosages reduced. In adults and adolescents, 52 percent had a significant reduction in seizure frequency, including 45 percent with ≥50 percent reduction in seizure frequency; 31 percent had no improvement, seven percent were unable to successfully initiate the diet, and ten percent had a >50 percent increase in seizure frequency. To be effective, the diet must be followed strictly. If it is discontinued seizures may return, even within hours. Unfortunately, there are long-term problems associated with the ketogenic diet. These include growth retardation in children, gallstones, metabolic abnormalities, recurrent infections, high cholesterol, high uric acid, vitamin deficiencies, and loss of bone mineral density. Kidney stones occur in five to eight percent of cases, as well.

A number of studies have found that PEMFs decrease seizure activity. PEMFs applied to the frontal, occipital, and temporal lobes resulted in rapid reduction of the electromagnetic brain activity of epileptics measured by magnetoencephalography (MEG). MEG is frequently used to identify the locations of seizure in the brains of epileptics prior to surgery, called seizure mapping. rTMS is being increasingly used in research for seizure treatment. rTMS reduces seizure frequency and/or epileptic discharges. In a patient with medically refractory partial seizures rTMS led to a 70 percent decrease in the occurrence of seizures and a 77 percent reduction in brain electrical spikes between seizures. rTMS applied to the top of the head with a round coil decreased the daily number of seizures in patients by 23 percent. rTMS in adults with medically intractable non-temporal lobe epilepsy for one week reduced the activity of all seizure types, complex partial seizures, and simple partial seizures by 19, 36, and 7 percent, respectively. A review of many studies found a 30 percent average rate of 50 percent seizure reduction with rTMS in the treatment of drug-resistant epilepsy. In general, rTMS is safe with minimal side effects experienced by only 18 percent of the study's participants. Side effects were mild, with headache or dizziness the most common. But, in about two percent of research studies, rTMS induced seizures, especially when rTMS was with faster pulses. The risk is small in children and similar to that in adults.

PEMF therapy for epilepsy or seizure disorder, targeted primarily to the brain, should also consider the possible causes of, or contributing factors to, seizures. These other causes or factors need to be managed, as well. Where there are no known or other contributing factors the focus of the treatment will be to the brain itself.

As with medication treatments for Parkinson's disease, PEMF therapy may make seizure medication even more effective. As a result, medications may produce more side effects. If this happens, the possibility of reducing the dose should be discussed with the treating doctor.

Intensity of the PEMF: 100-1000 gauss for "magnetic sandwich" application; 4000-7000 gauss for single coil local application.

Applicators: Portable small, battery-operated panels can be applied on both sides of the head as a "magnetic sandwich" when it is not known where the seizure focus in that area is. If the location of a seizure focus has been identified, then stacked applicators would be applied locally. A medium-intensity applicator can be applied to the side of the head and, if necessary, alternated. For high-intensity applicators, placements would depend on the type used: local applicators include a loop, butterfly, paddle, or pad. The loop coil may be placed over the top or side of the head. If flexible, it may be conformed into an elliptical form and placed over the top of the head and each side or the back of the head. The butterfly coil would be placed over the top of the head with a wing on each side. The paddle coil can be placed on the side of the head and moved from one side to the other. If the system allows two local applicators to be used as a "magnetic sandwich" and then place them on either side of the head.

Treatment Time: 30-60 minutes twice a day using a "low and slow" protocol. Treatment may be lifelong. With significant improvement, treatment times may be reduced for maintenance, guided by seizure activity. Repeat EEG and/or brain imaging may be useful to evaluate improvement in the seizure focus/foci.

Supplements: P5P 100-200 mg/D, magnesium citrate 500 mg/D, mixed tocopherols 400 IU/D, manganese 20 mg/D, L taurine 100 – 500 mg/D, thiamine 50 mg/D, methyl fully 3 mg/D, biotin 600 µg/D, D3 4000 IU/D, EPA/DHA 1 g/D and 0.7 g/D respectively. CBD 30-100 mg/D.

Erectile Dysfunction (ED)

Male sexual arousal is a complex process that involves the brain, hormones, emotions, nerves, muscles, and blood vessels. Erectile dysfunction can result from a problem with any of these. Likewise, stress and mental health concerns can cause or worsen erectile dysfunction. Common causes include heart disease, clogged blood vessels (atherosclerosis), high cholesterol, high blood pressure, diabetes, obesity, metabolic syndrome, Parkinson's disease, multiple sclerosis, some prescription medications, tobacco use, Peyronie's disease, alcoholism and other forms of substance abuse, sleep disorders, treatments for prostate cancer or enlarged prostate, or surgeries or injuries that affect the pelvic area or spinal cord. As men get older, erections can take longer to develop and not be as firm. Testosterone deficiency is also a common contributor (see **Testosterone** below).

Medications and supplements are the most commonly used treatments for ED. Injections can be useful for short-term benefit. Vacuum therapy has also been used with some success. PEMFs can be synergistic with any of these other therapies, increasing the benefit value of all of them.

PEMFs may help with ED by addressing many of ED's underlying factors or related health conditions. In addition, PEMFs help ED by direct stimulation of the pelvic nerves controlling erectile function, or to the pelvic blood vessels to provide adequate blood supply to erectile tissues. High-intensity treatment to the base of the penis has been found to improve tumescence and direction through a neural stimulation action, combined with improvement in blood flow. Treatment of the brain may help with anxiety and mood and assist in stimulating the production of testosterone. Stimulation of the penis directly will increase blood supply, allowing for a firmer erection. Stimulation of the testicles can increase the production of testosterone. Unless many of the underlying medical conditions behind the cause of ED are significantly improved the results are not likely to be sustainable. Most of the benefit for ED will come from stimulation at or near the time of need. The results are likely to be short-lived.

Intensity of the PEMF: Medium- to high-intensity local PEMF treatment with a focus on the genital area produces the best results. For any underlying medical conditions, including diabetes, vascular disease, etc., appropriate treatment of these conditions is necessary for better longer-term results. Review the relevant topics in this chapter for directions for these different conditions. For anxiety or to simply relax, review **Anxiety** above.

Applicators: For direct stimulation to the genital area a local applicator is used. For stimulation of the sacral nerves, a stronger local or regional applicator will be needed. For brain stimulation a high-intensity local applicator is needed, applied to the sides of the head slightly above the top of the ears.

Treatment Time: The treatment time needed will largely be determined through trial and error; 15 minutes may be all that is needed for a high-intensity system near the time of need. There is no risk in using much longer treatment times up to 30-60 minutes. For treatment time recommendations for related conditions, see the relevant topics.

Supplements: Some supplements to consider include vitamin B9 (folic acid), vitamin D, vitamin B3 (niacin), vitamin C, L-arginine, maca, tongkat ali, DHEA

50 mg, ginseng, and/or propionyl-L-carnitine. Be wary of "herbal Viagra" because they may contain unknown amounts of ingredients similar to the prescription medications, with the potential for significant side effects. I always emphasize the need for good nutrition and appropriate supplements.

Eye Conditions

The eye is composed mostly of fibrous connective tissue, thin epithelial cells, blood supply, and nerve type cells. Because of the arrangements of the tissues of the eyes, they are very responsive to PEMF stimulation. Considering the fact that eye tissues usually heal rapidly, PEMF therapy can enhance that healing and is a useful tool from both an effectiveness and safety perspective. Even extremely high-intensity PEMFs are routinely used on and around the head with no adverse reactions reported to the eyes.

A short list of eye conditions responsive to PEMFs includes:

- blepharitis
- chalazion/hordeolum
- conjunctivitis (redeye)
- contact lens issues
- corneal disorders
- corneal injuries
- dry eyes
- eye globe injuries
- floaters
- glaucoma
- macular degeneration
- orbital injuries
- post-procedure healing
- refractive errors
- retinal detachment
- retinal disorders
- retinitis
- uveitis

Because the eyes are not very deep into the body, low- to medium-intensity PEMFs will usually be sufficient. If somebody already has a high-intensity PEMF system, the lowest levels of intensity should be sufficient. The above conditions may be caused by infections, inflammation, blocked ducts, injuries, autoimmune disorders, vascular and nerve disorders, and muscle imbalances. Injuries and infections would be expected to resolve the fastest. Autoimmune disorders and retinal disorders should be considered to be systemic, whole-body problems even though they show up in the eyes as the only manifestation. That means that whole-body treatment may still be necessary to resolve the problem.

The recommendations for using PEMFs for eye conditions apply only to the eyes directly. For whole-body problems that may contribute to eye conditions see the relevant topics for guidance.

Intensity of the PEMF: Low- to medium-intensity PEMFs should be adequate if just treating the eyes. If high-intensity PEMFs are available for other reasons, use the lowest intensity settings.

Applicators: Local applicators. These can be placed directly over the eyes or to the orbital or temple bone at the side of the eye. Some PEMF devices have a small ring applicator which would encircle the eye and still allow a person to see. Local applicators, whether ringed or small flat pad, may be taped to glasses or the frames of glasses for convenience. If a larger local coil is used, it can be placed across the eyes, either coming down from the forehead or resting on the cheeks or placed at the temple next to the eye.

Treatment time: Most the time treatments would be between 15 to 30 minutes twice a day. For whole-body problems contributing to the eye condition, review the relevant topic(s) and guidance.

Supplements: Some supplements to consider include: Lutein, zeaxanthin, lycopene, L alpha-tocopherol or mixed carotenes, zinc, vitamin B1 (thiamine), omega-3 fatty acids, and vitamin C.
Fibromyalgia (see Chapter 9)

Fungal Skin Conditions

Skin conditions due to fungal infections can be local and regional. The most common fungal infections are toenail and groin, oral and vaginal yeasts, followed by skin. PEMFs increase the ability of the body to break down fungi and yeasts. Combining PEMFs with antifungal agents increases the effectiveness of killing the fungi. The combination treatment killed almost 90 percent of the fungi rapidly, versus only 43 percent with medication alone, even after a much longer exposure. Since antifungal therapies can be toxic, PEMF therapies combined with them could allow for much lower dosing with less risk of toxicity. In addition, while systemic therapies are often used for local tissue problems, PEMFs may allow for local tissue treatments, further reducing the risk of toxicity while improving benefit.

Fungal infections are much more common in those with immune issues, moist and warm local hygiene state and diabetes. Improving diabetes alone reduces the incidence of fungal infections.

PEMF therapy can be used for a fungal rash once it identified as a fungal infection. In the acute situation, medications probably are all that is needed. Once a fungal infection becomes chronic, especially to the hands, nails, and skin, PEMF therapy can be used alongside antifungal agents. Chronic fungal infections happen due to persistent environmental, genetic, immune, and metabolic host factors, as well as inadequate treatment.

Intensity of the PEMF: As with other skin conditions, local or regional PEMF therapy can be very effective because the skin is shallow. That means that a PEMF intensity of 50-100 gauss will be sufficient, when PEMF is applied directly to the affected area.

Applicators: Applicators are going to be local or large enough to cover an involved area. Larger area applicators may be best if having to treat all the toes and/or fingernails. PEMFs may need to be combined with antifungal medications or supplements for the best, fastest results.

Treatment Time: 15-30 minutes once or twice a day to the affected area until the infection is healed. Continue treatment until the tissues are healed. Once healed, if the conditions contributing to the infection are not removed, PEMF therapy may need to be started multiple times.

Supplements: The following supplements can help with fungal infections: caprylic acid, olive leaf extract, apple cider vinegar, undecylenic acid, grapefruit seed extract, garlic paste, colloidal silver, grapefruit seed extract, tea tree oil and neem, as they all contain antifungal properties.

Gall Bladder Disorders

Gallbladder disease (GBD) has a number of different facets to it. Most of the time it is associated with abnormal accumulation of cholesterol crystals, chronic inflammation, and challenges with gallbladder muscle function. If sufficient cholesterol crystals accumulate, over time, the gallbladder does not get rid of this concentrated bile (biliary sludge) appropriately and can lead to gallstones developing. Biliary sludge causes even more inflammation and pain in the gallbladder and doesn't allow the gallbladder to empty its contents properly, creating a vicious cycle. PEMFs may be the most helpful in the setting of biliary sludge. Biliary sludge is often associated with dysfunction of the sphincter of Oddi, a valve in the upper intestine that allows bile to be sent into the duodenum after a fatty meal. Sphincter of Oddi spasms can also lead to upper abdominal pain. Again, inflammation is the culprit. If inflammation progresses, gallstones are a common consequence. There can be recurrent gallstone attacks caused by spasms of the gallbladder and called biliary colic. Beyond biliary colic, gallstones can lead to cholecystitis, which is infection of the gallbladder. This does require surgery. Surgery is often required if the gallstones are ejected into the biliary system and lead to obstructions with jaundice or pancreatitis.

The proper management of GBD is to decrease the amount of cholesterol concentrating in the gallbladder, helping regular elimination of bile from the gallbladder, decreasing the concentration of the bile, and reducing the risk of inflammation. The basic approach to GBD is prevention, followed by reduction of progression of inflammation with PEMFs as aggressive nonoperative management. Gallbladder surgery should be a last resort except in the presence of a life-threatening condition.

Gallbladder surgery, even though it's a rescue therapy, creates its own complications long-term, which is why nonsurgical therapy approaches should be a priority. After a GB is removed, digestion is clearly affected because concentrated bile is no longer available to help with fat digestion. Fats are very important to physiologic and nutritional function, as they were before gallbladder disease and after removal of the gallbladder. In addition, one of the most common consequences of removing the gallbladder is bile reflux gastritis. Bile reflux into the stomach happens in about 80 to 90 percent of people after gallbladder surgery. Bile reflux is alkaline. Therefore, alkaline bile reflux is a contributing factor for chronic esophagitis or Barrett's esophagus. Esophageal reflux symptoms are seen in about 40 percent of people after cholecystectomy. Other symptoms include difficulty with swallowing and regurgitation. In addition, since bile reflux is alkaline, it reduces the normal acidity required by the stomach to do its proper tasks in breaking down food, destroying microbes in the stomach that produce vitamin B12.

PEMF therapy early in the course of GBD can be extraordinarily helpful in controlling symptoms and preventing progression. It is especially useful in gallbladder disease that does not involve gall stones. No matter whether stones are present or not, PEMFs will reduce inflammation and help gallbladder function. Once gallstones are present, it is not known whether PEMF therapies, along with other strategies, may decrease the gallstones. At the very least, with gallstones, PEMFs will help reduce pain and decrease GB irritability. PEMFs may also help to prevent or better control any infection. PEMFs are also more likely to help to prevent progression of stone formation, especially in the early stages of GBD.

Intensity of the PEMF: Treatment is local with a sufficiently high-intensity PEMF of a minimum of 100 gauss up to 4000 gauss. Lower-intensity PEMFs are expected to help the early stages and reduce symptoms. However, to be most helpful for reducing inflammation and improving gallbladder muscle function, higher intensities are likely necessary. A "low and slow" approach may be needed.

Applicators: Local or regional. Small, portable, battery-operated PEMF applicators can be placed over the surface of the upper right abdomen, at the right rib cage edge just before it slants to the side of the chest. Either two applicators can be used one above the other in the same area or two small applicators may be stacked one on top of the other over the painful area. A pad applicator may be used as well covering the whole area. With a high-intensity PEMF system, use a local applicator, either a butterfly coil, a paddle, or loop. If there is involvement of the pancreas or liver, these areas can be treated as well.

Treatment Time: Treatment time can be individualized. With smaller portable applicators treatments can be done for several hours at a time until symptoms subside for an episode of pain, 30 to 60 minutes two to three times per day at the beginning until symptoms have improved. Treatment time may be able to be backed off for maintenance. Maintenance treatments may need to be continued for one to two months. The only way to know that there is no inflammation in the gallbladder, other than symptoms, is to do ultrasound of the gallbladder to see if the gallbladder wall has shrunk or sludge is eliminated. Once GBD is diagnosed, the condition will be chronic unless removed surgically. That means that daily treatment is recommended, since the inflammation will be more or less permanent as long as cholesterol crystals or gallstones are present. If treatment is done in the early stages when there is only biliary sludge, repeat ultrasound three to six months later may be helpful to see if this has resolved. PEMF therapy is not likely to help with stones, except to reduce the pain from spasms of the gallbladder.

Supplements: Caffeine (two or more cups of coffee per day); five or more ounces of nuts per week; vitamin C 2000 mg twice a day, rowachol one capsule per 10 kg body weight/D, chenodeoxycholic acid 335 mg at bedtime or Jarrow Bile Acid Factors. Other supplements can also be considered, each having a different action on the whole biliary process: vitamin A, beet root, choline, vitamin E (mixed tocopherols), ginger, lecithin, magnesium, milk thistle, ox bile, psyllium husks, taurine, or curcumin.

Glaucoma

See the discussion above for **Eye Disorders**. The same rules and guidelines apply to glaucoma as with other eye conditions. The key for glaucoma and other eye conditions is that the earlier treatment is begun the better the results. Seeing improvements is more challenging when significant visual damage has been done already.

Heart Conditions

There are numerous heart conditions for which PEMFs can help significantly. Among the most common are atrial fibrillation, arrhythmias, cardiovascular, heart attacks, cardiomyopathy, heart failure, valvular heart disease, and pericarditis. These conditions are associated with inflammation, spasm of blood vessels, thrombosis, stenosis, and/or heart muscle strain. PEMFs help with atrial fibrillation and arrhythmias by reducing the sensitivity of the nerve or conduction pathways of the heart to stressful stimuli. PEMFs help with cardiovascular disease by opening the blood vessels of the heart to improve blood flow and helping with breaking down clot and formation of blood vessel plaque, most commonly through increasing nitric oxide production. PEMFs help heart attacks heal the damaged tissues by accelerating natural repair and increasing stem cell production. For cardiomyopathy and heart failure, PEMFs help with the function of the heart muscle by increasing ATP and general muscular energy, thereby helping with cardiomyopathy and heart failure. Whole-body PEMF therapy helps to dilate blood vessels in the whole body, decreasing the work of the heart. Pericarditis is inflammation of the lining of the heart, the pericardium. PEMFs decrease the inflammation of the pericardium helping to prevent scarring and constriction of the heart. Atrial fibrillation and arrhythmias are frequently caused by irritability of the heart's nerve conduction pathways caused by inflammation and vascular blockages.

The goal of PEMF therapy is to stimulate the heart directly and allow the PEMF to do the work it does naturally. The treatment of each one of the conditions causing heart problems is accomplished through the many actions of PEMFs. All of these actions are available to do the work the heart needs to function better and to heal. There is no specific magnetic field attribute unique for each function. General PEMF therapy to the heart is all that is needed. Since inflammation accompanies so many different aspects of heart conditions, this is the primary target for treatment. Therefore, guidelines for treatment will follow the intensities presented in Appendix A. How long treatment needs to be continued will depend on the condition of the heart and the overall condition of the person. PEMF treatment is likely to be needed for a long time, if not indefinitely, since people tend to start PEMF therapy late in the process of their heart disease. Atrial fibrillation, for example, most commonly takes years to develop because atrial fibrosis has to develop secondary to chronic inflammation.

Intensity of the PEMF: Given the dimensions of the heart and the chest, the minimum recommended PEMF is 4000 gauss. The going "low and slow" approach is necessary to determine the sensitivity of the heart to the stimulation. I have used a 200 gauss magnetic field over the heart for atrial fibrillation with some success in reducing the irritability of the heart to stimuli triggering the atrial fibrillation. Patients have reported significant reductions in stimuli triggering paroxysmal atrial fibrillation. In this case, the PEMF is worn over the heart for hours at a time, if not overnight. At that level of intensity, because of the natural decline of the magnetic field with distance from the surface of the chest, there is almost no likelihood of negative reactions.

Applicators: The most often recommended applicator will be local at a minimum intensity of about 4000 gauss. A butterfly coil with the wings pancaked or paddle applicators will be best, placed over the front of the chest. They can be held in place with an elastic wrap bandage, belt, or Velcro strap. A loop coil compressed to be elliptical can be wrapped horizontally around the chest from the side of the chest over the front to the breastbone. A high-intensity, whole-body PEMF system with "magnetic sandwich" capability may be useful without the need for local treatment. If necessary, a circular loop coil can be placed over the chest.

Treatment Time: A lower-intensity magnetic field may be used for extended periods of time, even hours a day. A medium- to high-intensity PEMF would be used for between 30 to 60 minutes twice a day. I have seen a non-PEMF, static, high-intensity magnetic field used 12 hours a day over the heart for a week at a time, for several weeks, with significant benefit for heart failure. In that case, a woman came in for treatments in a wheelchair due to severe heart failure. After several weeks of treatment, she was able to walk out and play golf.

Supplements: Supplements I frequently recommend to improve the function of the heart include: L-carnitine 1000 mg twice a day, magnesium 500 mg once or twice a day, L-taurine 1000 mg twice a day, CoQ10 1000 mg twice a day, and D ribose powder 3 g once a day. Many other supplements are available for heart treatment as well. As a result, I recommend consulting with a professional skilled in nutrition and supplements to give guidance on nutrition and the supplements that could be used. Doctors and cardiologists rarely make recommendations for supplements. I recommend reading the book "Metabolic Cardiology" by Dr. Stephen Sinatra.

Hepatitis, Viral and Autoimmune

Viral hepatitis is caused by a number of different viruses, some more severe than others. Much viral hepatitis is silent and the individual doesn't even know it's there. This is especially true for chronic hepatitis C, which long-term can turn into liver cancer due to the chronic inflammation caused by the virus. Autoimmune hepatitis can be triggered by viruses, food allergies, toxins, poisons, etc. It is not uncommon for chronic hepatitis to progress to a point of requiring a liver transplant. Aggressive PEMF therapy in these individuals could go a long way to extending life and liver function in preventing disability. Therapy would be even more aggressive if there is ascites.

To monitor results, liver function blood tests, including liver function tests (ALT, AST, alkaline phosphatase, bilirubin), fibrinogen, coagulation tests, albumin, ammonia, and immune markers, among others, could be followed regularly. Periodic ultrasounds and/or CT scans would be helpful as well. While it's possible, it's not certain that PEMFs would kill the virus. Viral load testing would have to be done to determine if that is happening. If the viral load returns to normal and liver function has also returned to normal, PEMF therapy may be scaled-back and used mostly for long-term health maintenance.

Research supports the possibility for PEMFs to help with severe liver inflammation, even viral infection, whether alone or with other therapies. I personally would not recommend relying solely on PEMFs in the setting of severe hepatitis. PEMF therapy alone can be used with good results in less severe cases of hepatitis, to limit the amount of liver damage caused by the viruses. The combination of viral therapy, steroids, and PEMFs would be expected to be synergistic. PEMF therapy should be able to be combined with medications to reduce viral load for even better, faster results. However, reducing viral load does not heal the liver. The body has to do that on its own, yet PEMF therapy would still be necessary to more completely heal the liver. The liver has a remarkable regenerative, healing capacity. PEMFs can stimulate regeneration of the liver by stimulating stem cells and fibroblasts to create new liver cells.

Intensity of the PEMF: Follow the intensity recommendations in Appendix A and, since the liver is a large organ, a magnetic field intensity of a minimum of 4000 gauss is recommended.

Applicators: A regional applicator can be used or a whole-body, high-intensity PEMF system. A regional applicator would include a half-body pad or an elliptical coil applied over the liver on the front of the lower chest and upper abdomen. Whole-body PEMF therapy should be done using a "magnetic sandwich" approach with the two pads or, if using a single pad and loop coil, apply the bottom of the two pads below the body as well as the loop coil on the front of the body.

Treatment Time: A "low and slow" approach should be used. The goal is to reach maximum intensity for an hour twice a day. Once significant results are achieved this may be able to be reduced to 30 minutes twice a day while monitoring test results. It is likely that treatment will be required for months followed by a maintenance protocol.

Supplements: Liver and antiviral supplements should be combined. At a minimum, liver supplements can include milk thistle, alpha lipoic acid, and acetyl cystine, acetyl l-carnitine, zinc, selenium, tocotrienols, licorice root, and vitamin C. There are many more possible antiviral supplements. As a result, I recommend consulting with a professional skilled in nutrition and supplements to give guidance on nutrition and the supplements that could be used.

Impaired Athletic Performance

In athletic competition, peak performance is the goal. To reach this optimal performance level, athletes train hard, sometimes harder than they should. Even if the training is appropriate, muscle fatigue results from the effort, and proper recovery and healing is important. When given adequate attention, recovery can allow athletes to thrive. But it can be difficult to allow enough time for recovery when participating in highly competitive sporting events.

After participating in competition, recovery usually takes between two and three days. Athletes push their bodies to the limit in competition, and that takes its toll. PEMF therapy is a safe, non-invasive treatment that can be used before injury to not only enhance athletic performance, but also reduce the risk of becoming injured through strenuous training and competition. PEMF therapy is also effective treatment when injuries do occur.

Years ago, people noticed that Eastern European and Russian Olympic athletes would be at the top of their game even after days of vigorous competition. These athletes were using PEMF devices to aid their recovery. Even by 1998, the Eastern Europeans had been using PEMFs for over 30 years, as I documented in my book *Magnetic Therapy in Eastern Europe: A Review of 30 Years of Research.*

Brain stimulation, including use of PEMF devices, is legal in the Olympics and most professional sports. Unlike doping, when PEMFs are used there are no chemicals added to the athlete's body. Instead, PEMF devices use the body's own natural electrical charges to heal cells and tissues, helping to relieve stress and soreness and reduce lactic acid in muscles. Many professional athletes worldwide use PEMF devices in their training and recovery.

With PEMF therapy, athletes can both enhance their performance and recover more quickly because PEMF therapy provides an energy boost and can also improve the condition of muscles, joints, tissues, and blood flow, as well as promote clear thinking. PEMFs also improve standing balance, indicating a more finely tuned and rapidly adaptive nervous system. All of these benefits can aid athletes in reaching their full potential.

PEMFs allow muscles to take in more oxygen, which in turn can significantly improve muscle performance and endurance. Muscle stimulation with PEMFs is stronger and less uncomfortable than electrical stimulation, allowing for higher peak torque muscle contractions with less discomfort—up to 215 percent higher. Some people have reported up to 60-70 percent improvement in overall performance after just a few weeks of using PEMF therapy. That's a huge difference, especially when you consider that at the competitive level, even a one percent improvement in performance can be the difference between winning and losing.

Muscles work harder and longer, and recover more quickly, with magnetic stimulation. Muscles that are used heavily during training and competition tend to spasm, and one classic action of magnetic field therapy is to reduce muscle spasms by stimulating the release of nitric oxide.

I've heard many stories firsthand about the power of PEMF therapy. One athlete I know of is able to continue performing at a world-class level into his 40s because of his regular use of PEMFs. A number of well-known professional and Olympic athletes, including football, baseball, and basketball players, also use PEMF therapy as a regular part of their training and recovery.

Studies have shown positive effects for athletes through the use of PEMF therapy, and research is ongoing to gain even more insight. Because PEMF devices stimulate the body's natural healing and self-regulating functions, they help optimize performance, accelerate recovery time, and reduce the risk of injury.

Research demonstrates that PEMFs stimulate a process called myosin phosphorylation, which produces energy in muscle. Phosphorylation produces ATP, which is crucial for cell energy. When ATP is depleted, muscles weaken. Strenuous training depletes ATP. That's why rest, which restores ATP, is so necessary after hard workouts. PEMFs help restore ATP quickly through stimulation of myosin phosphorylation, reducing recovery time.

Athletic training can also impact a protein called heat stress (sometimes called heat shock) protein, which is produced when cells are damaged through heating.

PEMFs can induce heat shock proteins before potential damage (such as before an intense workout) and reduce tissue damage.

Participation in any type of sport comes with some risk of injury. Most often, these injuries are caused by overuse of muscles and/or improper training methods. Many athletes push themselves to compete despite having an injury, which only make the injury more serious. Concussion is a common concern about many athletes. There is substantial research supporting the use of PEMF therapy for better and faster recovery from concussion. PEMF therapy does not leave the recovery from concussion to chance. Injury prevention is preferred, of course, and PEMF therapy can help with that. But if an injury does occur, PEMF therapy can help you heal sooner.

How PEMF Therapy Works to Enhance Performance: Your body's chemical reactions are stimulated by electrical signals, allowing cells to work more efficiently. PEMF therapy works at the cellular level to both boost energy production and protect against cellular breakdown, while simultaneously stimulating oxygenation of blood and tissues, and improving performance and endurance. PEMF therapy also induces proper reduction of lactic acid, which helps soothe sore muscles.

Injuries and stress on tissues produce swelling (edema), which delays the ability of tissues to receive the oxygen and nutrients they need. Ice is a common treatment for athletes, and ice will reduce superficial swelling, but it won't touch deep bruising or swelling in the muscles. PEMFs penetrate tissues deeply and completely, without risking harm to superficial tissues in the process, unlike ice, which can freeze these tissues, causing harm.

As PEMFs reduce swelling, blood is removed from a bruised area more quickly, leading to faster recovery and the ability to return to training or competition. Treatment before damage has settled into the tissue is preferred since, once this happens, healing takes longer. Another critical aspect to the function of athletes is adequate sleep. Battery-operated PEMFs applied under the pillow throughout the night help to ensure an adequate night's sleep.

Another benefit to athletes owning a PEMF device to use in their regular training routine is the versatility of use. Once you have the device, it can be applied to many different situations. This is why PEMF therapy can be considered the Swiss Army knife of health. This means that you'll already have what you need to use for enhancing performance, health maintenance, and injury recovery. Since there are always potential injuries, PEMFs' range of applications make a PEMF device ideal for athletes at any level.

Intensity of the PEMF: 100 – 7000 gauss. Lower-intensity PEMFs can be applied locally for mild, superficial injuries or problems and sleep using portable, battery-operated devices. Higher-intensity systems (4000-7000 gauss) will produce better/faster results with less treatment time needed. High-intensity "magnetic sandwich" systems would be the most efficient. Because of their weight and size, they may be less portable for use on the road. Ideally, athletes would have a combination of high-intensity and lower-intensity, portable devices.

Applicators: Small, portable local applicators. High-intensity local applicators for deeper/faster treatment and to target the brain to generate alertness and deal with any concussions. High-intensity regional applicators for treatment of larger areas, such as the back, hips, legs. High-intensity, whole-body PEMFs for maximum, rapid benefit before and after competition targeting large areas of the body for recovery, helping injuries and performance enhancement. The most efficient, cost-effective, high-intensity PEMF system would be a "magnetic sandwich" system.

Treatment Time: For basic health maintenance 30 – 60 minutes twice a day. For treatment of specific issues or areas of the body, typically, use a minimum of 30 – 60 minutes twice a day. Recommendations for very short treatment times, such as eight minutes, with very-low-intensity PEMF systems will produce very unreliable and limited results.

Supplements: This supplement list is a minimum and is additional to an adequate diet. Micronutrient deficiencies are common in intense physical performance. Multivitamin/mineral. For iron deficiency during intense competition 105-180 mg ferrous sulfate/D, magnesium citrate 4 mg/Kg/D, vitamin C 3000 mg 2X/D; glutamine 10 g after a marathon run; L arginine/L or anything 1 g each/D during intense training; calcium citrate 2000 mg/D during active competition with significant sweating; l-carnitine 4 g/D during periods of strenuous exercise; CoQ10 300 mg/D during fatigue-inducing workouts; zinc 30 mg/D plus copper to milligrams/D during periods of athletic performance; phosphatidylserine 750 mg/D during exhaustion-producing activity; wheat germ oil at 5 ml/D may be helpful for endurance.

Interstitial Cystitis/Bladder Pain Syndrome (IC/BPS)

Interstitial cystitis/bladder pain syndrome (IC/BPS) is a chronic pelvic pain syndrome (CPPS) of unknown cause and with no generally accepted treatment. There is no clear pathology associated with it. Symptoms of IC/BPS frequently overlap with other conditions, including irritable bowel syndrome, fibromyalgia, chronic fatigue syndrome (CFS/ME), anxiety disorders, and a number of other conditions not directly related to the bladder. Sometimes there are ulcerative lesions in the bladder. There may also be alterations in the lining of the bladder, the sensory/barrier functions of the bladder wall, nerve inflammation, possible autoimmune involvement, and perhaps "crosstalk" between different pelvic organs.

Chronic stress may be involved in the development, maintenance, and enhancement of IC/BPS. More than half of the people with IC/BPS have daily or constant pain and urinary frequency exacerbated by stress. Stress can induce exaggerated pain responses in many parts of the body, including the bladder.

Evidence shows that there is often reduced vagal activity resulting in sympathetic nervous system dominance that is a chronic fight/flight response. Just as chronic stress can create gastritis and gastric ulcers, the focus of the stress response can show up in the bladder. Because of the impact of the stress on the lining of the bladder, and even the rest of the urinary tract, water, urea and other toxic substances and infectious agents in the urine abnormally pass into the underlying tissues of the bladder. These substances may then affect the bladder muscle and nerves, setting up chronic inflammation and irritation.

The lower part of the bladder and urethra contain the largest density of bladder nerves. The irritability and inflammation present then activates these nerves to become overly sensitive to stimuli, which then create pain and the urge to empty the bladder, effectively causing a vicious cycle. In addition, this chronic irritability of the bladder and urethra, with the accompanying constant pain signals, sensitize the spinal cord and the brain. The sensitization of the spinal cord and the brain then leads to additional sensitization of the perception of filling and actions of the intestines in a vicious cycle. Hence the "crosstalk" from the intestines to the bladder and vice versa. These types of brain sensitization changes are also seen in fibromyalgia and prostate disorders.

The fact that numerous treatments are used for this condition suggests that there are no good answers. The results of treatment are frequently unsatisfactory. Spontaneous improvement happens in a significant percentage of cases. The goal of PEMF therapy is to decrease inflammation in the bladder, reduce spasticity, improve pain, help other pelvic inflammation causing "crosstalk," and help with stress and anxiety.

Intensity of the PEMF: Full distention of the bladder measures about 15 cm (~6 inches) from front to back. Then one has to add the distance from the skin over the lower abdomen to the front part of the bladder wall. Based on the goal of delivering about 15 gauss throughout the bladder to reduce inflammation, at least a 4000 gauss magnetic field is necessary. This level of intensity would be sufficient as well for treating the sacral nerves and the brain. Also see **Anxiety** and **Pain**.

Applicators: A local/regional PEMF applicator will work. Even better would be a "magnetic sandwich" approach, applying an applicator to the front of the abdomen above the pubic bone and one over the sacrum. This will stimulate both the bladder and the sacral nerves. An alternative set up would be to treat over the bladder and the brain at the same time. This type of double stimulation will make treatment times more efficient. An even more efficient approach would be to use a whole-body, high-intensity "magnetic sandwich" system, combining whole-body therapy along with whole-body/local therapy at the same time. This may be the most effective in reducing the general stress response in the tissues of the body.

Treatment Time: Each area should be stimulated for about 30 minutes twice a day. Once significant improvement in symptoms is seen, maintenance could be accomplished by 15 minutes twice a day. The body will tell you how much treatment time is needed and how often, once an initial course of treatment at the 30 minute level is done for at least a month. It may take weeks to months of twice-a-day treatments to determine whether this level of treatment time needs to be continued. If symptoms return any time treatments are cut back, this tells you that more treatment time is needed. Your body will tell you what your maintenance program needs to be to maintain the benefit. There is a chance that treatments will need to be continued indefinitely.

Supplements: L-arginine 500 mg 3X/D, quercetin 500 mg 2X/D, bromelain 200 – 400 mg/D, CystoProtek 6 capsules/D, magnesium 500 mg/D, mixed tocopherols 500 mg/D.

Intestinal (Bowel) Function

The intestinal tract includes the mouth, esophagus, stomach, small bowel, large bowel, and anal-rectal area. The tissues of the intestinal tract comprise most of the tissue types of the body, especially muscle, soft tissue, blood vessels, nerves, veins, lymphatics, secretory tissues, and valves. The intestinal tract is the largest absorptive and excretory organ of the body. It has more nerve cells in it than the brain, numbering in the trillions. The largest percentage of the immune system is housed in its walls. It is home to more non-human organisms than the whole-body itself has cells. This is the microbiome. PEMFs easily affect the intestinal tract. Some examples include relieving cramping of abdominal contractions, regulating bowel function, whether to slow it down or speed it up, healing bowel wall damage, improving circulation to the bowel itself, reducing inflammation, balancing immune function, and balancing stomach acid production. PEMFs increase the removal out of the body of stress hormones.

Treating the intestinal tract is not done in isolation. Any treatment of the abdomen will affect all organs in the abdomen, equally as easily and beneficially. In addition, any treatments to the abdominal wall will affect all the many acupuncture points and meridians in the area of the magnetic field to also give the multiple benefits of acupuncture, without the needles.

Intensity of the PEMF: Because of the effects on acupuncture points and meridians, a lower-intensity PEMF system can often work quite well for stimulating bowel function. However, to deal with inflammation, tissue healing and the microbiome directly, deeper in the belly, higher-intensity PEMFs would be necessary. The ideal would be at least 4000 gauss.

Applicators: A regional applicator would be best unless using a whole-body pad. Local applicators may provide some benefit but if results are not being seen, then applicators covering a wider area would need to be used.

Treatment Time: Treatment time will vary with need. It's possible to get results with even 10 to15 minutes, especially with higher-intensity PEMFs. For chronic problems, this should be done twice a day and carried on indefinitely until permanent results are seen. Treatments on and off over time are common as bowel function waxes and wanes. Part of this process will depend on underlying conditions in the abdomen at the time of treatment, including conditions such as Crohn's disease, irritable bowel syndrome, etc.

Supplements: The supplements for bowel function will depend on underlying causes of poor bowel function. A partial list to improve bowel function includes fiber, apple cider vinegar, probiotics, digestive enzymes, lactase, licorice, peppermint oil, ginger, chamomile, L-glutamine, aloe vera, artichoke, and/or bovine derived immunoglobulin concentrate. There are many more possible for bowel function. As a result, I recommend consulting with a professional skilled in nutrition and supplements to give guidance on nutrition and the supplements that could be used.

Joint Replacements and Implanted Prosthetics

Joint replacements and implanted prosthetics are becoming very common. Joint replacement prosthetic implants need to be integrated into the pre-existing bone. Implants are believed to cause faster osteoblast proliferation that can better promote osteo-integration. Surgeons doing an original joint replacement or implant often have to wait until a person is older to do the procedure because of the possibility that in ten to fifteen years the procedure will have to be redone. Revisions (also called re-dos) are usually more surgically complicated and challenging, with an increased risk of breakdown and complications. Loosening of the prosthesis inside the bone, whether due to loss of blood supply (avascular) or infection (septic), remains the main complication of joint replacement and is the cause of most revisions.

Revision prostheses have poorer outcomes compared with the primary joint replacement because the quality of the bone tissue where the next prosthesis is to be implanted is poor, with loss of bone mass and osteoporosis of the surrounding bone. Breakdown of bone around the implant, bone loss, poor natural bone-healing capability, and local inflammation are the main problems in reconstructive hip surgery and reduce the lifespan of revision implants even more than the primary implant. Inflammation produces enzymes that degrade tissue at the bone implant interface.

Because of the value of PEMFs in healing bone (see **Bone Healing and Repair**), PEMF stimulation has been found to significantly enhance the integration of implant materials, including titanium, stainless steel, and ceramic implants.

Even nails or rods implanted long before into the bone marrow of large bones for fractures, such as the femur, which became movable or unstable, improved and were integrated better into the bone.

Because of the impact of PEMFs on inflammation and strengthening the bone around the implant, it makes sense to consider PEMFs even before surgery is considered because PEMFs can stimulate the bone to prepare it for the surgical process. If the tissues are optimized prior to surgery, they would be expected to recover faster and the prosthesis would be placed into bone that is healthier. Many considering joint replacement already have a predisposition to problems by having osteopenia or osteoporosis. Since PEMFs clearly help with loosened prosthetics and in revision surgery, they would help to maintain the lifespan of a prosthesis, by keeping inflammation at a lower level.

PEMFs are best considered at an early stage of aseptic prosthetic loosening. Daily long-term use of PEMFs are needed to complete healing and, especially, to avoid revision surgery, as long as the prosthesis remains in the bone.

Most PEMFs, except for very-high-intensity fields, do not react with bone or metallic implants negatively. PEMFs at very high intensities should be used with caution because of the risk of aggravation of pain, usually due to significant inflammation still present in the area the prosthesis and to surgical damage to nerves anywhere along the prosthetic, from above to below. This is a reason to use the "low and slow" approach to magnetic stimulation.

Intensity of the PEMF: One of the primary goals of using PEMF therapy in the setting of joint replacements is to decrease inflammation while at the same time increasing bone formation around the prosthesis. The magnetic field intensity at the bone is 15 gauss. See Appendix A for the necessary magnetic field intensity. Smaller joints, such the hands, feet, and shoulders, would need less magnetic field intensity; 200 to1000 gauss would work. For knee replacements a minimum of 2000 gauss is needed. Hip replacements involve a bigger area and are deeper into the body. At four to six inches into the body a PEMF of 2000 to 4000 gauss would be best. High-intensity PEMF applicators are not contraindicated with prosthetics. **Caution should be used by gradually increasing the magnetic field to tolerance, using the "low and slow" approach.** If there is sufficient irritation in the area of the prosthesis, maximum intensity may not be able to be achieved, especially at the earliest stages of PEMF stimulation. As healing occurs and inflammation decreases, intensity may be able to be gradually increased.

Applicators: For most joint replacements, a local magnetic field applicator is all that is needed. If there is osteoporosis, many areas of the body with arthritis, diabetes, or other health conditions needing it, a whole-body PEMF system of at least 4000 gauss, preferably a "magnetic sandwich" type, would be best. (See **Osteopenia/Osteoporosis.**) If a lower-intensity PEMF system is used, extended treatment times may be needed and therefore a portable, battery-operated system may be best to allow more freedom of activity.

Treatment Time: For lower-intensity PEMFs extended treatment times may be needed, even as much as up to six hours per day, especially with fresh replacements or joint revisions. It would be easier to determine the treatment time if there are significant symptoms. As symptoms improve, treatment time may be gradually reduced. It's possible to do around three hours twice a day instead of six hours all at once. For high-intensity PEMFs, treatment time should be between one to two hours twice a day initially, followed by regular use for an hour twice a day, depending on tolerance. For long-term management, 30 minutes twice a day would probably suffice, depending on symptoms and tolerance. Ultimately, the amount of PEMF stimulation will be determined by clinical and/or imaging evaluations, which may indicate that more extended treatment time is needed.

Supplements: Bone can't be built without adequate nutrients to support bone development. At a minimum these would include vitamin D3 5000 IU per day, a general bone building formula, DHEA 25 mg per day, Ultra K2, Osteo-sil, Fructoborate 6 mg, and curcumin 3000 mg/day.

Kidney Disease

There are many kidney diseases, including autoimmune, hypertensive, diabetic, polycystic kidney, kidney stones, glomerulonephritis, nephropathy, nephrotic syndrome, pyelonephritis, hydronephrosis, among others. The end result of kidney diseases that is of concern is end-stage kidney failure or chronic kidney disease (CKD). The primary goals of using PEMFs for kidney disease is to improve circulation, decrease inflammation, improve kidney function, and heal damaged kidney tissue. As with most other health conditions, the sooner treatment is started in the process of chronic kidney disease the better. One of the goals in the treatment of polycystic kidney disease is to decrease inflammation, improve tissue health, and reduce the damage caused by recurrent infections. PEMF treatment of kidneys will be limited by the degree to which the underlying causes are controlled, especially for hypertension, diabetes, autoimmune disease, and kidney stones.

Intensity of the PEMF: Intensity is important because the depth of the kidneys in the body, which is typically from 5 to 7 cm (2 to 2.8 inches) from the front of the abdomen. The thickness of the kidneys is typically about 5 cm (2 inches) from the center of the kidney to the back of the kidney. If a PEMF applicator is placed over the anterior abdomen and the expected depth to reach the back of the kidney is about 4 inches, with the goal intensity being 15 gauss, the PEMF intensity would need to be at least 2000 gauss. This means that a PEMF system would need to be selected that can deliver at least this much magnetic field intensity to adequately target the kidneys. In adults, the kidneys are situated at a depth of 5-9 cm. (2-4 inches) from the skin of the back, and in two thirds of all persons the right kidney is higher than the left. Again, 2000 gauss or more would be optimal.

Applicators: The kidneys are located in the abdomen just along the spinal column. Local or regional applicators may be applied either over the abdomen or over the back. In the front of the belly, they would be placed on either side of the bellybutton, between the bellybutton and the bottom of the breastbone. In the back, they would be placed just below and over the lowest ribs. If a high-intensity, half-body pad is used it can be placed over the back, making sure that it reaches the lowest edge of the ribs. In the front, it would be placed in the center at the bottom edge of the breastbone. A butterfly coil may be opened out to be placed in the right locations. A circular coil bent into an elliptical shape may also be used over the front or the back. High-intensity, whole-body magnetic systems can be effective, including a "magnetic sandwich" system.

Treatment Time: The recommended treatment time, using the "low and slow" approach, is 30 to 60 minutes twice a day. Up to 60 minutes twice a day early in the course of treatment may be needed and then the time backed off as lab test results, symptoms, and imaging studies show improvement. Treatments should be considered indefinitely unless the underlying cause is removed or the kidney specialist says the kidneys are fully recovered. Even if the kidneys are not fully recovered, but are at least stable, PEMF therapy should continue in order to support and maintain kidney function. When PEMF therapy is discontinued, kidney function will often decline again.

Supplements: Supplements for kidney diseases include L-carnitine, methyl folate, B12, B6, thiamine, zinc, vitamin C, N-acetylcysteine (NAC), mixed tocopherols, omega-3 fatty acids, selenium, and CoQ10. For proper combinations, dosing, and use, I recommend consulting with a nutritionist skilled in working with chronic kidney diseases to give guidance on nutrition and the supplements that be used.

Lyme Disease, Chronic

Acute Lyme disease is notable by the bull's-eye rash, with or without other symptoms. If treated and symptoms last beyond six months, it is considered Post-treatment Lyme Disease Syndrome (PTLDS). Unfortunately, a large percentage of the time people have not realized they had a bite and therefore did not receive treatment. They can present to their doctors with many obscure and challenging symptoms. During their workups, they are discovered to be Lyme positive through antibody testing. These individuals can have more obvious damage to specific organs, especially the brain, the heart, and joints. Most often, symptoms are vague and nonspecific, and can be very debilitating. Fatigue, weakness, and brain fog are very common. Almost everybody has EBV antibodies. They can also have multiple co-infections with other organisms.

I call this syndrome chronic Lyme disease (CLD). Treatment of CLD is complex, controversial, and frustrating. Many people who are debilitated seek care from "Lyme-literate doctors," that is, doctors who specialize in Lyme disease. CLD is not recognized by conventional medicine at this time, so conventional medicine has little to offer these unfortunate individuals. Unfortunately, long-term use of antibiotics creates a new set of issues for these individuals. Since it is becoming increasingly recognized that a major part of CLD is autoimmune, this, and the presence of significant inflammation in the body, is the focus for the use of PEMFs. Additionally, PEMFs can help the body to better combat various kinds of infectious problems that may be persistent by enhancing immune function. PEMFs can safely help with many of the symptoms caused by CLD and help organs specifically and obviously affected, and help and augment any other therapies being used for CLD.

Because the nervous system is so frequently involved, I tend to approach CLD similarly to fibromyalgia. Please review the section on fibromyalgia. When specific organs are involved review the relevant organ sections, such as heart disease, kidney disease, hepatitis, arthritis, autoimmune conditions, etc.

The goals with PEMF therapy are to decrease inflammation, improve function and symptoms, whether overall or organ-specific, and to promote healing of the body.

Intensity of the PEMF: The intensity of the PEMF should be based on the target organs or symptoms. Going "low and slow" is very important in managing CLD because of the risk of aggravations. The ultimate goal is to get to the highest intensities tolerable in order to decrease inflammation throughout the body generally and the most significantly affected organs.

Applicators: Applicators depend on the specific areas of the body being targeted for treatment. Targeting specific organs may be the first stage of approaching the problem. Ultimately, CLD should be considered a whole-body condition, as would be the case for any autoimmune condition. Because of the risk of aggravations and the challenge in being able to tolerate higher intensities, I frequently recommend a whole-body PEMF that allows control over intensities, frequencies, and treatment time. This allows the greatest control for going "low and slow." Sleep is a common problem with CLD so the system chosen should be able to help with sleep. Another option would be to also add a portable, battery-operated PEMF system with multiple programs, that can be used for brain tuning throughout the day as needed, for example for brain fog and alertness, to help with anxiety, and at nighttime to help with sleep, etc.

Treatment Time: 30 to 60 minutes twice a day, as tolerated. Some people may need several hours a day to get the best results. The need for treatment is likely to be long-term until the various treatment strategies being implemented are effective.

Supplements: See the supplement recommendations for **Autoimmune, Fibromyalgia,** and the specific organs involved.

Memory Loss

About 40 percent of people over age 65 experience some memory loss. It is known as "age-associated memory impairment" if there is no medical condition that causes this loss of memory. Then, it is considered part of normal aging. Alzheimer's disease and other dementias are not part of normal aging.

Age-associated memory changes are often seen as:

- not being able to remember the details of a discussion or incident that took place a year earlier
- not being able to remember the name of a friend
- forgetting stuff and incidents
- occasionally have trouble finding words
- you're concerned about your memory, but your family isn't.

The hippocampus is responsible for memory and is known to shrink with age. It is an area of tissue deep into each side of the brain at the level of the bottom part of the ear. The hippocampus links two unrelated things together into a memory, like the place you left your keys or your new neighbor's name. The hippocampus plays an important role in the formation of new memories about experienced events. When the hippocampus is not functioning normally, spatial orientation is affected; people may have difficulty in remembering how they arrived at a location and how to proceed further. Getting lost is a common symptom of amnesia. Research found that dysfunction of these connections increases with age, explaining the causes of memory loss as we get older.

Research shows that high-intensity PEMF stimulation of the parietal area of the brain impacts the memory associated with the hippocampus. The magnetic field penetrates deep enough into the brain through the parietal area into the hippocampal area to improve memory. Research found that recollection improves by about 31 percent with high-intensity rTMS PEMF stimulation for five days. Memory tasks of the older individuals improved so much that they appeared similar to the younger control group. In other words, memory loss was reverse-aged with active PEMF stimulation. But memory improvement did not last for a week afterwards. It is not known whether longer episodes of stimulation would work better, whether stimulation beyond five sessions would work better, whether high-intensity PEMF stimulation to other areas of the brain would produce similar or better results, whether stimulation with lower-intensity PEMF systems would be as effective, and whether similar memory improvements could be seen in dementia or early-stage Alzheimer's disease. Other high-intensity brain stimulation research has already found benefits for Alzheimer's disease. But, as is seen with many other conditions, the sooner treatment begins relative to memory loss the better the results. Waiting until Alzheimer's disease has clearly been established is less likely to produce the same benefits as treating age-related memory loss earlier. Nevertheless, these results are exciting, not only assuring that high-intensity PEMF stimulation is safe, but also that this PEMF therapy actually improves age-related memory decline.

Based on the results of this research, I recommend daily use of a home-based PEMF system, preferably of high intensity, to encourage not only temporary improvement in memory but also to rebalance the brain tissues, hopefully reversing the age-related decreases in function of the hippocampal area. For convenience, a portable PEMF unit may be able to help as much, is likely to be used regularly, and is certainly more affordable. Otherwise, if someone already has a higher-intensity PEMF system, this can be used regularly to the parietal area of the brain, preferably daily.

Intensity of the PEMF: Medium-intensity 100-1000 gauss or 4000-7000 gauss. **Applicators:** For medium-intensity devices, place a coil on each side of the head just above the top of the ear and slightly to the back of the head. For high-intensity systems, use the local applicators, including loop, butterfly, paddle, or pad. The loop coil can be placed over the top or side of the head. If flexible, it can be conformed into an elliptical form and placed over the top of the head and each side or the back of the head and each side. The butterfly coil would be placed over the top of the head with a wing on each side. The paddle coil can be placed on the side of the head and moved from one side to the other. For a high-intensity, whole-body PEMF with or without "magnetic sandwich" capability, a coil in the whole-body pad may be placed under the head.

Treatment Time: 15 to 30 minutes twice a day.

Supplements: B12 5000 µg/D, P5P 100 mg/D, methyl fully 3 mg/D, niacin 50 mg 3x/D or 1.5 g/D, thiamine 100 mg/D, magnesium citrate 500 mg/D, acetyl l-carnitine 2000 mg/D, beta-carotene 50 mg/D, phosphatidylserine 300 mg/D, ginkgo biloba 120 mg/D and/or DHEA sulfate 10 – 25 mg/D.

Migraine (See **Headache and Migraine** in Chapter 9)

Multiple Sclerosis (MS)

Individuals with MS have inflammation, destruction of the myelin sheath covering nerves in the brain and spinal cord (demyelination), scarring of brain tissue, nerve cell degeneration, and dysfunction resulting from immune system imbalances. Inflammation causing demyelination predominates in the relapsing/remitting phase of MS and is seen as recurrent episodes of worsening and improvement (exacerbation and remission). Neurodegeneration, leading to extensive brain nerve cell (neuronal) damage, occurs at the same time as inflammation in progressive stages of the disease.

PEMFs act as a potential antibacterial, anti-inflammatory, and general brain tissue regenerative treatment method, among all the other known benefits of PEMFs when it comes to managing MS. PEMFs, although not creating a cure (there is no known cure for MS), can alleviate many of the major symptoms, including spasticity, fatigue, cognitive function, mood changes, and other impaired physiologic functions, as well as improve quality of life. Even though MS starts in the brain and spinal cord, it ultimately affects the functioning of the whole body. Because PEMFs act at such basic cellular and physiologic levels throughout the whole body, including the brain and spinal cord, they become a valuable tool to improve function and enhance the quality of life of individuals with MS.

Most of the recent research on MS has been done using high-intensity PEMFs applied to the brain and/or spinal cord. Bladder and bowel control issues associated with MS are best treated by targeting the brain, since that's where the spasticity is caused. Whole-body PEMF is especially helpful to keep the vitality of the tissues healthy and to reduce the progression of the MS process. Ideally, PEMFs should be started as soon as MS is diagnosed. The sooner treatments are begun, the better the results and the likelihood of a reducing the progression. Most medications for MS decrease the severity of flares and symptoms but they do not help much to stop progression. Treatment of MS will be lifelong.

Intensity of the PEMF: Since the whole brain and upper spinal cord are typically involved, high-intensity PEMF is best, with a minimum intensity of 4000 gauss for the brain. While lower-intensity brain and whole-body PEMFs can provide some benefit, they are probably acting primarily through the acupuncture system. As a result, they can help with symptoms and function to some degree but will not help to decrease inflammation deep in the brain or the spinal cord, or help to repair brain and nerve tissue. Also, since bacteria have been implicated in the brain as a cause of MS, the PEMF needs to be deep enough to target those areas, typically around the areas where the plaques are. A "low and slow" approach is recommended.

Applicators: High-intensity local applicators will be able to target the brain and spinal cord. A butterfly coil may be optimally placed with each wing of the butterfly on either side of the head with the connecting part over the top. Another alternative is to place the butterfly coil over the back of the neck with the wings coming around to the sides of the neck and head, especially for upper spinal cord lesions. A loop coil may be conformed to be elliptical and wrapped from the back of the head around to the sides of the head. The preferred treatment would be a high-intensity, whole-body "magnetic sandwich" system with a loop coil. The two larger pads would be used for one session, followed by treatment with the lower body pad combined with the loop coil applied to the brain. If either local or whole-body high-intensity treatments do not help with sleep, a portable PEMF system with a sleep mode is recommended for treatment all night long. This would also help with the brain as well as the sleep.

Treatment Time: Early in the course of treatment, a total treatment time of 60 minutes twice a day is recommended. If significant symptoms are still present in the middle of the day, an extra session can be added then. As symptoms improve, total treatment time may be reduced to whatever is needed without symptoms returning. Treatment will be lifelong.

Supplements: Supplements to consider include omega-6 fatty acids, omega-3 fatty acids, vitamin B12, L-carnitine, acetyl L-carnitine, vitamin D3, vitamin B3, L-threonine, curcumin, CBD, palmitoylethanolamide (PEA) 600 mg twice a day, methyl folate, and melatonin. Though not a supplement, I frequently recommend the compounded prescription of low dose naltrexone (LDN) 3 mg per day. Other supplements can be added as needed depending on symptoms. For this reason, I recommend consulting with a professional skilled in nutrition and supplements, preferably with expertise in MS or neurology, to give guidance on nutrition and the supplements that could be used.

Obesity

The causes of obesity are complex. PEMFs are not normally thought of as helping this problem because obesity is considered caused by sluggish metabolism, hormone imbalances, lack of exercise, and poor nutrition. For many people, food addiction is another major cause of obesity. The reward pathway in the brain is the same for food addiction as for other addictions. Another underlying cause of obesity may be impaired gut bacteria (microbiota) composition, an imbalance in the complex mix of beneficial and harmful microorganisms that inhabit the digestive tract. Impaired gut microbiota can alter the brain's signals for appetite and satiety (fullness). Stress hormones affect the gut microbiome to contribute to obesity. Since PEMFs help with stress reduction they can also help with restoring the microbiome, as well as helping to reduce the size of fat cells, thus helping with reduction of waist size. PEMFs may also help to reduce the production of fat cells by changing the stem cells in the abdominal tissues to not produce fat cells.

Abdominal obesity is also associated with a significant amount of inflammatory molecule production. These inflammatory molecules circulate into the body affecting the brain and the rest of the body. They create sluggishness, depressing the drive to move and exercise.

PEMFs can help with obesity in many different ways, especially when combined with appropriate nutrition, behavioral modification, and increased physical activity.

Intensity of the PEMF: One strategy is to target the brain with high-intensity local PEMF therapy to reduce stress and stimulate the reward centers. Because of the production of inflammatory cells by the fatty tissue, PEMF treatment of the abdomen may be very helpful to reduce inflammation. In addition, treatment of the abdomen with a higher-intensity regional PEMF system will help with the microbiome aspects that lead to increased weight, as well as decreasing fat cell size. The optimal PEMF therapy would be to use a high-intensity, whole-body "magnetic sandwich" system which would allow all these components to be treated at the same time. In addition, many people with obesity have many other health issues, including body aches and pains, diabetes, vascular disease, and arthritis, all of which a whole-body PEMF system would help, as well as the whole-body in general. Lower-intensity whole-body PEMF systems may also help by stimulating the acupuncture system, producing a greater sense of wellness. Unfortunately, this would not help with many of the other problems present and would not do that well with inflammation, unless the system was producing at least 15 gauss.

Applicators: See above. High-intensity local and/or regional or high-intensity whole-body, preferably a "magnetic sandwich" system.

Treatment Time: Unless there are other significant health issues, treatment time should be 30 minutes twice a day to each area being treated. A whole-body system will decrease the total time needed for treatment.

Supplements: Calcium 600 – 1000 mg per day, vitamin C 3000 mg per day, borage seed/evening primrose oil (GLA) 2 – 4 g per day, L-carnitine 3 g per day, curcumin 3000 mg per day, and/or CBD. Supplements can also be used for stress-reduction, anxiety, addiction, sleep, calorie-burning enhancers and appetite stimulants. Because of the complexity of managing obesity, I recommend consulting with a professional skilled in nutrition and supplements, preferably with expertise in weight loss and obesity, to give guidance on nutrition and the supplements that could be used.

Osteopenia and Osteoporosis

Osteopenia and osteoporosis are caused by reduction in bone mineral density. Bone loss is most common in women and is common enough that it is recommended to screen women at age 50 with bone-density testing. Bone mineral density in women begins to change in their 40s. By age 50, a significant percentage of women show the beginnings of bone loss, osteopenia, or actual osteoporosis. Even women who are very active can still develop reduced bone mineral density. Most bone loss happens because of a significant reduction in hormones, especially estrogen, progesterone, and testosterone. Hormone treatment should really involve replacement of all of these hormones using bioidentical hormone replacement therapy. Women who do not have an adequate "bone bank," are the most vulnerable to the natural loss of hormones as they enter into perimenopause and menopause. The "bone bank" is the reserve of bone developed in the teens and early 20s. The more active women were at these ages, the better preserved their bones will be as they go through the menopausal transition.

There are many other causes of osteopenia and osteoporosis, including steroid use, being bedridden, chemotherapy, celiac disease, autoimmune disease and chronic inflammation, cigarette smoking, excessive alcohol, genetic factors, hyperthyroidism, diabetes, and aluminum-containing antacids, among other factors.

The medications used to treat osteopenia and osteoporosis create numerous problems years after use. Initial approval by the FDA of these medications only followed two years of use. Women are frequently placed on these medications for many years. Among the problems caused by bisphosphonates and immunotherapy is an increased risk of fractures several years later, since these agents limit the bones' ability to heal itself and withstand stress. Moreover, they do not do a good job of restoring bone. Basically, all they do is to restrict the amount of breakdown naturally seen with hormone withdrawal or hormone blockade but do nothing to help to build bone. Unfortunately, once bone loss happens, it is very difficult using any method to restore it completely.

Most therapies simply stop further bone loss. As a result, it is very important to start treatment for bone density issues as early as possible after it is identified. All women should have bone density measurements at age 50 and treatment strategies should begin as soon as possible to prevent any further bone loss. Bone density testing just evaluates bone loss locally, that is, either the heel, the wrist, or the lumbar spine and a hip area. Osteopenia/osteoporosis are whole-skeleton problems, requiring whole-skeleton treatment.

PEMFs are an ideal treatment for maintaining and modestly restoring bone density. As discussed earlier in **Bone Healing and Repair**, PEMFs have been found to be important tools to help build bone. Low-intensity PEMFs, between 12 to 18 gauss, were approved by the FDA over 20 years ago to treat local bone lesions following nonunion fractures and help preserve bone implants used in spinal fusions. These were applied locally over the bone but were not designed for whole-body skeletal treatments. Even applied locally, these PEMFs were used for between 4-12 hours per day to heal the nonunion in three to twelve months, depending on severity and physical factors.

The goal with PEMFs is to treat the whole skeleton with at least 12 to 18 gauss and even higher intensities applied over the hips and spine. With higher intensities, treatment times can be significantly shorter. The results will depend on the control of other factors contributing to the osteopenia/osteoporosis, such as lack of exercise, control of inflammation and autoimmune disease and use of a gluten-free diet.

Intensity of the PEMF: Since the whole skeleton is being treated and the magnetic field has to penetrate throughout the body, high-intensity whole-body PEMF system is needed of at least 4000 gauss. The PEMF therapy along with bone-building supplements is expected to halt the progression of osteopenia/osteoporosis, with some possible mild improvement in the bone density as well.

Applicators: A whole-body "magnetic sandwich" system will produce the best results, not to mention the general whole-body benefit for other health needs. An inadequate fallback position would be to simply treat the lumbar spine and hips.

Treatment Time: For osteoporosis the ideal treatment time would be 60 minutes twice a day. For osteopenia, 30 minutes twice a day could suffice if underlying factors are removed.

Supplements: Bone can't be built without adequate nutrients to support bone development. At a minimum, these would include vitamin D3 5000 IU per day, a general bone-building formula, DHEA 25 mg per day, Ultra K2, Osteo-sil, Fructoborate 6 mg, and curcumin 3000 mg/day. Other possible supplements for bone building are copper, strontium, vitamin C, and vitamin A.

Pain Management

Pain management with PEMFs is discussed in detail in Chapter 9. The treatment of the brain is vital for effective management of pain conditions. Treating the brain with PEMFs is essentially the same as discussed in other conditions where the brain is the target of treatment. (See **Chronic Fatigue Syndrome, Fibromyalgia, Concussion** and **TBI**.)

Pancreatic Conditions

Some of the more common pancreatic conditions include diabetes, exocrine pancreatic insufficiency (EPI), pancreatitis, pancreatic cancer, and cystic fibrosis.

EPI is a deficiency of pancreatic enzymes, resulting in the inability to digest food properly, or maldigestion. The pancreas produces three main types of enzymes—amylase, protease, and lipase—that help with food digestion, especially starches, protein, and fat. The primary causes include pancreatitis, cystic fibrosis, pancreatic duct obstructions, diabetes, celiac disease, Crohn's disease, and gastrointestinal surgical procedures.

This discussion will focus on pancreatitis, which has two forms, acute and chronic. Mild cases of pancreatitis can be very painful, but can go away without treatment, but severe cases can be life-threatening. Causes include alcoholism, gallstones, high calcium levels, high triglyceride levels, infection, significant obesity, abdominal surgery or injury, certain medications, cystic fibrosis, and pancreatic cancer, as well as endoscopic retrograde cholangiopancreatography (ERCP), a surgical procedure that combines upper gastrointestinal endoscopy and X-rays to treat problems of the bile and pancreatic ducts. Episodes of pancreatitis can lead to pancreatic cysts and infections, diabetes, EPI, and pancreatic cancer.

There are no specific medical therapies for pancreatitis. Most of the time, general support and fasting, pain medications and intravenous fluids are the therapies used. PEMF therapies can be very important for pancreatitis. Unfortunately, PEMF therapies are not allowed in the hospital setting. That means that people with a history of pancreatitis, whether one episode or multiple, should be using PEMF therapy daily to decrease the destruction of the pancreas by its own enzymes and infection. The pancreas' own enzymes "auto-digest" the pancreas. The purpose of PEMF therapy is to decrease the inflammation which is the cause of the leakage of auto-digesting enzymes. In addition, PEMF therapy can be extraordinarily helpful with the pain associated with pancreatitis, both acute and chronic. Clearly, the underlying conditions need to be managed, if possible, to prevent recurrence, for example alcoholism and gallbladder disease. (See **Gallbladder Disease**.) Anybody with pancreatic cysts has chronic inflammation and should be doing regular PEMF therapy.

Intensity of the PEMF: The pancreas is not that deep in the body so higher medium-intensity or lower high- intensity local PEMF devices should be adequate. Intensities should range from 1000-4000 gauss to provide adequate anti-inflammatory and healing action.

Applicators: The pancreas is about six inches long, sitting just below and behind the stomach, so the applicator should be wide enough to treat this area. A butterfly, paddle, or loop coil (shaped into an ellipse) will work.

Treatment Time: The "low and slow" approach should be used because of the amount of inflammation that may be present. Intensity and treatment time should be adjusted as tolerated. Ultimately, in the initial stages, treatment should be gradually increased until 60 minutes is tolerated twice a day. Once control of pain is achieved, and normal nutrition is resumed, treatment may be able to be used long-term daily over months for at least 30 minutes twice a day. Pancreatic enzyme lab tests, including amylase and lipase, would be followed by the doctor to see if they improve. Imaging with ultrasound of the pancreas may be needed to determine if there is a reduction in the size of cysts or swelling or inflammation.

Supplements: Raw soy flour 30 Gm 3X/D4 30 days, enteric-coated pancreatic enzymes 1–2 with each meal for one to two months, selenium 600 µg/D, mixed tocopherols 400 IU/D, vitamin C 2000 mg, beta-carotene 5.4 mg/D, methionine 2 g/D, magnesium citrate 500 mg/D, zinc 50 mg 3X/D + copper 1-4 mg/D (not if there is cirrhosis), glutamine 30 g/D glutamine, omega-3 fatty acids 3.3 g/D, CBD 25-100 mg 1-3X/D. Other supplements and nutritional advice may be needed for EPI. As a result, I recommend consulting with a professional skilled in nutrition and supplements to give guidance on the nutrition and the supplements that should be followed.

Paraplegia and Spinal Cord Injury (SCI)

One of the most important uses of PEMFs in spinal cord injury is general support, including especially the reduction of spasticity and neurogenic or overactive bladder, and improvement of bowel function. This is covered in other topics in this chapter, specifically, **Multiple Sclerosis** and **Bladder Conditions**. Spinal cord injury is often associated with pain, the general vitality of tissues in the body below the level of the injury, functional problems in the organs that do not receive adequate spinal cord nerve support, pressure sores, joint and ligament laxity, mood changes, and inability to maintain muscle mass, among many other issues, requiring special care to facilitate physical therapy and rehab.

PEMFs will not reverse the spinal cord injury. Spinal cord injury is a complex problem that varies tremendously from person to person. From this perspective, it is hard to generalize the benefits from one person to the next.

PEMFs may help the body to regenerate spinal nerves, however, at least based on animal research. In addition, in a human study, non-invasive stimulation using a technique called paired associative stimulation (PAS) was studied as a long-term treatment for chronic, incomplete SCI of traumatic origin. PAS is a noninvasive neuromodulation approach using transcranial magnetic stimulation (TMS) of the motor cortex combined with peripheral nerve electrical stimulation (PNS). After about six months of the stimulation, a paraplegic could bend and flex both ankles. The new voluntary movements could be performed by other patients for at least one month after the last stimulation session. PEMFs to the brain (TMS) aim at sparing or restoring at least part of spinal nerve function at the acute stage by strengthening weak spinal cord connections that are spared or restored. In fact, frequent home-based use of high-intensity PEMF stimulation to the brain and spinal cord may reveal the degree to which function still exists and what further improvement may be discovered with continuing stimulation.

Intensity of the PEMF: 4000-7000 gauss is necessary for adequate penetration of the spinal cord and brain, to reduce inflammation in the area of the spinal cord lesion, and to provide additional stimulation for enhancing brain plasticity, reduce spasticity, and improve bowel and bladder function. This level of intensity is also adequate for helping to improve the general vitality of the body and to help with mood.

Applicators: The most benefit will be gained with whole-body stimulation using a "magnetic sandwich" system. If this is not feasible, a local high-intensity PEMF system would still be of significant benefit, although several areas of the body would have to be targeted separately.

Treatment Time: Treatment time will depend on the level of damage and how many areas of the body need to be targeted. At the very least, the brain and the area of the spinal cord lesion will be targeted. A minimum of 30 minutes per area is recommended, using a "low and slow" approach.

Supplements: Suggested supplements include thiamine, magnesium, pyridoxal-5-phosphate (P5P), vitamin B 12 (methylcobalamin), methyl folate, pantothenic acid, acetyl l-carnitine, alpha-lipoic acid - 600 mg, L-glutamine, Agmaset, ubiquinol CoQ10, omega-3 fish oil, astaxanthin and/or vitamin D3. Other supplements and nutritional advice may be needed as well. As a result, I recommend consulting with a professional skilled in nutrition and supplements to give guidance on the nutrition and the supplements that should be followed.

Parkinson's Disease

Parkinson's disease (PD) is primarily a chronic and progressive movement (motor) disorder, the symptoms of which continue and worsen over time. The cause is unknown, and there is no cure. Conventional treatment options include medication and surgery to manage symptoms. Neither treatment approach reduces PD progression.

PD most obviously involves the malfunction and death of vital nerve cells (neurons) in the brain, primarily in an area of the brain called the substantia nigra. These neurons produce dopamine, a neurochemical that sends messages to the part of the brain that controls movement and coordination, and a broad array of behavioral processes such as mood, reward, addiction, and stress response.

The intestines also have dopamine cells that degenerate in Parkinson's, and this may be important in the gastrointestinal symptoms that are part of the disease. Dopamine is also produced in other areas of the body, including the autonomic nervous system, gut epithelial cells, and immune cells (dendritic cells, regulatory T cells, B cells, and macrophages). About 50 percent of dopamine in the body is produced in the gastrointestinal tract by enteric neurons, intestinal epithelial cells, and by gut microbiome bacteria, including bifidobacteria and Bacillus species. This dopamine then ends up in the liver and into the rest of the body. There is crosstalk between the gut and the liver.

Besides its brain functions, dopamine has also been shown to regulate immune responses in the body, and has been related to tumor immunity and several autoimmune diseases, including inflammatory bowel diseases, multiple sclerosis, and rheumatoid arthritis. As PD progresses, the digestive tract will slow down and function less efficiently, leading to increased bowel irritability and constipation. These facts are important in deciding where PEMF should be targeted in Parkinson's disease.

The amount of dopamine produced in the brain also decreases as PD progresses, leaving a person unable to control movement normally. Loss of cells in other areas of the brain and body contribute to Parkinson's. For example, researchers have discovered that the hallmark sign of PD—clumps of a protein, alpha-synuclein, which are also called Lewy bodies—are found not only in the mid-brain but also in the brain stem and in scent function cells. These areas of the brain correlate to non-motor functions such as sense of smell and sleep regulation. The presence of Lewy bodies in these areas could explain the non-motor symptoms experienced by some people with PD before any movement (motor) signs of the disease appear.

Standard medication treatment of PD is only 50 percent effective overall. As the dose of taken medication is wearing off there can be a decline in benefits. For example, in the morning, shortly after taking it, the medication may be 90 percent effective, in the afternoon only 50 percent effective, and in the evening only 30 percent effective. This is why PEMFs should be considered.

Twice-weekly treatments with extremely-low-intensity PEMFs applied to the head for ten weeks has been shown to eliminate the daily declining benefit symptoms. At ten weeks after starting the PEMFs, there was 40 percent improvement in response to medication with minimum change in benefit during the course of the day or evening. PEMFs appeared to enhance response to medication. Since decline in the response to medication is a phenomenon associated with progression of the disease, these results suggest that daily use PEMFs may reverse the course of progressive PD.

Intensity of the PEMF: 4000 to 7000 gauss in order to target the whole brain and the abdomen.

Applicators: Either local or regional high-intensity applicators for the brain and abdomen. These would be applied separately to the brain and abdomen. This could include a butterfly coil opened up to treat the whole brain, by placing the wings of the butterfly coil on the sides of the head above the ears with the connecting part at the top of the head. It could be placed opened up over the middle of the abdomen. If the loop coil is used, it would be formed into an ellipse or dumbbell shape and placed horizontally across the middle of the abdomen at the level of the bellybutton. A whole-body, "magnetic sandwich" system would be the most efficient. Individuals with PD often have other health issues, all of which could be managed best by this type of whole-body system.

Treatment Time: Treatment of the brain itself may require between 30 to 60 minutes twice a day. The abdomen itself may only require about 15 minutes unless there are other abdominal needs. The time can be adjusted based on the results. With the high-intensity whole-body system total treatment time would be about 30 to 60 minutes twice a day. The loop coil can be used separately if needed over the brain and/or abdomen.

Supplements. Supplements to consider include CoQ10, B6, riboflavin, B3, NADH, D3, mixed tocopherols, vitamin C, octocosanol, D-phenylalanine, L-tryptophan, methionine, L-tyrosine and/or glutathione, and probiotics which include bifidobacteria and Bacillus species.

Premenstrual Syndrome and Dysmenorrhea

Premenstrual syndrome (PMS) is a combination of symptoms that many women experience about a week or two before their period. Over 90 percent of women report they get some premenstrual symptoms, such as bloating, headaches, and moodiness. The symptoms of PMS are usually mild or moderate, but 20 to 32 percent of women report moderate to severe symptoms that affect some aspect of life and 3 to 8 percent have premenstrual dysphoric disorder (PMDD). The severity of symptoms varies by individual and by month.

PMDD causes severe irritability, depression, or anxiety in the week or two before your period starts. Symptoms usually go away two to three days after your period starts. Symptoms may include:

- anger or irritability
- anxiety and panic attacks
- depression and suicidal thoughts
- difficulty concentrating
- fatigue and low energy
- food cravings or binge eating
- headaches
- insomnia
- mood swings

The goal of PEMFs is to decrease or eliminate the pelvic symptoms and, for those who have PMDD, to reduce the severity of the PMDD. It is expected that

PEMFs would decrease inflammation and swelling that contribute to the bloating and pain. It's possible with regular pelvic therapy and brain stimulation that there may not only be a reduction in symptoms but also, potentially, a stop to PMS and PMDD from occurring altogether. PEMF treatment may also decrease or eliminate the need for birth control pills or hormones. More severe PMDD is often treated with SSRIs, through the whole cycle or only after ovulation. These drugs may have undesirable side effects and be difficult to withdraw. PEMFs would be applied between days 17 to 28 of the cycle.

Intensity of the PEMF: 1000 to 4000 gauss in order to adequately treat the pelvis and the brain. If the correct intensity is chosen this may be the only PEMF system needed. With lower-intensity systems, a portable battery-operated PEMF system may be needed to improve mood, sleep, brain fog, food cravings, etc., by applying treatment to the brain, including the ability to use it throughout the night.

Applicators: A local applicator to the brain for PMDD symptoms and to the pelvic area, just above the pubic bone, during the same session. Portable battery-operated PEMF pads would be applied across the head, just above the ears and slightly behind the midline of the ears. If used to help with sleep, the applicators would be placed under the pillow and run all night long at 3 Hz.

Treatment Time: PEMFs would be applied between days 17 – 28 of the cycle. Treatment time would be between 30 to 60 minutes once or twice a day depending on results, both to the brain and the pelvic area.

Supplements: Evening primrose oil 500 – 1000 mg three times per day, days 17 through 28 of the menstrual cycle. Chaste tree berry 30 – 40 mg per day, days 17 through 28 of the menstrual cycle. Aromatherapy oils, such as chamomile, clary sage, lavender, neroli or rose. Other supplements may include calcium 1200 mg/day, magnesium 360 mg/day, mixed tocopherols 400 IU/day, or B6 50 – 100 mg/day, and/or L-tryptophan 500-1000 mg/day taken at bedtime during the last half of the cycle.

Prostate Hyperplasia—Benign Prostatic Hypertrophy (BPH)

Benign prostate hypertrophy (BPH), also called prostate hyperplasia, is a progressive urinary tract condition in men associated with aging. There appears to be an age-related impairment of the blood supply to the lower urinary tract in the development of BPH. Chronic inflammation is also a significant cause of BPH and lower urinary tract symptoms (LUTS). Almost 50 percent of men with BPH have overactive bladders (OAB). The overactive bladder may be a bigger contributor than the BPH to frequent urination or difficulty with urination.

Medications may slightly reduce prostate size and improve symptoms but have less benefit as the prostate gets larger. A definitive solution for BPH is surgical, among other invasive interventions, to reduce the size of the prostate and improve the flow of urine. The common treatments used for BPH, which include medications and prostatectomy, fail in one-third of the men who have OAB. Surgical or invasive procedures often also lead to major complications, including lifetime urinary incontinence and impotence. Because of the complications of these invasive procedures, men will often try to live with their obstruction symptoms as long as possible.

Because inflammation, reduced circulation, and OAB are identified as causes or major parts of BPH symptoms and progression, PEMFs become an ideal therapy for BPH. The challenge with treatment of the prostate with PEMFs is the depth of the prostate in the body. The prostate is a little bigger than a golf ball and a little smaller than a tennis ball. It is tucked behind the pubic bone and sits under the bladder and in front of the rectum, deep inside the lower abdomen. The dimensions of the prostate itself are 3 cm long, 4 cm wide, and 2 cm deep. The distance of the prostate from the anus to the top is ~10.3 cm (4 inches), range 7.3–15.7 cm (2.8-6.2 inches).

The goals for prostate treatment are to target inflammation and reduced circulation to the prostate directly and to combine this with treatment of overactive bladder. The earlier treatments are begun, the better the results, usually. For OAB bladder treatments, see the **Bladder Conditions.**

There is no concern that PEMFs may cause or contribute to prostate cancer. Research has shown that PEMFs can induce cancer cell death in prostate cancer cells. And, because inflammation is a common contributing factor to prostate cancer, it is expected that PEMF therapy may reduce this risk factor. What is the probability of developing prostate cancer at different ages? From ages 50 to 59, one in 57 men will develop prostate cancer, from ages 60 to 69, the probability increases to one in 21, and from 70 to 79, it goes to one in 12. In men dying after age 81, 59 percent will have prostate cancer. The lifetime risk is for one in nine men to get prostate cancer. This means that prevention is an important aspect of controlling prostate cancer and PEMFs are an important tool in this prevention strategy.

Intensity of the PEMF: Follow the intensity guides in Appendix A. For targeting a depth of 4 to 6 inches, the PEMF intensity needed is between 2000 to 4000 gauss. Since it is hard to be certain of the distance of the prostate from the anus to the top of the prostate, it would be best to use the longest distance of about 6.2 inches. For this distance, 4000 gauss is recommended. Distance of the back of the prostate from the pubic bone is greater than from the anus, so sitting on the PEMF coil or laying it against the perineum when sitting on one's side with the knees pulled up will produce the best magnetic field intensities at the level of the prostate. A "low and slow" protocol is recommended, aiming for the maximum intensity.

Applicators: Local PEMF applicators would be best. Either the butterfly coil can be used with the coil sitting at the anus. Taking a loop coil and putting the leg inside the loop and bringing it up the leg into the groin could work, as well. Lying on one side and putting a paddle applicator against the perineum would work too. Using a "magnetic sandwich" system with one pad underneath the body and the second applicator in the groin area may be most efficient.

Treatment Time: Minimum 30 minutes per day. Best would be 30-60 minutes twice a day until improvements in symptoms are seen. Then treatment time may be cut back to 30 minutes twice a day until symptoms are gone. Then, maintenance should be 15-30 minutes per day for cancer prevention and to maintain symptom management.

Supplements: Ground flaxseed 30 g/D, zinc sulfate 50 mg/D, beto-acids (glycine, alanine, glutamic acid) 400 mg one capsule three times per day, saw palmetto, stinging nettle, pygeum Africanum hundred – 200 mg per day, beta sitosterol/phytosterols, and/or pumpkin seed oil 500 – 1000 mg/D.

Scleroderma or Progressive Systemic Sclerosis (PSS)

Scleroderma or progressive systemic sclerosis (PSS) is a complex condition with a major autoimmune component. Raynaud's disease or syndrome is also common in scleroderma. PEMFs may be effective for controlling certain aspects of scleroderma but would not be expected to cure the condition. Basically, PEMFs would be helpful to control some of the complications and side effects of the scleroderma and may actually slow down its progression. There is no reason that it could not be used alongside any other therapies, including disease-modifying medical regimens.

PEMFs facilitate clinical as well as immunological improvements in scleroderma/PSS. It may be necessary to continue traditional disease-modifying agents (DMARD treatments) at the beginning, depending on the severity of the scleroderma, and then gradually taper them off with continued PEMF use and monitoring of clinical parameters. Physical therapy and stretching following PEMF therapy would aid in releasing some of the contractures seen with this condition.

The goal of PEMF therapy is to decrease inflammation in the body, repair damaged tissues, slow progression, and balance immune function. Because this is an autoimmune condition, whole-body therapy is recommended. Because the immune issues create inflammation in blood vessels, leading to Raynaud's disease/syndrome, this further supports the need for systemic treatment. Since Raynaud's disease manifests most commonly in the hands and feet, these areas can be targeted with local treatments, especially if there is cellular or tissue damage and/or more severe symptoms, especially with cold exposure.

Intensity of the PEMF: High-intensity PEMF therapy (4000 to 7000 gauss) using a "low and slow" protocol, whether local and/or whole-body.

Applicators: Whole-body PEMF therapy, with a "magnetic sandwich" system preferred. Local applicators to hands and feet for Raynaud's disease and areas of significant scarring/fibrosis. Applicators can be applied to the spine from the neck through the chest to help with opening blood vessels in the case of Raynaud's disease. Similarly, for esophageal involvement, regional applicators may be used to the neck and chest from the neck down to the stomach.

Treatment Time: Minimum of 30 minutes twice a day for the whole body. Additional time of 30 minutes for hands and feet and/or esophagus. Treatments are likely to need to be continued lifetime. Once symptoms are significantly controlled, a maintenance protocol will need to be started to keep symptoms and progression at bay. This will be highly individual.

Supplements: Para-aminobenzoic acid (PABA) (also called potassium para-aminobenzoate – KPAB) 12 g/D, mixed alpha tocopherols 800 IU/D orally and, if needed, 50 IU/mL to the hands and/or feet daily, D3 5000 IU/D, evening primrose oil 6 g/D, N-acetylcysteine (NAC), IV, oral 600 – 1200 mg twice/D, S-adenosylmethionine—consider IV therapy, zinc 50 mg/D combined with copper to milligrams/D, 1,25 –hydroxyvitamin D3 (calcitriol).

Shingles

Shingles has elements of a number of topics in this book, including virus infection, skin lesions, pain, and an assault on nerves. Shingles result from reactivation of dormant herpes zoster virus living in the body following a previous exposure to chickenpox virus. PEMFs are expected to decrease the inflammation and pain, help heal the skin lesions related to shingles attacks, and shorten the overall course of the attack. The potential for benefit will depend on how soon treatment is started after the attack becomes apparent. PEMFs are somewhat antiviral, but most of their activity is expected to be through the modulation and strengthening of the body's own immune responses to these infections.

PEMFs should be applied not only to where the pain is being experienced, but also to the spinal column at the level where the virus lives. For example, if the pain is in the mid chest or under the breasts, then the treatment area should be in the upper back just below the level of the shoulder blades. If the problem is in the abdomen, then the treatment area should be in the lower back. Part of the treatment time should be spent where the pain is or where the lesions appear, and the rest of the treatment time should be spent where the virus actually lives, which is usually along the spinal column.

In the case of acute lesions, patients typically need to be on either an antiviral, steroids, or both to reduce the level of inflammation. I would never use PEMFs in this case without using some kind of an antiviral, anti-inflammatory, or immune-modulating treatment protocol. We do need to quiet down the acute and uncomfortable situation using standard medical therapies while at the same time beginning to stimulate the process of natural healing with PEMFs. In this situation, the PEMFs will also be helpful for reducing the level of neuropathic pain (See **Neuropathies** in Chapter 9). This will allow better rest, which also gives the body's immune system a better fighting chance.

In the later stages of shingles, we are dealing with nerve pain, called post herpetic neuralgia. In this situation, mid- to high-intensity, low-frequency PEMFs are likely to reduce the level of pain substantially, even from the earliest days of treatment, primarily by reducing nerve cell and tissue inflammation, as well as the natural pain-reducing benefits of PEMFs. Post-herpetic neuralgia is by definition chronic, although it can also be spikes of pain, like bolts of lightning. In this case, treatment of the brain is also necessary.

Shingles in the face is likely to involve the trigeminal (Gasserian) ganglion, which is inside the skull, inward from the area of the temporomandibular joints (TMJs). There is a ganglion on each side of the head. That's why the shingles neuralgia (trigeminal neuralgia) is often one-sided. This ganglion has three branches: ophthalmic, maxillary, and mandibular. The ophthalmic division involves the forehead, the eye, and the nose. The maxillary involves the cheek and the upper teeth. The mandibular involves the jaw, tongue, and lower teeth. With facial, eye, or forehead pain, treatment can be directed not only to where the pain is experienced but also to the trigeminal ganglion.

Once you have had shingles, the risk of recurrence is increased, even despite shingles shots. In that instance, it is easy to remember to use PEMF therapies since there is still likely to be some discomfort. The challenge comes when the pain and rash go away. This does not mean the virus is dead or gone from the body. Typically, it still survives in the nerves feeding the area in which the pain was experienced in the first place. It may also survive in other parts of the body, creating the potential of additional shingles outbreaks elsewhere in the body. For this reason, once you have had a shingles attack, regular therapy with PEMFs is recommended to the area of the spine or brain where the shingles is likely living, increasing the natural immune functions of the body in the local tissues to keep the virus quiet.

Intensity of the PEMF: 100 to 1000 gauss applied to local lesions. 2000 to 7000 gauss applied to the spine and face. 4000 to 7000 gauss applied to the brain for the effects of severe and chronic pain on the brain. Going "low and slow" is important.

Applicators: Local applicators can be used for facial or very local blisters or pain areas. Applicators covering a larger area are needed for painful rashes on the trunk or chest. A local high-intensity applicator would be used on the painful side of the head with trigeminal neuralgia, applied over the local TMJ, just in front of the ear. It is recommended to treat the brain as well to generally reduce the sensitivity of the pain and prevent centralization.

Treatment Time: Using the "low and slow" approach gradually build up the treatment time to tolerance. Treatments can be between 30 to 60 minutes twice a day. If needed and results require, 10 to 15 minute treatments may be applied to each area multiple times a day to control the pain if the pain returns after a treatment session.

Supplements: Intravenous vitamin C 2–3 g as often as every 12 hours +1000 mg orally every two hours, if available in your area. Mixed tocopherols 1200 – 1600 IU/day, vitamin E cream 30 IU/gm applied as often as needed, capsaicin cream 0.025 or 0.075 percent applied 3-4 times per day (use the lower concentration for mild to moderate pain and the higher concentration for moderate to severe; there may be a burning sensation for the first few days but that decreases with continued use). Topical peppermint oil with 10 percent menthol applied 3–4 times/D (you may experience stinging sensation before pain relief). Also consider curcumin 1000 – 3000 mg twice a day, CBD 50 – 200 mg (of the pure CBD, not the total hemp) three times per day. Caution needs to be used with topicals applied around the eyes.

Sickle Cell Disease

Sickle cell disease (SCD) is a genetic disorder of hemoglobin synthesis occurring mostly in those of African descent. The hemoglobin forms abnormally in red blood cells (RBCs) that turn into a sickle shape. These sickled RBCs can block blood vessels, causing the pain of ischemia. The blockages may be bad enough to cause death of tissues and organs supplied by those blood vessels. This is called a sickle crisis. Sickled RBCs also do not carry oxygen well and break down quickly (hemolysis), resulting in sudden anemia, increasing risk of infection. There are many other aspects to SCD. There is an increased risk of early death caused by infection, organ failure, and stroke. The conventional medical therapy for SCD includes hydroxyurea, which also causes numerous adverse effects.

The goal of PEMFs therapy in SCD is to improve oxygenation, decrease sludging of the abnormal RBCs, decrease the risk of infection, decrease any associated inflammation, and help with tissue repair and recovery. Since the whole vascular system is involved, whole-body PEMF therapy is needed. No clinical trials been found on the use of PEMFs in the setting of SCD for any aspect of it. But, because SCD is so dangerous and there are no safe and very effective therapies for it, PEMFs should be considered to help with this condition. PEMFs are not expected to reverse it. However, they may be helpful with various aspects of the effects of the sickling process, particularly pain, ischemia, thrombosis, organ damage, infection, oxygenation, and inflammation.

It is not expected that PEMFs would be dramatically helpful in the setting of sickle cell crisis. Many of these unfortunate individuals are in chronic pain between crises and need continued narcotic support. If PEMFs can help to reduce the dependency on narcotics, reduce the complications of infections, and decrease the severity of organ damage by increasing some elements of circulation, then the risk/benefit profile appears to be well worth it.

Intensity of the PEMF: 2000 to 7000 gauss local and regional applicators. High-intensity whole-body "magnetic sandwich" device.

Applicators: Local, regional, and whole-body "magnetic sandwich" applicators. It's likely that all three applicator types will be necessary for local, regional, and whole-body use. Whole-body use is especially important for ongoing health maintenance to prevent crises. Local and regional applicators would be used for pain areas that are specifically active and present. Local high-intensity PEMF therapy is important for brain treatment because the pain in these situations is frequently chronic and narcotic-dependent. When first starting with PEMF treatment, the "low and slow" approach should be used. It's likely that a combination of whole-body/regional/local electrically powered devices need to be combined with a portable battery-operated system that can be used for extended periods of time without limiting activity.

Treatment time: Most treatment times with a higher-intensity system are likely to be between 30 – 60 minutes at a time. Treatment times may need to be adjusted based on results and needs. If PEMF therapy is initiated when a person is much younger, there is a higher probability of needing less treatment time. Once significant and serious consequences of SCD occur, for example, some degree of organ damage, longer treatment times may be needed multiple times a day.

Because of the complexity of the levels of issues caused by SCD, all therapy needs to be individualized. Since the risk of PEMFs is considered to be lower than the progression of the SCD, extended use of the PEMFs is not likely to be a problem.

Supplements: Zinc – ages 4-10, 10 mg/D; ages 14-17, 15 mg twice a day; adults 30 mg 2-3 times/D (zinc picolinate or zinc citrate), reducing the dose after several months to 30 mg 1-2 times/D. Long-term zinc use should be accompanied by copper 1-4 milligrams/D. B6 (P5P form) 50 mg twice a day. Mixed tocopherols 400 IU/D. Methyl folate 1 mg/D. B12 5000 μg/D sublingual form. Magnesium citrate 500 mg/D. L-carnitine 50 mg/kilogram/D. L arginine for pulmonary hypertension 100 mg/kilogram of body weight three times per day.

Sleep and Insomnia

Sleep disturbances are common but not easily diagnosed as a single condition. Insomnia, for example, is not a disease, as there is no single definition of it that applies to all people reporting the condition. Multiple aspects are at play in any given person's sleep problem, including stress and anxiety levels, and the use of caffeine and alcohol.

Sleeplessness itself varies dramatically from person to person, with some people struggling to fall asleep (latency) and others struggling to stay asleep, alongside physiological urges like needing to go to the bathroom in the middle of the night or suffering with pain.

PEMF therapy has positive effects on calming the brain and on regulating circadian rhythms. Disturbed circadian rhythms have an important role in controlling sleep patterns and cycles, and stresses, whether physiologic or emotional, can affect circadian rhythms.

Sleep patterns can also be disrupted significantly by background high-frequency EMFs coming into the sleep environment (see Chapter 2). Wi-Fi in the room or building is often broadcast 360° and penetrates through walls. The room in a house with a router is broadcasting to other rooms in the house, and even beyond to other surrounding homes and to the street.

Even low-intensity PEMFs may enhance the effects of sleep medications and psychotropic drugs. This may result in a hangover-like effect in the morning. If this should happen, then the dosing of the medications may be able to be decreased, under appropriate supervision.

Normal sleep has well-defined brainwave frequency patterns. These include theta (4-7 Hz - when you first fall asleep) and delta (1-4 Hz - about an hour into sleep—this is the deepest, most restorative sleep). Theta can also be defined into non-REM and REM (dreaming) sleep; 75 percent or more of our sleep is in theta. The brain has to go through the theta state to get down to delta.

Brain entrainment to help facilitate sleep is commonly done using "ramping." Ramping means that various frequencies are presented to the brain in either descending or as sending patterns. The brain usually does its own ramping as we fall asleep. However, every brain has its own unique ramping patterns, which vary every day. So PEMF ramping may be artificial to the brain and not considerate of the brain's own ramping process. Having tried many different ramping systems over the years, I have found that presenting the brain with one frequency is less confusing, allowing the brain to do its own ramping. The key is the strength of the signal. The brain will frequency-follow faster with the single, higher-intensity signal, rather than being confused with multiple frequency signals.

I have also found that there is no absolutely effective and safe sleep-inducing and maintaining single approach to helping with sleep. Multiple approaches may need to be "stacked" depending on how successful any given strategy is. Stacking means that individual approaches are added one to another. One might start with PEMFs for brain entrainment for sleep, then melatonin may need to be added, and/or theanine, 5HTP, St. John's Wort, CBD, Palmitoylethanolamide (PEA), magnesium, etc., in no particular order. Enhancing sleep hygiene should always be the first place to start. Two other approaches I have added to stacking include delta binaural beat frequencies and a magnetic necklace. The magnetic necklace helps to balance all the acupuncture points and meridians in the neck area through the night, "softening" the neurologic activity the brain and body.

Sometimes the brain needs to be coaxed into sleep. If the brain has been particularly activated in the evening it may need some quiet time to be able to slip into the theta level. Sometimes a brain in a beta state may have difficulty transitioning into alpha and then theta, so it needs to be stimulated in theta first for a while, perhaps 15 to 30 minutes before using delta waves when falling asleep.

Some PEMF manufacturers recommend placing their magnetic coils under the mattress. The magnetic field will have to travel through the mattress, a mattress cover and one or two pillows and then into the brain to stimulate brain waves. Since magnetic fields drop off in intensity according to the inverse square law, a magnetic field starting at 1000 gauss will have dropped to 15 gauss within about three inches; 15 gauss will barely penetrate the skull and not go deeper into the brain. Because of this rapid loss of magnetic field, I always recommend placing the PEMF applicator under the pillow. If for some reason this is not tolerated, then a better solution would be to use a thicker pillow or two pillows, to create more distance separation of the head/brain from the magnetic coil.

In addition to targeting the brain for treatment, there are two other considerations. One is the belly and the other includes other parts of the body that may disturb sleep due to pain, such as arthritis, or the bladder. Since the belly is considered the second brain, it may be useful to activate the parasympathetic system by stimulating the vagal nerve activity in the abdomen. To this end, a coil could be used over the belly, which in some people may actually be more useful than even treating the brain. Combining an all-night coil treatment under the pillow with an all-night lower-intensity PEMF pad to the abdomen may work better still.

Some people may need to not only treat under the pillow with an appropriate Delta frequency local applicator, but also may need to have a separate PEMF applicator applied to an area of pain or over the bladder. It is safe to combine the use of a PEMF coil under the pillow and a low-intensity whole-body PEMF system or a local applicator to a painful area or the bladder through the night.

Many people using PEMF systems for other reasons will often notice significant improvements in sleep without the need for a PEMF approach through the night when PEMFs are used just before bedtime.

Some PEMF systems can be programmed to run for 90 or more minutes while sleeping. The risk of using whole-body PEMF systems during sleep is that they may not be that comfortable. Also, movements during sleep will tend to create stress on the coils in a whole-body system and therefore may shorten the lifespan of the whole-body applicator.

Intensity of the PEMF: While low-intensity PEMFs (10 to100 gauss) may work, they may not be consistent in their benefit and not effective for everybody, depending on life circumstances. I found the best benefit comes from 200 to1000 gauss. A whole-body PEMF system can be used through the night at the same time as treating the brain. A minimum of 10 gauss is recommended and 200 gauss or more is preferred. With a whole-body system, more of the nervous system is being activated and lower intensities may still be effective.

Applicators: Local medium-intensity under the pillow. Local medium- to high-intensity under the abdomen. Whole-body system that can run through the night. A local PEMF system that would allow two applicators to be used at one time or two separate systems of more than one area is going to be treated.

Treatment Time: Before sleep, 15 to 30 minutes. During sleep, 60-90 minutes at the beginning of sleep. The preferred approach is to treat throughout the night using the delta frequency. If treatments are used before sleep or in the early part of the night, then if needed, treatments may be done again during the night for as much time as available in the PEMF system.

Supplements: L-tryptophan 1-2 g at bedtime, melatonin (short-acting if trouble falling asleep and extended-release with early waking) 3-12 mg, niacinamide 1-2 grams at bedtime, magnesium citrate 500 mg, B12 5000 mcg sublingual, and theanine, 5HTP, St. John's Wort, CBD, and/or palmitoylethanolamide (PEA) with various dosing patterns.

Smoking Cessation

Various brain stimulation techniques for tobacco addiction were reviewed in one scientific paper. High-intensity local PEMF (rTMS) was found to be the most well-studied method with respect to tobacco addiction. Results indicate that rTMS to the left side of the upper forehead (dorsolateral prefrontal cortex) was the most effective in reducing tobacco cravings. This is likely due to stimulation of the brain reward system involved in tobacco addiction. In the reviewed studies, rTMS was shown to reduce the amount of smoking, but no brain-stimulation technique at this date has been studied for abstinence rates. PEMF therapy helped about 44 percent of those treated quit smoking. At six months between 28 and 33 percent were still not smoking. Nicotine substitution (patches and chewing gum) only have a 15-20 percent quit rate at six months.

More recent, limited research, has shown a significant impact on addiction using gamma waves at medium intensities.

Intensity of the PEMF: 200 to1000 gauss with gamma frequencies. 4000 to 7000 gauss with high-intensity PEMF.

Applicators: Local medium- or high-intensity butterfly or paddle coil applied to the left upper forehead. A butterfly coil may be tried with one wing on each side of the head and the peak of the butterfly in the center of the top of the head.

Treatment time: 15 – 20 minutes twice a day for between two weeks to one month. Repeated as necessary if cravings return.

Supplements. Niacin 500 mg/D time release or 500 mg niacinamide 2-3 times/D, glutamine 1-6 grams/D, magnesium 500 – 1000 mg/D, P5P 100 mg/D, B12 5000 MCG/D, thiamine 100 mg 2-3 times/D, taurine 1 g 2-3 times/D, evening Primrose oil 4 g/D.
(See also **Addiction.**)

Stem Cell Therapies

Currently, the only stem cell (SC) products that are FDA-approved for use in the United States consist of blood-forming stem cells (also known as hematopoietic progenitor cells) that are derived from umbilical cord blood. These products are approved for use in patients with disorders that affect the production of blood (i.e., the "hematopoietic" system) but they are not approved for other uses.

Despite lack of FDA approval, the number of centers advertising stem cell therapies for just one indication, osteoarthritis (OA) of the knee, are increasing in the United States. These centers claim an 80 percent success rate, success being undefined, according to research presented at the 2018 Annual Meeting of the American Academy of Orthopedic Surgeons (AAOS). For OA of the knee, costs ranged from $1,150 to $12,000, with an average of $5,000 per injection, with prices varying from $1,150 to $12,000. The claim of "stem cell" therapy carries a high level of expectations for the potential benefits, but research is still many years away from providing clear evidence of effective treatment to patients.

Stem cell therapies are currently being offered for anti-aging, brain, COPD, diabetes, neurological, osteoarthritis, CRPS, stroke, arthritis, heart failure, kidney disease, liver disease, inflammatory bowel disease, ED, Lupus, PD, stroke, Alzheimer's, autism, Lyme, autoimmune, hair loss and shoulder conditions, among others. There are SCs in almost all tissues in the human body with various developmental potential. SCs control homeostasis, regeneration, and healing.

The effects of EMF stimulation on SCs depend on intensity and frequency, and the time of exposure. Other factors affect these processes, including growth factors, reactive oxygen species (ROS), etc. EMFs have been successfully used for stem cell-based therapies for SC proliferation and differentiation. Proliferation means increasing the number of stem cells growing. Differentiation means that they will turn into the stem cell type of the tissue into which they are being placed. Finally, both the SCs and the differentiated new cells have to survive and function in their new home.

A wide range of EMF parameters have been used in research, depending on the desired effect. For example, 5 mT, 50 Hz (for sinusoidal EMF), 1.8 mT, 15 Hz or 1.8–3 mT, 75 Hz (for PEMF) have been used to stimulate the number of stem cells. To enhance differentiation varied from 1 to 5 mT for sinusoidal EMF and from 0.1 to 3 mT for PEMF; the frequencies varied from 15 to 100 Hz for sinusoidal EMF and from 15 to 150 Hz for PEMF. Most of these studies would have been done in the laboratory setting with the PEMF and the tissue very close to each other. As a result, the inverse square law has to be considered when thinking about working with stimulating stem cells deeper in the body. See Appendix A for recommendations for peak intensities related to reducing inflammation.

SC functions rely on intrinsic genetic programs, extrinsic signals from their niche, and also the interaction between the two. And differentiation PEMFs can influence SC fate decisions by alteration of ROS generation and intracellular ion concentrations. It's known that PEMFs regulate cellular processes and affect the fate of SCs. PEMFs also participate in the SC niche and impact SC fate since SCs sense and respond to these fields. However, further research is needed. Stem cell therapy is a complicated process with many opportunities for failure, considering its expense and the fact that it is still largely an investigational therapy. The other factor to consider is the health of the tissues into which the stem cells are being encouraged to be in, grow in, and survive. I frequently say, "you can't grow a garden in a swamp." That means that the tissue needs to be made healthier before stem cell therapy is used. PEMF therapy and improving nutritional and general health status should be done before expensive stem cell therapy is initiated. A plastic surgeon with whom I spoke once, said that he found that he obtained the best results with his surgical patients if he had them on a nutritional program and general health program for at least three months before doing plastic surgery. He wouldn't do surgery on people who were not willing to make this effort.

The goal of PEMF therapy is to prepare the tissue for stem cell therapy, help with increasing the number of stem cells, protect and encourage them during their development, and maintaining their viability after development is completed. After that it's a matter of maintaining the tissue long-term into which they are placed. If the causes of the problems in the tissue leading to the need for stem cell therapy are not resolved, then the previous pattern that became the problem in the first place will repeat itself. This is yet another reason to treat the problem tissues with PEMFs long enough to make sure the old pattern is reversing or improving, before considering or doing stem cell therapy. I have heard too many stories of people who paid significant amounts of money to do stem cell therapy without getting any significant long-term benefits.

Intensity of the PEMF: 10 to 50 gauss at the target tissue. Use the Table in Appendix A as a guide when dealing with deeper tissues, such as lung, heart, brain, gut, etc.

Applicators: Local, regional, or whole-body. Whole-body, preferably, and regional at the least, is recommended to prepare the body or organ/tissues to be healthier before the stem cell treatment is started. Local or regional treatment would be continued before, during and after stem cell treatment.

Treatment Time: 30 – 60 minutes twice a day, or more depending on the condition of the body and the organ/tissue. Once treatment of the organ/tissue has been successful treatment time may be able to be reduced to a maintenance level.

Supplements. See the recommendations for the specific organ for which the stem cells are being intended. Also consider the recommendations for support for regeneration of wounds.

Stomach Problems

For the purposes of this section, the stomach will include the esophagus, the stomach itself, and the duodenum. Some of the more common stomach problems, starting from above, include gastroesophageal reflux disease (GERD), gastritis and gastric ulcer, duodenitis and duodenal ulcer, and celiac disease. Most of these problems, except for celiac disease, are caused by excessive acid in the stomach and an inadequate mucosal barrier. Celiac disease is an immune disorder caused by gluten sensitivity. Excessive acid in the stomach can reflux into the esophagus, which does not have the tissue barrier to deal with it. The same can be said of the upper part of the duodenum.

The biggest cause of excessive acid production in the stomach is stress. So, stress reduction strategies are paramount and PEMF therapy may be able to help with decreasing anxiety and improving relaxation.

GERD, is caused by a combination of excessive acid entering the esophagus and hiatal hernia. Everybody has hiatal hernia to some degree. The more severe forms of hiatal hernia create an open highway for acid to travel up into the esophagus. The lower esophagus has a sphincter which is more functional than physical, the end of the stomach leading into the duodenum has a sphincter which is more physical. The analogy is turning off a garden hose. You can turn off a garden hose by using a valve or kinking the hose. A valve won't let the water out but a kinked hose can still allow water to leak past it. A valve creates a tighter closure and a kink is looser. A loose closure is more likely to allow fluid to get past it when the fluid is under pressure.

A hiatal hernia evolves as a result of pressure on this lower esophageal sphincter/valve. A full stomach under pressure will cause the hiatal hernia to stretch. If this happens frequently enough and with enough pressure, the hiatal hernia becomes bigger and more permanent. With the constant refluxing of acid into the lower esophagus, this sets up a situation of chronic esophagitis, or chronic inflammation of the lower esophagus. Not only will this produce constant discomfort at the lower end of the esophagus (heart burn), but it could also lead to Barrett's esophagus and esophageal cancer.

The goal in treating GERD is to reduce the pressure and help to reduce the inflammation. As far as PEMFs are concerned, their primary role in this situation is to reduce inflammation. Otherwise, nutritional guidance is needed to deal with the other aspects, such as weight reduction and helping with digestion of food, to have it leaving the stomach faster.

Chronic gastritis leads to stomach ulcers, both of which cause pain and may result in gastric bleeding. Chronic gastritis is often accompanied by chronic duodenitis. All of these may be further caused or aggravated by gluten sensitivity. The solution for gluten sensitivity is to eliminate all gluten from the diet.

Gluten sensitivity is a milder aspect of celiac disease. The diagnosis of celiac disease can really only be made by doing an endoscopy and a duodenal biopsy. Gluten sensitivity CAN be diagnosed by food allergy testing, primarily IgG and IGA. Sensitivity to other foods, including dairy, eggs, and many others, can also contribute to gastritis. Removing these foods from the diet is the best solution, along with local application of the PEMF to the stomach area. When the proper approach to solving these issues is taken, PEMF therapy may help to decrease pain and discomfort. I have found PEMFs to help with gastric pain many times over the years. It works very quickly.

Intensity of the PEMF: Local application of 100 to 1000 gauss minimum. Higher intensities will help as well if a system is handy, but higher intensities are not needed.

Applicators. Local or regional. Small, portable battery-operated PEMF applicators can be placed over the surface of the upper abdomen in the upper half of the area between the lower end of the breastbone and the bellybutton. Either two applicators can be used, one above the other in the same area, or two small applicators may be stacked one on top of the other over the painful area. A pad applicator may be used as well covering the whole area. With a high-intensity PEMF system, use a local applicator, either a butterfly coil, a paddle, or loop. Since stress is a major contributor to stomach issues, local applicators may be used to the brain in addition, preferably using 7 Hz or 10 Hz frequencies. Often, treatment of the upper abdomen over the solar plexus, with any PEMF helps reduce stress anyway by activating the vagal nerves in the abdomen.

Treatment Time:15 – 60 minutes at a time as needed or, for more chronic problems, twice a day until the pain and discomfort have been resolved.

Supplements: DGL chewable tablets, chew two tablets two hours after each meal and bedtime. Apple cider vinegar to help digestion of food if symptoms tolerate, 2 tablespoons in 4 ounces of water with each meal. If not tolerated, do DGL for several days and try again. GI Revive or other similar gastric support supplement. For GERD: calcium carbonate (Tums EX); chew two tablets as needed, beta-carotene 25 mg/D, and sodium alginate one hour after meals and bedtime.

Stroke and CVA

A stroke happens when the blood supply to part of your brain is interrupted or reduced, preventing brain tissue from getting oxygen and nutrients. Brain cells begin to die in minutes. There are two types of strokes: ischemic and hemorrhagic. Ischemic stroke happens when the blood supply becomes blocked, either through the natural development of plaque in the blood vessels or when a plaque or clot travels from other blood vessels leading from the heart (embolic stroke). Two of the most common sites of embolic strokes are the carotid arteries and the heart. Atrial fibrillation is a common cause of stroke due to the production of clots coming from the heart.

Hemorrhagic stroke happens when an artery in the brain ruptures. Blood coming out of the blood vessel into the brain causes damage because the brain develops a reaction to it. There are two types of hemorrhagic strokes: intracerebral and subarachnoid. The first one happens when an artery bursts, surrounding the brain tissue with blood. These are most commonly associated with either trauma, a ruptured aneurysm, or with anticoagulants. The second type happens when there is bleeding between the brain and the coverings of the brain. This most commonly occurs from a head injury. Either type of stroke leads to significant amounts of inflammation, which then cascades into a series of events that create further damage to the brain if not immediately controlled.

A third category of "stroke" is what can be called pre-stroke or mini stroke, also called transient ischemic attacks (TIAs). This happens when the blood supply in a blood vessel is shut off either wholly or partially for no more than five minutes. More than a third of people who have a TIA suffer a major stroke within one year. As many as 10-15 percent will have a major stroke within three months. People can have many tiny unrecognized TIAs as well as symptomatic TIAs. The goal with managing TIAs is prevention and healing the small amount of damage they cause.

Before PEMF should be used for treating hemorrhagic stroke, it needs to be certain that the bleeding has stopped. In any treatment program for stroke, the cause of the stroke needs to be determined in terms of where and how the brain blood vessel was affected.

The goal in using PEMFs for the treatment of stroke is to reduce the extent of damage, improve symptoms and function, heal as much of the damaged brain as possible, help with rehabilitation, and prevent future strokes. These goals are the same as anyone treating any condition causing damage to the brain, including traumatic brain injury (TBI) or concussion. Strokes are usually emergency events and require hospitalization. Most people who seek PEMF therapy after stroke have already been through their hospitalizations and rehabilitation. Often, it's a waiting process to see how much recovery happens during that time. Strokes can be mild, moderate, or severe, with varying degrees of loss of function and disability; 35 percent of stroke victims almost completely recover or only have mild problems and 40 percent have moderate to severe impairments.

When recovering from stroke, the brain may be able to resume functioning by changing the way tasks are performed. This is called neuroplasticity. One area of the brain takes over tasks from another area. If blood flow to the affected area is restored quickly, some of the brain cells may be damaged instead of destroyed. These damaged cells may be able to resume functioning over time. This is why the sooner PEMF therapy is started after a stroke, the faster these damaged cells may be able to recover and prevent other vulnerable cells from dying. PEMF therapy does not restore the function of cells that have died, but it can help to improve the function of cells and areas of the brain.

The brain is in a constant dance between inhibition and excitation. When there's too much inhibition other parts of the brain react by trying to wake those areas up. When there's too much activity then other non-hyperactive parts of the brain try to dampen the hyperactive parts. In stroke the damaged part of the brain cannot perform this dance at all or as well. As a result, the non-involved part of the brain will often become overactive in inhibiting brain function. So, counterintuitively, in stroke rehabilitation and improving function, treating the opposite side of the brain can be a very effective strategy, even long after a stroke. The chances of helping to heal the damaged parts of the brain long after a stroke become less possible. At the very least, in this situation, PEMF therapy may help to improve function by treating the opposite side of the brain as well. Therefore, with PEMF therapy, treatment would be focused on the damaged part of the brain, the opposite side of the brain, and the source of the stroke, either the carotid arteries or the heart.

Intensity of the PEMF: Because of the depth of the brain, higher-intensity magnetic fields are needed, between 4000 to 7000 gauss.

Applicators: High-intensity local applicators would include a loop coil, butterfly coil, pad, or paddle. The loop coil may be placed over the top or side of the head. If flexible, it can be conformed into an elliptical form and placed over the top ahead and each side, or the back of the head and each side. The butterfly coil would be placed over the top of the head with a wing on each side. The paddle coil can be placed on the side of the head and moved from one side to the other. A whole-body PEMF system may help with other health issues and/or with general vascular benefits. If there is significant spasticity, the treatment would be focused on the brain and/or the spinal cord in the neck. If a whole-body system is used, I recommend using a local applicator as well.

Treatment Time: Using the "low and slow" approach, the treatment time would be 30 – 60 minutes to the brain, adding other time that is needed to other parts of the body. If both sides of the brain are treated, 30 minutes can be devoted to each side. Treating any other areas of the body would be on top of the brain treatments. Once significant benefits are seen with PEMF treatment, maintenance may be able to be reduced to 15 minutes to each side of the brain and adjusted, depending on response when treatment is cut back.

Supplements: Magnesium citrate 500 mg once or twice/D, methylfolate 5 mg/D, homocysteine factors or another homocysteine-reducing formula per the suggested dosing. For hemorrhagic stroke, rutin 20 mg three times/D, hesperidin 250-500 milligrams three times/D, quercetin 30-50 mg/D, curcumin 1000-3000 mg/D, CoQ10 300 mg twice/D.

Tendinitis/Tendonitis and Tendinosis/Tendinopathy

Tendinitis is an acutely inflamed swollen tendon that doesn't have microscopic tendon damage. The underlying culprit in tendinitis is inflammation. Tendinosis, also called tendinopathy, is a chronically damaged tendon with disorganized fibers and a hard, thickened, scarred and rubbery appearance. Some people use the terms tendinopathy and tendonitis interchangeably. While the two have almost identical symptoms, they're different conditions. Tendinopathy is a failed healing response of the tendon, with haphazard proliferation of tenocytes, intracellular abnormalities in tenocytes, disruption of collagen fibers, and a subsequent increase in non-collagenous matrix. The term tendinopathy is a generic descriptor of the clinical conditions (with both pain and pathological characteristics) associated with overuse in and around tendons. The oxygen consumption of tendons and ligaments is 7.5 times lower than skeletal muscles. The low metabolic rate and well-developed anerobic energy-generation capacity are essential to carry loads and maintain tension for long periods, reducing the risk of ischemia and subsequent cell death. However, a low metabolic rate means slow healing after injury. Tendinopathy is usually seen in lateral epicondylitis (tennis elbow), medial epicondylitis (golfer's elbow), patellar tendon, Achilles tendon, rotator cuff, and rotator cuff tendinopathy. Established tendinopathy consistently shows either absent or minimal inflammation. Inflammation is only present at the beginning of the process, but not in its progression.

In very early tendinopathy, pain may be present at the beginning of an activity and then disappear during activity itself. The pain may reappear when cooling down if the activity is prolonged or be more severe on subsequent activity. The pain is localized clearly and described as "severe" or "sharp" during the early stages and sometimes as a "dull ache" once it has been present for some weeks. Once tendinopathy has developed, it is usually going to be lifelong, often waxing and waning, depending on activity or the load of placed on the tendons. Conventional treatments include steroid injections, physical therapy, shockwave therapy, low-level laser, iontophoresis, friction massage, ultrasound, or hyperthermia. All of these require application by a professional and are often effective only for short periods of time. This means they need to be repeated many times over the years. Steroid injections are effective for short-term benefits but are worse than no injections for intermediate and long-term outcomes. In addition, steroid injections can create their own damage and weaken the tendons long-term. This is why they are recommended to be done only once or twice in the same location.

The goal of PEMF therapy in tendinitis is to decrease the inflammation and help with tissue repair. The goals for tendinosis/tendinopathy are to stimulate metabolic activity in the tendons, promote healing, and provide pain relief. A home PEMF system is recommended so that treatments can be extended over longer periods of time and repeated as necessary without the need for the inconvenience and cost of professional therapy.

Intensity of the PEMF: 100 to 2000 gauss, depending on the depth of the tendon. Tendons in and around the hip area tend to be deeper and need the higher intensities.

Applicators: Local or regional applicators. Local applicators would be applied to more superficial tendons, such as the hands, elbows, shoulders, knees, ankles, and feet. Regional applicators may be needed around the hip area or lower back.

Treatment Time: 30 – 60 minutes twice a day to begin with. As improvement is seen, the treatment time may be reduced to what works best. The most common mistake is to not continue treatment beyond the time when symptoms are gone. Even though symptoms are gone, healing may not have been completed. Resumption of activity too soon will cause symptoms to flare up again. A rule of thumb would be to continue treatment for at least a month after symptoms are gone.

Supplements: Curcumin 1000-3000 mg 2-3 times/day, hyaluronic acid oral 200-1000 mg/D, topical DMSO, glucosamine and chondroitin sulphate, vitamin C, hydrolyzed type 1 collagen (Col 1), L-arginine, alpha-keto-glutarate, boswellic acid, methylsulfonylmethane (MSM) 3000-5000 mg powder, bromelain, Vinitrox, and/or CBD gel or oral. Doses will have to be individually tailored.

Testosterone ("Low T")

Testosterone is an androgen hormone produced in both men and women, though in much higher amounts in men. It helps maintain a variety of essential functions in the body, including affecting levels of body fat, muscle mass, sexual health, disease prevention (by improving insulin sensitivity, among other things), mental function, depression, cardiovascular and musculoskeletal health, and bone strength. Women in perimenopause and menopause may also have an interest in increasing testosterone to support their bones, muscles, connective tissues, cardiovascular system, and cognitive function. Since the ovaries also produce testosterone, it makes logical sense that PEMF stimulation over that area of the abdomen, would also increase testosterone production for women, and at the same time also increase estrogen production.

Intensity of the PEMF: 100 gauss or more applied to the testicles, 2000 to 7000 gauss applied to the lower abdomen over the ovaries.

Applicators: Local applicators for the testicles and local/regional applicators applied to the lower abdomen.

Treatment Time: 15-30 minutes once a day for the testicles and 30 minutes once a day to the lower abdomen to stimulate the ovaries.

Supplements: D-Aspartic Acid 2352 mg/day. vitamin D3 1000 IU/D, tribulus terrestris, fenugreek 40 mg/D, ginger, DHEA 25-50 mg/D, zinc 10 mg/D, nettle leaf 40 mg/D, Korean red ginseng 40 mg/D, K1 20 mcg/D, boron 8 mg/D and/or ashwaganda 5 gm/D.

Tinnitus

Tinnitus is commonly described as a ringing in the ears, but it also can sound like roaring, clicking, hissing, or buzzing. It may be soft or loud, high-pitched or low-pitched. You might hear it in either one or both ears. Roughly 10 percent of the adult population of the United States has experienced tinnitus lasting at least five minutes in the past year.

Tinnitus is a sign that something is wrong in the auditory system, which includes the ear, the auditory nerve that connects the inner ear to the brain, and the parts of the brain that process sound. Something as simple as a piece of earwax blocking the ear canal can cause tinnitus. But it can also be the result of a number of health conditions, such as noise-induced hearing loss, ear and sinus infections, diseases of the heart or blood vessels, Meniere's disease, brain tumors, hormonal changes in women, or thyroid abnormalities.

Tinnitus is sometimes the first sign of hearing loss in older people. It also can be a side effect of medications. More than 200 drugs are known to cause tinnitus when you start or stop taking them.

People who work in noisy environments, such as factory or construction workers, road crews, or even musicians, can develop tinnitus over time when ongoing exposure to noise damages tiny sensory hair cells in the inner ear that help transmit sound to the brain. This is called noise-induced hearing loss.

Service members exposed to bomb blasts can develop tinnitus if the shock wave of the explosion squeezes the skull and damages brain tissue in areas that help process sound. In fact, tinnitus is one of the most common service-related disabilities among veterans returning from Iraq and Afghanistan.

Pulsatile tinnitus is a rare type of tinnitus that sounds like a rhythmic pulsing in the ear, usually in time with your heartbeat. A doctor may be able to hear it by pressing a stethoscope against your neck or by placing a tiny microphone inside the ear canal. This kind of tinnitus is most often caused by problems with blood flow in the head or neck. Pulsatile tinnitus also may be caused by brain tumors or abnormalities in brain structure.

Even with all of these associated conditions and causes, some people develop tinnitus for no obvious reason. Most of the time, tinnitus isn't a sign of a serious health problem, although if it's loud or doesn't go away, it can cause fatigue, depression, anxiety, and problems with memory and concentration. For some, tinnitus can be a source of real mental and emotional anguish.

Although we hear tinnitus in our ears, its source is really in the networks of brain cells (called neural circuits) that make sense of the sounds our ears hear. A way to think about tinnitus is that it often begins in the ear, but it continues in the brain. It's not certain what happens in the brain to create the illusion of sound when there is none. Some think that tinnitus is similar to chronic pain syndrome, in which the pain persists even after a wound or broken bone has healed. Tinnitus could be the result of the brain's neural circuits trying to adapt to the loss of sensory hair cells by turning up the sensitivity to sound. This would explain why some people with tinnitus are oversensitive to loud noise.

Tinnitus also could be the result of neural circuits thrown out of balance when damage in the inner ear changes signaling activity in the auditory cortex, the part of the brain that processes sound. Or it could be the result of abnormal interactions between neural circuits. The neural circuits involved in hearing aren't solely dedicated to processing sound. They also communicate with other parts of the brain, such as the limbic region, which regulates mood and emotion. Although medication and non-medication treatments have become available, they are unable to eliminate the sensation in most sufferers. So, at this point, most treatments are aimed at symptomatic relief. Non-invasive, nondrug, stimulation treatment of the brain, including PEMFs, is now being found as a way of helping with the problem.

rTMS not only affects the directly stimulated area of the brain, but it also has an effect on remote areas that are functionally connected. This means that parts of the brain producing the perceived sound which may be overactive (excitable) can still be quieted down or inhibited by many positions of application to reduce the production of the perceived sound. Higher-intensity, lower-pulse-rate stimulation is better at reducing neural overactivity and can reduce tinnitus. This seems to be true whether it is applied to the movement area the brain or the auditory cortex, again suggesting that effects in one stimulated area of the brain spread to other areas, such that tinnitus is still impacted. Repeated daily treatments can significantly improve tinnitus complaints. It is unknown how many daily treatment sessions are required to produce long-term benefits. It's also possible that combining stimulation of the auditory cortex with TMS treatment of the front of the brain may produce even better results.

If the source of the tinnitus is the ear itself, treatment should be directed to the ear. Your ear doctor would be able to tell you if that is the source of the problem.

Intensity of the PEMF: 100 to1000 gauss for ear problems causing the tinnitus; 4000 to 7000 gauss for direct brain stimulation of the frontal lobes of the brain and/or the auditory cortex. The auditory cortex is slightly above and slightly back of the top of the ear.

Applicators. For problems starting in the ear, see the **Ear Problems** for the right applicators. For brain stimulation, portable small, battery-operated panels can be applied on both sides of the head as a "magnetic sandwich" to the auditory cortex on both sides of the head slightly above and slightly back of the top of the ear. Stacked 100 to 1000 gauss applicators could be tried locally. A medium-intensity applicator can be applied to the side of the head and if necessary, alternated between the two sides of the head. For high-intensity applicators placements would depend on the type used: local applicators include a loop, butterfly, paddle, or pad. The loop coil may be placed over the side of the head. If flexible, it can be conformed into an elliptical form and placed over the top of the head or the back of the head and each side. The butterfly coil would be placed over the top of the head with a wing on each side or over the back of the head and each side. The paddle coil can be placed on the side of the head and moved from one side to the other in successive treatments. If the system allows two local applicators to be used as a "magnetic sandwich" then place them on either side of the head. Some research shows that even treating one side of the head, regardless of which side the tinnitus is on, can still help.

Treatment Time: 30 minutes total treatment time or 15 minutes to each side of the head when using separate applicators. Some research shows that it may take upwards of six months to produce results before treatments are suspended. Otherwise, treatments are likely to be long-term if the symptoms recur.

Supplements: Zinc citrate 25 – 30 mg two – three times/D, plus copper 1-4 milligrams/D, B12 sublingual 5000 mcg/D; melatonin (short-acting) 3-9 mg ~1 hr. before bedtime, if trouble falling asleep, and extended release 3-12 mg at bedtime if there is early waking; ginkgo biloba 120 mg/D.

Tremor

Neurological disorders or conditions that that can produce tremor include multiple sclerosis, stroke, traumatic brain injury, and neurodegenerative diseases that damage or destroy parts of the brainstem or the cerebellum. Other causes include the use of some drugs (such as amphetamines, corticosteroids, and drugs used for certain psychiatric disorders), alcohol abuse or withdrawal, mercury poisoning, overactive thyroid, or liver failure. Some forms of tremor are inherited and run in families, while others have no known cause. There are two types of tremor: resting and action (intentional). In resting tremor, the hands are shaking even without any movement. With intentional tremor, the hands do not shake at rest but only begin shaking when movement or actions are attempted. Essential tremor (sometimes called benign essential tremor) is the most common of the forms of abnormal tremor. The hands are most often affected and tremor is typically present as an action or intention tremor. These often run in families. Parkinsonian tremor is caused by damage to structures within the brain that control movement. This tremor is mostly a resting tremor.

There are fundamentally two medical approaches to the treatment of these tremors. One is medication. The medications most commonly used are for seizure disorders, anxiety medications, or beta blockers. All of these can have significant side effects, particularly in the elderly. Another option is neurosurgery to destroy (ablate) the brain tissue causing the tremor, or doing deep brain electrical stimulation (DBS), an electrical procedure with electrodes implanted into the brain.

PEMFs ranging from low-, medium- or high-intensity applied to the brain can be helpful for the treatment of tremor, without the need to resort to invasive procedures. PEMFs should be attempted first before considering an invasive approach. It is also possible that medications combined with PEMFs may work better than either one alone and perhaps allow for lower doses of medications. Even though there may be spasticity peripherally or stiffness of movement, treating the brain is much more likely to provide benefit than whole-body treatment.

PEMFs are expected to only provide control over the symptoms and unlikely to produce a cure. This means that lifetime treatment may be necessary.

Intensity of the PEMF: Low-, medium-, or high-intensity applied to the brain. Low- and medium-intensity PEMFs are likely to have an indirect effect on the brain, and can be tried first to see what the level of benefit is. High-intensity PEMFs are expected to help heal the brain tissue and provide better and more obvious control, with faster more sustainable results. High-intensity magnetic field would be between 4000 to 7000 gauss, using a "low and slow" protocol.

Applicators: Local applicators, including loop, butterfly, paddle, or pad. The loop coil may be placed over the top or side of the head. If flexible, it can be conformed into an elliptical form and placed over the top ahead and each side or the back of the head and each side. The butterfly coil would be placed over the top of the head with a wing on each side. The paddle coil can be placed on the side of the head and moved from one side to the other. A whole-body PEMF system may help with other health issues and/or with general vascular benefits. If there is significant spasticity, the treatment would be focused on the brain and/or the spinal cord in the neck. If a whole-body system is used, I recommend using a local applicator as well.

Treatment Time: 30 – 60 minutes twice a day. Once significant benefits are seen with PEMF treatment, maintenance may be able to be reduced to 15 minutes to each side of the brain and adjusted, depending on response when treatment is cut back.

Supplements: Safflower oil 2 g twice/D combined with mixed tocopherols, magnesium citrate 500 mg/D, zinc 25 mg/D, and/or B12 5000 µg/D.

Vascular Disease

Vascular disease is primarily caused by atherosclerosis. Atherosclerosis is a chronic, slowly progressive arterial disease that is the most common cause of death in Western societies. It consists of endothelial dysfunction, arterial inflammation, and formation of plaques within the blood vessel wall which contain cholesterol, lipids, and calcium. As the plaques increase in size, they progressively obstruct the blood vessel and restrict blood flow, which can then lead to angina, peripheral vascular disease, and intermittent claudication. Atherosclerotic plaques can rupture, leading to the formation of a clot (thrombus) which may lead to partial or complete obstruction of the artery. Acute obstruction may cause unstable angina, myocardial infarction, transient ischemic attack, stroke, or blockages of other blood vessels.

Ischemia is caused by insufficient blood flow to a particular tissue or organ to meet that organ's needs for oxygen, glucose, and other nutrients. Ischemia is usually caused by and is a primary symptomatic manifestation of atherosclerosis.

Endothelial injury is the initial stage of the long-term process of atherogenesis. Endothelial injury leads to a cascade of events including vascular inflammation, activation of platelets, arterial smooth muscle thickening, and deposition of foam cells which are macrophages with low-density lipoprotein (LDL) cholesterol. Endothelial injury is largely caused by oxidized LDL. LDL is very susceptible to oxidation and in this state, is highly atherogenic, whereas native LDL is relatively innocuous.

Conventional therapy usually involves statin drugs designed to lower lipid levels and/or by diet plus exercise, to lower elevated lipid levels and improve other risk factors. Statin drugs work by lowering LDL and inhibiting inflammation. The benefits of statins may be mostly due to their anti-inflammatory as opposed to their cholesterol-lowering properties.

The goal of PEMF therapy is to reduce vascular inflammation, and reduce activation of platelets and the thickness of smooth muscle. In addition, PEMF therapy is fibrinolytic, meaning it not only helps to prevent the development of clots, but also helps break down clots in blood vessels. Thus, whole-body PEMF therapy is a long-term strategy to reduce or reverse the development of vascular disease, especially when combined with diet and exercise. This means that PEMF therapy can be used not only for prevention, but to help with existing cardiovascular and systemic vascular disease.

Intensity of the PEMF: 10 to 7000 gauss. The lowest-intensity PEMFs will improve circulation and decrease vascular disease mostly superficially. These PEMFs may be more useful in the prevention of vascular disease, but may not be as effective when there is significant vascular disease present. When there is significant vascular disease, especially if significant symptoms are present, then much higher-intensity whole-body PEMF treatment is necessary. See Appendix A for guidance on the intensity of the PEMF field needed to treat vascular problems deeper in the body.

Applicators: Local or regional applicators for local vascular problems such as the brain, heart, the kidneys, the skin, for intermittent claudication, for vascular ulcers, etc. Local therapy should always be accompanied by daily whole-body therapy, since the problem is systemic and not just local. A whole-body "magnetic sandwich" system would be more ideal.

Treatment Time: 30 – 60 minutes twice a day, and more often depending on the severity of the underlying problem.

Supplements: Since this is a complex subject, consultation with a nutritionist is especially important. Consider magnesium, potassium, vitamin C, methyl fully, P5 P, B12, niacin, omega-3 fish oil, mixed tocopherols, tocotrienols, selenium, zinc, copper, antioxidant combinations, l-carnitine, CoQ10, chromium, silicon, vitamin K2, vitamin D, lutein, flavonoids, choline, and/or lecithin.

Wounds

Many of the actions of PEMFs responsible for healing have already been discussed throughout this book, including decreased inflammation, improved oxygen levels, reduced swelling, increased growth factors, production of collagen and fibroblasts, stimulation of regeneration and stabilized electrochemical gradients across cell membranes and stimulation of stem cells. There is plentiful research evidence showing benefits of PEMFs on wound healing. Skin wounds respond well with a medium-intensity PEMF applied directly over the wound, whether covered with a dressing or not.

Wounds typically involve many tissue types, including connective tissue, blood vessels, nerves, skin, and, often, muscle and bone. Each tissue type responds differently with the speed of repair. Connective tissue, skin, and muscle respond the fastest.

Most wounds to which this topic applies are the superficial wounds involving connective tissue, skin, and muscle, and include bruises, scrapes, cuts, and gouges. These may be accidental wounds or wounds made on purpose in the setting of surgery. Accidental wounds are more likely to be contaminated and potentially ragged. The deeper the wound the longer it will take to heal. PEMFs can also improve the healing of wounds deep in the body, for example surgical wounds of the intestines, liver, lung, kidneys, bladder, etc.

Other factors, including age, nutritional status, circulation, general debility, immune deficiencies, and genetics also affect successful and rapid wound healing. While PEMFs accelerate wound healing in general, all these other factors that affect wounds will determine the rate of wound healing.

Acute inflammation is a necessary part of wound healing. While PEMFs decrease inflammation, they enhance so many other factors involved in the healing process that, overall, they provide more benefit than harm.

Intensity of the PEMF: Medium-intensity 100 to 1000 gauss for superficial wounds. Higher-intensity PEMFs, 2000 to 7000 gauss, for wounds deep in the body.

Applicators: Local or regional are necessary most the time. If a whole-body PEMF systems is available there will still be some benefit to the body from using that system, but more likely to be helpful would be the smaller applicator(s) that come with the system. Applicators may be applied over bandages, dressings, or clothing, even shoes or boots.

Treatment Time: 30-60 minutes twice a day at a minimum. The wider and deeper the wound, and the more factors present that would inhibit wound healing, the more treatment time may be needed, especially early in the healing process.

Supplements: Collagen, vitamin C 2000-5000 mg twice a day, zinc citrate 25 mg twice a day (begin treatment 2-4 weeks prior surgery and continue four to six weeks after surgery) combined with copper 2-4 mg/D; magnesium citrate 500 mg/D, vitamin A 25,000 IU/D (begin treatment 2-4 weeks prior surgery and continue 4-6 weeks after surgery), mixed tocopherols 400 IU/D (begin treatment 2-4 weeks prior surgery and continue 4-6 weeks after surgery), B12 5000 IU/D sublingual, P5P 100 mg/D, pantothenic acid 20-100 mg/D, L-arginine 1000-6000 mg/D, citrus flavonoids 500-1000 mg 2-3 times/D.

When PEMF Therapy Won't Work and What You Can Do About It

As this book, along with a solid amount of scientific research supporting it, makes clear, most people will gain health benefits from PEMF therapy most of the time, especially if they use it consistently and for the necessary amount of time needed to meet their health concerns. However, no single therapy or therapeutic systems can possibly solve all human health problems. It's important to acknowledge the limitations of any therapy or therapeutic system. Even though a single therapeutic approach, PEMFs for example, may solve so many problems better and safer than many other systems, there are times when PEMF therapy may not work or not work well. In this chapter, I explain why and offer tips about what you can do to avoid and resolve such problems, should they occur.

In order to improve the likelihood that you will benefit from PEMF therapy you need to understand the PEMF field being used, the nature of the health condition you are treating (see Chapters 9 and 10 for my recommendations for using PEMFs to treat a wide range of health conditions), the overall condition of your body at the time you begin treatment, and how well you prepared yourself and your body for healing work, including being able to set aside the necessary amount of time you can devote to each treatment. In addition, even if all of these factors are optimized, your expectations for results also need to be set properly.

The body is fallible, has limitations, and has an expiration date. The soul may not, but the body does. The body is a physical instrument and has to follow physical laws. PEMF therapy also follows physical laws. The two acting together amplify each other's healing and life-extending possibilities. While PEMF therapy can often seem miraculous, in terms of the results it can provide, gaining benefit depends on taking the right amount of time and using the right PEMF equipment properly, per the guidelines I provided in Part One of this book.

What follow are the most common reasons why some people fail to benefit from PEMF therapy.

Not Understanding PEMF Field Characteristics

Understanding the PEMF field produced by the system you use is critical to getting good results. This includes understanding the size of the PEMF field, based on the configuration of the applicators, the intensities of the field or fields, and the frequencies or programs being used, if any. Please review the guidelines in Chapters 4 and 5 if you are uncertain about these issues.

The PEMF Field Is Too Weak for the Tissues Being Treated

Based on Faraday's Law, dB/dT, the energy charge induced in the body by the PEMF system is one of the most important factors that drives the effects of PEMFs. As I discussed earlier in this book, all magnetic fields dramatically drop off in intensity the further away the PEMF applicator is from the body, according to laws of physics. For best results, you need to be sure the applicator is placed on or near the area of your body being treated.

The depth of the part of the body being treated also drives the value of PEMF therapy and the level of the magnetic field necessary to produce sufficient results. Treating superficial areas of the body, such as a wrist, hand, elbow, knee, feet, or toe, requires less of a magnetic field to have a benefit. On the other hand, a much stronger PEMF field is needed to achieve results when treating problems deeper in the body, such as inside the brain, the heart, the lungs, the liver, kidneys, bowel, bladder, hips, deeper bones, or the spine. This means that the peak intensity of the PEMF field needs to be taken into account when deciding which PEMF system to use. This important concept in the law of physics may run counter to the marketing claims of many companies promoting and selling PEMF systems.

If your intention is to use a PEMF system on all parts of your body to treat a multitude of different conditions, a higher-intensity PEMF system will likely be needed. Almost all whole-body PEMF systems produce intensities that are significantly weaker than many currently available high-intensity systems. The trade-off is that most of these high-intensity systems tend to be more local and only capable of treating a smaller area of the body at a time. However, newer systems are available that combine high-intensity and whole-body therapy.

The PEMF Field Is Too Far From the Body Part Being Treated

When a PEMF system produces results on superficial tissues, but doesn't help for problems deeper in the body, it usually does not mean that the system doesn't work. Rather, it means the PEMF field is wrong or too weak for its intended purpose. As a result, there will be no significant benefit or much longer treatment times will be needed. Even moving the magnetic field applicator two to three inches away from the surface of the body by placing applicator coils under cushions, blankets, or mattresses, as some manufacturers recommend, can dramatically decrease the PEMF field intensity at the point of the tissue being targeted, as well as decreasing the intensity of the magnetic field on the body. In addition, what may work when PEMFs are applied to the back, won't be as strong on the other side of the body. For treating the brain, for sleep, putting a magnetic field under the mattress will result in a dramatically lower magnetic field at the brain. It may have some effect, but not as good as placing it much closer to the brain.

No matter what the intensity of the magnetic field, a PEMF field applied at the skin of the back will be much less at the front of the body. That means that some people need to apply their applicators to both the back and the front of the body, whether simultaneously or over separate treatment times. Likewise, when lying on your side, the magnetic field has to cross through your whole-body from side to side. This is farther than going from back to front. The same thing is true when going from front to back. This is why you need to always consider this decrease in PEMF field strength when treating deeper areas of your body.

Wrong Entrainment Frequency

Sometimes PEMF fields make people feel sleepy or more relaxed. Conversely, at other times, they can make people feel more alert, "buzzed," or over-stimulated. Both types of responses have to do with the frequencies of the PEMF system being used and their entrainment effects on the nervous system.

Different PEMF entrainment frequencies influence the state of brainwave frequencies and how they affect human function. Entrainment frequencies range from the extremely low, delta frequencies, up through theta, alpha, beta to gamma frequencies and higher. The higher the frequencies, the more alerting and stimulating the actions are on the brain waves. Deep sleep corresponds to delta waves, lighter sleep to theta, relaxation to alpha, and alertness to beta and gamma, both of which affect higher brain functions, such as learning, memory, and conscious integration of information. For sleep, higher frequencies such as beta and gamma should not be used close to bedtime as they may make the brain more alert. If one wants to have a high level of alertness, then beta or gamma frequencies would be better at that time. For deep sleep, delta is probably the best frequency, followed by theta.

Many PEMF systems have built-in programs that run through different frequencies. Sometimes they use concepts called ramping, for example, using higher frequencies to start with and then gradually running descending frequencies in a stair step fashion. Programs may also be designed to work in the opposite direction. The starting state of the brain needs to be considered when using ramping frequencies or preprogrammed frequencies. If one is already in a very relaxed state before going to sleep, using programs with ramping frequencies that are start in beta will tend to wake you up first before bringing you back down again. This does not always work because the timing of these stairstep frequencies may not change brainwave frequencies adequately or quickly enough. Ramping may work, but you will first have to determine whether that's true for you personally, at any given time, which may vary.

When one starts PEMF field therapy, the brain is going to be in whatever brainwave state it is in. There are many brainwave states in different parts of the brain at any given time. Experience has shown me that when the brain is presented with a single given frequency, brain regions entrain themselves at their own pace and time. Once the brain gets used to a specific frequency, it becomes easier for the brain to move faster and better into the entraining frequency during future entrainment sessions. However, it is always necessary to determine which entrainment frequencies are most appropriate to use each time that you use PEMF entrainment frequencies.

Problems with the PEMF Applicator

Another reason why PEMF devices may not be providing benefits is because their applicators may not be working. You can test your system's applicators to determine if that is the case.

People frequently say they can't hear or feel the PEMF applicator. This is most especially true for very-low-intensity PEMF systems and the highest-intensity systems at the lowest settings. The easiest way to know the that the applicator is working is by putting your ear to the applicator with the system running at the highest intensity and the lowest frequency. Very high frequencies, typically, over 100 Hz, are harder to hear because intensity drops normally with frequency.

Once you hear the highest intensity you can dial down the intensity to see at which level you stop hearing it. That could give you a gauge in the future for knowing how to test the applicator. Generally, the smaller applicators are going to produce the strongest magnetic fields and may be the most likely to give you an indication of operation.

Some PEMF systems provide their customers with a test device to show that it's working. They will usually give instructions on how to use the tester. It's almost always better to use the equipment provided by the manufacturer, because it will have been designed for the signal of their specific device.

These are samples of some of the test devices manufacturers provide.

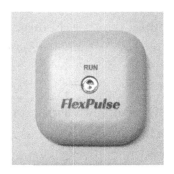
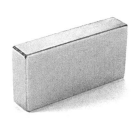
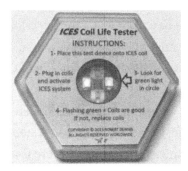

| FlexPulse tester | Magnet for Parmeds | MicroPulse tester |

The FlexPulse and MicroPulse testers have electric circuits in them that are activated by the pulsing magnetic field. When that happens the lights on these testers begin to flicker.

You can also purchase a mini amplifier (Mini Amp) and a suction cup pickup microphone, or use a sensitive microphone. I've found these on Amazon and have used them occasionally. These will detect the PEMF signal when set at the highest intensity and lowest frequency. The suction cup microphone is plugged into the MP3 in port. Use the headphone pieces to listen to the amplified sound.

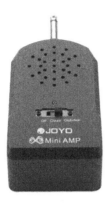

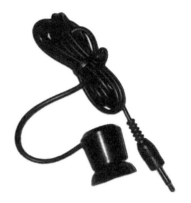

JOYO JA-01 Mini Amplifier Guitar Amplifier

Telephone Pick-Up Coil with Suction Cup with big sound Headphone Output

Mobile Phone Apps: There are many mobile phone apps that also detect magnetic fields. For the iPhone, the Magnetometer app will show a significant jump in the intensities detected. Many of the mobile phone apps are designed to detect ambient EMF magnetic fields. These may not be able to detect PEMF magnetic fields because their frequencies are very low and often these ambient magnetic field testers are not designed for the level of intensity used with PEMFs. They may work for very-low-intensity PEMFs—for example, the tri-field meter range; however this meter detects magnetic fields with intensities varying from 0.1 – 100.0 milligauss (mG) or up to only 0.1 gauss.

Magnets and PEMF Field Testing: Several PEMF systems supply magnets for testing. The Parmeds systems are supplied with a rare-earth test magnet enabling the user to know if there is a pulsed magnetic field or not, without the need for an additional electronic detection device. Rare earth magnets are permanent strong magnets, also called neodymium magnets, and consist of neodymium, iron, and boron, with nickel coating to prevent corrosion.

With the help of the test magnet the user is able to establish if there is any PEMF or not. This means that the goal of the magnet is to know if the device works or not (yes/no), but by no means will this magnet enable the user to establish the precise strength of the magnetic field because the pulsed magnetic fields disturb the magnetic field lines of the test magnet itself, which is "translated" into mechanical movements in sync with the pulsing frequency.

Of course this method can only be used for higher-intensity PEMF devices because low-intensity devices do not have sufficient power to disturb the magnetic field lines of a test magnet. So, if the test magnet moves when exposed to a higher-intensity PEMF, it means that the magnetic field is strong enough to move the magnet.

The mechanical movements of the pulses can be felt while holding the test magnet in the hand over the coil locations in the PEMF applicator. The actual movements of the test magnet are dependent on the pulsing repetition rate (frequency), intensity, location in relation to a specific coil in the applicator, direction of the magnetization of the field lines of the test magnet itself in relation to the current through the applicator coil, distance from the coil (in the middle or at the side), the degree of direction of the magnet held towards the coil, etc.

Some people think that the full-body mattress might not work optimally because they do not feel the pulses with the test magnet at the edges of the mattress as strong, or not at all, versus directly above the coils inside the mattress. It should be clear that the test magnet is only supplied as an indicator to test if the system works correctly.

However, the pulsing magnetic field even extends beyond the edges of the mat. The field will generally be weaker there since it's farther away from the actual coil. In order to feel the Parmeds PEMF pulses, simply hold the test magnet loosely in the palm of the hand directly above one of the coils, whether in a small pad or in the mattress. Because the repetition rate of the pulses depends on the pulsing frequency, for feeling the PEMF pulses, better results can be obtained by choosing program number 8 for the home system (one pulse per second), program number 4 for the Parmeds Pro system (two pulses per second), and program number 5 for the Parmeds Super and Ultra 3D systems (two pulses per second). After pressing the start button of the PEMF control unit, the above pulse repetition rates will be clearly felt for the first five minutes in movements of the test magnet. After five minutes the frequency changes and the pulsations will be reduced or not felt at all.

Professional Magnetometers: For many of the high- or very-high-intensity PEMF systems, the signal reaches a very high peak extraordinarily rapidly, often as fast as a one microsecond (a millionth of a second). Even 1000th of a second (millisecond) is extraordinarily fast. The magnetometer has to be specifically and technically precisely designed to be able to detect a magnetic field peak in such an incredibly short period of time. These get to be very expensive and often are unique to each individual PEMF system. An improperly designed magnetometer will significantly underestimate the true peak intensity of the magnetic field.

The Wrong System for the Job

Many people prefer to purchase PEMF systems that treat the whole body. Such systems are good for health maintenance and treating many areas of the body at the same time. A good part of the time this works. But, clearly, this whole-body approach does not work well for significant health problems or problems deeper in the body as shown by research. This is because whole-body PEMF systems, unless they provide very high intensity, tend to only have intensities that are inadequate for reaching deeper into the body.

There have previously been three levels of intensity of whole-body systems: low, medium, and high. We are starting to have available very-high-intensity systems, with little risk of harm if used properly. Knowing the peak intensity of the PEMF system you are purchasing or using is critical to getting this right. Always ask for the peak intensity of the PEMF system you're looking at. You can always go down in intensity but you can't go up if the system is not capable of higher intensities.

Most higher-intensity PEMF systems, unless they are whole-body, tend to treat smaller areas of the body. Such systems are very useful when dealing with significant health issues in specific parts of the body. But when there are multiple parts of the body that need fairly intense treatment, a higher-intensity whole-body PEMF system may be needed to not only achieve the right intensities at the tissue being treated, but also to decrease the treatment time needed. If a whole-body system is not used, then treatment will need to be divided between the different areas being targeted. Then the issue becomes one of having enough treatment time for each of the targeted areas.

One of the biggest mistakes people make, even if the intensity chosen is correct, is to devote too little treatment time to any given body area needing treatment. If you have multiple areas that need treatment, I recommend that you choose one or two key areas that really need your attention, devote significant treatment time to those areas, and when they are better, move to one or two other areas for intense treatment, and so on. It may be that previously treated areas will still need some "touchup" time periodically for maintenance of benefit.

Health Condition Characteristics

The best results with PEMF therapy in healing various health conditions depend on your understanding of the severity and acute/chronic state of the problem, the healing times of the various types of tissue and the ability of the body to respond to treatment.

There are different levels of severity of health conditions: mild, moderate, or severe. These can further be considered in terms of acute, or recent onset, and those that are chronic or expected to be permanent. While not always true, the more severe the problems are, especially when it comes to impairing function, the more treatments and time will be necessary to recover, resolve symptoms, and restore function. Chronic problems may be made to be better over time by using PEMFs, but not necessarily completely resolved.

The removal of symptoms and the improvement of function doesn't necessarily mean the problem has been reversed. A good example of this is a bone fracture. Acutely, a fracture is very painful, but over time the pain reduces. It may feel well enough for you to feel like you can use the body area again. Even so, on X-rays or even with physical examination, the fracture may still be shown to exist. If the fracture is still present even after the pain it causes is reduced, it remains vulnerable to not healing properly or to being reinjured or broken anew. The same concept applies to many other tissues. Always remember: lack of symptoms does not always mean complete healing. Less compromised deeper tissues do not always "talk" to you to let you know their level of health.

In addition to their severity and whether they are acute or chronic, the type of tissue involved with health problems also need to be considered. Different tissues heal in different time frames, depending on the severity the problem. For example, under optimal circumstances, the cornea of the eye can heal in 24 hours, gastrointestinal cells can heal in three days, skin and muscle can heal in two to three weeks, and tendons, ligaments, nerves, brain, and bones can take several years to fully heal, if ever. Bones may be usable in eight to 12 weeks but that doesn't mean that the fracture site in the bone is completely healed. Tendons and ligaments take a long time to heal because they have a very poor blood supply. Nerves and brain cells also tend to heal very slowly.

Understanding the above is very important in terms of having properly set expectations, determining the amount of treatment time necessary, knowing how long to wait to see results, and recognizing the likely eventual outcome of any therapy, including PEMF treatments. In some cases, problems may not be completely resolved with PEMF therapy, or, quite possibly, with any other therapy, yet PEMFs can still be used on a regular basis to reduce or minimize symptoms and gain whatever healing is possible. This should be expected when one understands the nature of the condition being treated.

Many problems require at-home therapy on an ongoing basis compared to attempting in-office professional treatments, which is why I recommend you own your own PEMF system if at all possible, for chronic conditions. Many people schedule professional PEMF treatments to see how their bodies react and then proceed to purchase their own home system for regular long-term use.

Acute Versus Chronic Problems

With acute problems, meaning problems that have occurred recently, PEMFs have the best chance of stimulating the body's repair capability, often speeding healing and recovery time by as much as 50 percent. This is one more reason why having your own PEMF system on hand can be so helpful. Already owning your own system will allow you to treat new onset acute health problems as soon as they arise, rather than having to wait to schedule an appointment with a healthcare professional while the acute problem progresses and potentially becomes chronic. The sooner you can treat an acute problem, the sooner you are likely to be able to heal it. With acute problems, it is often prudent to consult with your health professional to determine if your PEMF treatment is appropriate and whether other approaches might be needed, whether combined with PEMF therapy or not. An example of this, is if you already own your own PEMF system, and you start to develop a new abdominal pain, it is important to know what that abdominal pain is from, because PEMFs are often able to mask the pain of an evolving serious intra-abdominal problem that may require more aggressive treatment, such as surgery for a rupturing appendix.

Should healing stall or be delayed, an acute health condition can become chronic. Health conditions such as pain, arthritis, diabetes, autoimmune disease, and cardiovascular disease are examples of chronic problems which people may have to cope with for the rest of their life. People often start using PEMF therapy late in the process of a health problem becoming or being chronic. Given the level of severity of the problem and the type of tissue involved, the longer the time that will be necessary for stabilization, repair and recovery to occur. In some cases, full healing may never occur, and the partial yet still noteworthy improvements that PEMFs can provide to reduce symptoms may have to be accepted as a reasonable outcome beyond what conventional medical approaches can provide. This does not mean that PEMF therapy isn't working, only that it is only capable of providing symptom relief benefits for certain chronic health problems.

Sensitivity

There are individuals who are in such a delicate state of balance that it is challenging for them to receive and benefit from PEMF therapy. Individuals with multiple chemical sensitivities, or who suffer from excessive inflammation or toxicity, often perceive PEMF field stimulation as a physical or psychological threat. The same can be true of people who are in a chronic state of fight and flight, have extraordinary anxiety, or who experience major mental/emotional disorders. Any change, whether positive or negative, can be perceived as a change that is or may be a threat for their current state of instability. Even very weak, barely perceptible PEMFs can overwhelm the nervous system responses of such people.

Unfortunately, healing in these individuals may not be able to happen without the PEMF field stimulus, so these individuals are caught between a rock and a hard place. They would need to be able to access other health services that can help them to restore and recover their ability to heal and accept stimulation and support of almost any kind of therapy, including sound, light, temperature change, supplements and herbs, nutrition, and PEMF fields.

Fortunately, research has shown that healthy cells tend to ignore the PEMFs. Cells that can benefit from PEMFs will accept the support PEMFs provide, while the healthy cells basically continue to go on about their normal business. On the other hand, of the trillions of cells in the body, a large percentage can still benefit from PEMFs therapy even though it's not obvious that they need help. This allows these healthy or nearly healthy cells to be further optimized in their function, given that all of life is subject to entropy and breakdown over time, even though this breakdown process is gradual and barely discernible. Entropy is a gradual loss of energy in any physical system over time. Some might call this aging. There is slow, average, and rapid aging. PEMFs help to support the slowing down of the aging process while helping to keep overall health optimized.

Poor State of Health of the Body

For PEMF therapy to be effective, the body has to have the proper tissue support to do regeneration and healing. For someone in a very poor nutritional state, with protein and lipid (fat) malnutrition, the body has little fuel for tissues to make the PEMF field therapy able to heal. Poor nutritional status affects far too many people these days due to their unhealthy dietary habits, and can be exacerbated due to chronic starvation, major illnesses causing cachexia or wasting, prolonged gastrointestinal or kidney fluid and electrolyte losses, tissue damage from treatments, such as chemotherapy and radiation, destruction of the gut microbiome, as well as other health issues. Restoring nutritional and fluid and electrolyte states become critical to being able to obtain the full extent of the benefits that PEMFs can provide.

To ensure that your body's overall health is optimized, I recommend that you follow the dietary, nutritional, and other healthy lifestyle guidelines I shared in Chapter 6 and some of the supplement recommendations at the end of each condition in Chapter 10. Consulting with the appropriate nutritional specialist may also be required.

Inadequate PEMF "Dose"

The "dose" of PEMF treatment is not unlike the dosage use of a medication. This includes the strength of the magnetic field, the length of action, and how often treatments need to be repeated for benefits to be achieved. When any of these are inadequate, the results of the PEMF treatment will be inadequate, as well, notwithstanding factors affecting the tissue and underlying condition, mentioned above.

The most common problems with PEMF "dosing" are:

- inadequate intensity
- treatment time that is too short for the given problem being treated
- inadequately repeating treatments, whether daily or other time frames
- stopping treatments too soon
- restarting activity or intensity of activity too soon.

The most common dosing problem is the intensity of the PEMF field. Research has shown that the PEMF field intensity at the tissue being targeted to reduce inflammation is optimally around 15 gauss (see Appendix A). If the depth of the problem being treated is not taken into account, the PEMF field intensity is usually going to be too low. Lower than optimal intensity PEMF fields, even if they do help, will almost always require much more treatment time to produce effective healing.

Symptom improvement helps but it is not healing. PEMFs can be fairly dramatic in improving symptoms, but the symptoms will recur if the underlying condition is not truly healing. This is why the PEMF field intensity and the treatment time needed are so closely tied together. If the optimal intensity is provided for the problem being treated, then the treatment times can be much more efficient and effective.

Many people expect and are told by salespeople that all they need to do is to treat themselves for eight minutes a day to produce benefits. While such short treatment times may be effective in improving superficial circulation, this usually only improves for a short period of time unless the underlying cause of the circulation problem is also improved. The rule is that the body will tell you what it needs. Start treatment. See what the response is. Then readjust the time and intensity. People need to go into PEMF treatments with the expectation that they will do what is needed to make the benefits of the PEMFs maximized for their investment to be worth it.

The above considerations need to be applied to how many times a day to treat, over what period of time to expect results, when PEMF treatment can be cut back, and what the therapeutic maintenance requirements will be. Most people don't realize that PEMF therapy may take some work and effort. That's because PEMF therapy doesn't take over the body, it makes the body do the work needed. In certain respects, PEMF therapy can be considered to be similar to athletic training in that it too is providing a form of cellular training, as well as protocols for both performance enhancement and recovery. Just as athletic training routines are adjusted based on the health of the body, results, and the intensity of the training, so do PEMF therapy adjustments need to be made as treatments and healing progress over time.

Most research studies with PEMFs are not conducted over long enough time periods to see how effectively PEMF therapy has been to resolve health issues. Instead, most studies are simply looking for measurable temporary/short-term improvements because of the costs and need for continuing participant involvement. In addition, most studies are inconvenient for the participants, since they are conducted outside people's individual home environments and lifestyles. This is one of the reasons why home PEMF therapy becomes very important. It allows treatment to be under much more direct individual control to produce long-term benefits.

The general rule of thumb is that the higher the intensity of the PEMF field, the less treatment time will be required and the faster the results will happen. Although there are exceptions to this rule, this is the place to start.

Other complicating factors to the above "dosing" considerations include the starting point of PEMF therapy relative to the severity of the problem (how late in the tissue damage process therapy is started), the healing capacity of the tissue or tissues involved, the symptoms and/or functional limitations caused by the problems, and the healing capacity of the individual both in terms of vitality, nutritional and lifestyle support, and age.

Conditions Being Treated That Are Unlikely to Respond

Despite the fact that PEMFs are proven to facilitate healing and improved function of the body, as with all other therapies, for some conditions there are still natural limitations to what they are going to be able to help, at least to a significant extent. Not all health conditions respond equally well. This is especially true of very severe conditions that have little chance of being impacted to improve function or result in healing. Some examples include:

- vascular malformations
- congenital disorders
- congenital or traumatic blindness
- sepsis
- structural/mechanical problems in the body
- benign tumors
- valvular heart disease
- organ failure
- physical loss of a whole or part of an organ
- a person being too depleted to marshal a positive response, such as in end-of-life care
- scars which can't be reversed or turned into normal tissue.

As mentioned, in some cases, PEMF therapy can only be helpful for improving symptoms without fully healing a specific health condition, depending on the person's overall health status. While PEMFs stimulate the body to repair and heal itself, the body still has to have the capacity to be able to do that, whether in whole or in part. In other words, the body has to have enough vitality to repair and rebalance tissue and cellular function. This explains why PEMF treatments may be able to bring the body into a better level of function while not being able to restore function completely. It's a matter of finding the best balance achievable in the presence of imbalance.

Expectations

Everyone wants and would love to obtain the best results immediately and permanently from PEMF therapy, with the least amount of effort, time, and inconvenience. Such hopes and expectations are only natural, yet most health issues did not arise overnight; they occurred over months and even years. Therefore, it's unrealistic to expect that your health problems, especially if they are chronic or severe, will be miraculously and rapidly improved to normal. Hope springs eternal, but understanding the basic considerations of the technical aspects of the PEMF signal, including the intensity and the area of treatment, the starting point relative to the severity of the problem, the likely benefit that can be achieved, your body's capacity to maximally use the stimulation provided by the PEMFs, and what is needed to be done with the PEMF, all determine what will happen. Your body will let you know. Your body is in control.

When people start using PEMF therapy, setting realistic expectations is critical. One of the reasons I provide so much information on DrPawluk.com and why I wrote this book and my previous book, Power *Tools for Health*, is to help you to be able to set reasonable expectations, both in terms of the PEMF system that will best meet your needs, and also what you can expect from using it, so that you will achieve the most optimal benefits. People who properly educate and inform themselves about PEMFs and how they work are more likely to have reasonable expectations and will put in the work necessary to get the results they want. PEMFs are not magic pills, and one size does not fit all. You typically get what you pay for. If you don't have the PEMF system most suitable for your needs, don't use it properly, and don't support the body otherwise to be as healthy as possible, the results you achieve with it will be less than what you would hope for. They may be better than before but still not optimal.

On the other hand, if you put in the time to give yourself regular PEMF treatments at the right intensity and overall applications for long enough time periods, you will achieve a variety of benefits and experience steady improvements in your health and overall quality of life, with less pain, more energy, and greater overall physical and even mental/emotional control and function. You may also find that you achieved benefits that you never even expected.

Since the benefits of PEMF therapy for many conditions can be slow to happen as the body heals itself, you may look back after a year of use and see what the real changes have been from the time it was started. Also, people will often see what PEMFs have been doing when they stop them for a week or two after going on vacation. When they come back, they will begin to see what they were missing by generally feeling better once PEMF therapy is restarted.

People often ask me what the biggest risk factor is with PEMFs. With a smile, I will say that if sometime after using PEMF therapy you have the urge to put on a cape. You can do that, just don't try to jump over tall buildings!

After 30 years of working with PEMFs, this book is the culmination of the wisdom, knowledge, and experience I've garnered. Hopefully, you'll find what I've shared with you within is helpful for your own journey of healing.

All the best in your health journey.

Pain, Inflammation, Adenosine, and PEMF Therapy

A critical consideration for selecting and applying pulsed electromagnetic field (PEMF) therapy is the strength of the magnetic field needed to affect the tissue being treated. For the most effective results, the individual seeking to do PEMF therapy needs to determine three factors:

1. The goal magnetic field intensity
2. The length of treatment
3. The number of sessions needed for the target tissue to be treated.

PEMF Therapy is a developing medical field and there are no clear-cut guidelines available for the myriad of conditions and circumstances for which people can and are likely to want to use PEMF therapy. One thing is clear though: one "size" does not fit all.

Another critical consideration is the intensity of the magnetic field at a distance from the applicator. For this calculation, apply the inverse square law. This law dictates that the magnetic field, normally, rapidly reduces in intensity with distance from the source of the field, that is, by the inverse square root. (For more information about this, please see my Intensity Matters video, available at www.DrPawluk.com/videos/intensity-matters-video)

Treating Chronic Inflammation with PEMF Therapy

One of the most common uses of PEMFs is to reduce chronic inflammation. Inflammation is at the root or a major part of a majority of health conditions in humans and animals. This Appendix provides an example of the magnetic field intensities required to adequately treat inflammation throughout the body. Because of their actions on inflammation, PEMFs have been found to help with a number of other health conditions as well: infection, pain, sleep problems, arthritis, bone stimulation (fractures and bone surgery), cancer, ischemia, wound healing, and problems with the eyes, liver, lungs, heart, and nervous system, among many other tissues.

Adenosine: The Inflammation 'Guardian Angel'

A very important part of control of inflammation is through a molecule in the body called *adenosine* acting through its receptor, the *adenosine receptor (AR)*. Adenosine is a building block for RNA/DNA and a part of the energy molecule ATP (Chen). Adenosine regulates the function of every tissue and organ in the body and is considered a "guardian angel" in human disease (Borea).

All cells release ATP at low levels. Release is enhanced with PEMF stimulation, inflammation, pH change, hypoxia, tissue damage, or nerve injury in all the tissues of the body. The mitochondria need adenosine to make ATP in all the cells of the body. Through various metabolic processes, adenosine is released by the breakdown of ATP to create energy and then is re-used to create more ATP in a perpetual cellular cycle.

How Adenosine, Inflammation and Pain are Linked: The concentrations of adenosine are naturally at physiologically low levels in body fluids between the cells of unstressed tissues. These concentrations increase rapidly in response to cell injury-causing stress conditions such as low oxygen (hypoxia), lack of blood supply (ischemia), inflammation, or trauma. Adenosine has a short half-life in the blood (a few seconds) and in spinal cerebrospinal fluid (10 to 20 minutes) (Antonioli). Adenosine is released from within the cell after production of ATP by mitochondria inside the cell (intracellular space) and then passes through the cell wall into the spaces between cells (extracellular space). Once released into the extracellular space, adenosine functions as an alarm or danger signal; hence a "guardian angel." It then activates specific adenosine receptors, causing numerous cellular responses that aim to restore tissue homeostasis.

Adenosine acts through four subtypes of adenosine receptors: A1, A2A, A2B and A3. These receptors are widely distributed throughout the body and have been found to be part of both physiological and pathological biological functions. They affect, at the least, cardiac rhythm and circulation, breakdown of fat, kidney blood flow, immune function, regulation of sleep, development of new blood vessels, inflammatory diseases/inflammation, blood flow, and neurodegenerative disorders. ARs are found in many types of immune cells, including neutrophils, macrophages, dendritic cells, and mast cells.

PEMF Therapy for Inflammation and Pain

PEMFs appear to primarily influence A2A and A3 ARs. They do not appear to influence A1 or A2B ARs (Varani, 2002). PEMFs stimulate the activation of adenosine receptors, increase their functionality, and augment chemical agents that also stimulate these receptors.

Stimulation of A2A and A3 ARs by PEMFs in cells throughout the body results in reduction of inflammation by lowering many pro-inflammatory tissue cytokines, including reduction of:

- The levels of tumor necrosis factor-α (TNF-α)
- Interleukin (IL): IL-1β, IL-6, and IL-8 in microglial cells (Vincenzi, 2017)
- IL-6 and IL-8 in cartilage and bone cells (Vincenzi, 2013)
- IL-8 and NF-kappa B in skin cells (Vianale)
- Synovial fibroblasts (Ongaro)

But very-low-intensity PEMFs between 3 and 5 microTesla (μT) do not affect IL-1β, IL-6, TNF-α, IL-8, or IL-10 production (de Kleijn).

Most research to date has been done on PEMF stimulation of A2A ARs. PEMF stimulation of A3 ARs specifically could benefit bone marrow and lymphatic disorders and gastrointestinal and various skin conditions.

The Anti-inflammatory Effect of PEMF Therapy

PEMFs stimulate the production of adenosine by stimulating A2A receptors, being especially helpful in chronic inflammation (Palmer). A2A receptor stimulation and adenosine produce most of their immune benefits through the T cell immune system. A2A receptors' inhibitory effects on immune and inflammatory processes are very complex. Basically, the A2A receptor is, normally, naturally stimulated by acute inflammation-producing molecules to inhibit or control the inflammation. When adenosine production drops off or is low, inflammation persists and produces chronic inflammation.

In fact, PEMFs, by increasing ARs, enhance the functional efficiency of adenosine, resulting in a stronger physiological action than the use of drugs. The anti-inflammatory effect of adenosine enhanced by PEMF is less likely to have the side effects, desensitization, and receptor resistance than drugs used to act on adenosine receptors. Prolonged stimulation of adenosine receptors with a drug can dampen the ability of the receptor to function. Prolonged use of drugs decreases the quantity of receptors, thereby reducing the effectiveness of the drug over time.

The role of adenosine receptors and adenosine in modifying inflammation is well accepted (Varani, 2017). A2A receptors are plentiful in the membranes of neutrophils. Neutrophils play a major role in inflammation and tissue repair. Neutrophils are about 40 percent to 70 percent of white blood cells in most mammals. They form an essential part of the innate immune system. The innate immune system is one of the two main immunity strategies; the other is the acquired or adaptive immune system. Like the innate system, the acquired system includes both circulating and cell-based immunity. Neutrophils are recruited to a site of injury within minutes following trauma and are the hallmark of acute inflammation. Neutrophils are one of the first responders of inflammatory cells to migrate toward the site of inflammation.

The Best PEMF Therapy for Pain and Inflammation

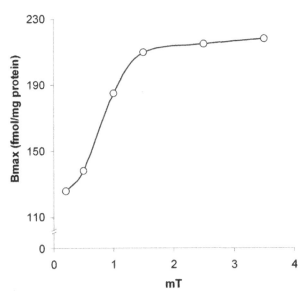

Figure 1. From *Saturation binding of A2A adenosine receptor as a function of magnetic field peak intensity (mT) in human neutrophil membranes. Bmax = receptor binding capacity. Adapted from Massari (2007).*

Stimulating the A2A adenosine receptor on the neutrophil is essential for controlling inflammation. Because PEMFs stimulate the A2A receptor, determining the appropriate dose of the magnetic field is critical for optimal benefits. PEMFs applied in the lab at the surface of neutrophils have been found to significantly increase the binding of adenosine to the A2A receptor. This effect was time, intensity, and temperature dependent. PEMF dose-response studies have found that after 30 minutes of exposure, the receptors became saturated with a 1.5 mT magnetic field (Massari). The effect plateaued with intensities greater than 1.5 mT (Figure 1). This means that intensities above 1.5 mT produce no additional benefit, although they do not appear to have any negative actions either.

The PEMFs used in this research had an intensity range from 0.1 to 4.5 mT; frequencies ranged from 10 Hz to 120 Hz. The most-used peak intensity of the magnetic field was 1.5 mT (15 gauss) at 75 Hz.

Armed with this information, 1.5 mT would be the optimized intensity of a magnetic field needed to help with reducing inflammation, at least as far as neutrophil involvement is concerned. When considering individuals applying PEMFs for various problems associated with inflammation, the need is to be able to reduce inflammation at various depths in the body, depending on the target organ and tissue. Therefore, the intensity of the magnetic field of the applicator always needs to be considered in the decision-making.

To achieve the 1.5 mT goal, PEMF intensity acting on neutrophils at various distances from the applicator—that is, at various depths into the body—the clinician must be aware of the inverse square law governing the loss of magnetic field intensity with distance from the applicator.

Table 1 was calculated for the 1.5 mT goal intensity at various depths in the body, using Newton's inverse square rule.

From the table, it can be seen, for example (in the blue areas), that to deliver 1.5 mT (15 gauss) to the target tissue 2 cm (0.8 in) from the applicator, a 14 mT (140 gauss) intensity magnetic field would be required. At 20 cm (8 in), 662 mT (6620 gauss) would be required to deliver 1.5 mT (15 gauss) at the target tissue.

Targeted PEMF Therapy for Specific Conditions

To give an example, the kidneys may be a target for PEMF treatment. Inflammation in the kidneys is common, and the kidneys have been found to have adenosine receptors. We know that neutrophils are present within the kidney circulation

Target Depth (in)	0	0.4	0.8	1.2	1.6	2	2.4	2.8	3.2	3.6	4
Target Depth (cm)	0	1	2	3	4	5	6	7	8	9	10
Intensity needed (mT)	1.5	6	14	24	38	54	74	96	122	150	182
Intensity needed (G)	15	60	140	240	380	540	740	960	1220	1500	1820

Target Depth (in)	4.4	4.8	5.2	5.6	6	6.4	6.8	7.2	7.6	8	8.4
Target Depth (cm)	11	12	13	14	15	16	17	18	19	20	21
Intensity needed (mT)	216	254	294	338	384	434	486	542	600	662	726
Intensity needed (G)	2160	2540	2940	3380	3840	4340	4860	5420	6000	6620	7260

Target Depth (in)	8.8	9.2	9.6	10	10.4	10.8	11.2	11.6	12	12.4	12.8
Target Depth (cm)	22	23	24	25	26	27	28	29	30	31	32
Intensity needed (mT)	794	864	938	1014	1094	1176	1262	1350	1442	1536	1634
Intensity needed (G)	7940	8640	9380	10140	10940	11760	12620	13500	14420	15360	16340

when there is inflammation. The depth of the center of the kidneys into the body is typically from 5 to 7 cm (2 to 2.8 in) from the front of the abdomen (Xue). The thickness of the kidneys is typically about 5 cm (2 in) from the center of the kidney to the back of the kidney (Moorthy). If a PEMF applicator is placed over the anterior abdomen and the expected depth to reach the back of the kidney is 9.5 cm—or rounding up, 10 cm (3.9 in)—with the goal intensity being 1.5 mT, the maximum PEMF intensity would need to be 182 mT (1820 gauss). This means that a PEMF system would need to be selected that can deliver at least this much magnetic field intensity to adequately target the kidneys.

Similar calculations can be done for any organ or tissue in the body to determine the optimal PEMF intensity needed. All one needs to figure out is the depth of the tissue, not only at the surface of the organ but also across the diameter of the organ or tissue farthest from the PEMF signal. In treating the brain, for example, the skull may be 15.2 cm (6 in) front to back and 12.7 cm (5 in) side to side. That means to treat the brain from front to back would require a magnetic field intensity of around 384 mT/3840 gauss, to deliver 1.5 mT/15 gauss to the back of the brain. Side-to-side treatment would require about 294 mT/2940 gauss.

Targeting the anti-inflammatory effects of adenosine receptor stimulation is only one possible consideration for selection of magnetic field intensity in judging magnetic field intensity needs. Because there are so many different physiologic effects and actions of PEMFs (see Chapters 3 and 4 of this book), dosing calculations for each of these effects are not available for the PEMF user. In addition, it is unlikely that any specific physiologic action—for example, enhanced circulation, accelerated healing, pain reduction—can be uniquely and specifically selected in considering actual applications in the clinical environment. Experience suggests that multiple actions are at play any time a PEMF is used.

Effects of PEMF Therapy on The Body Through Indirect Action

A recent study (Cañedo) showed that diabetic foot ulcers could be helped by treating parts of the body other than the foot ulcers directly. (www.DrPawluk.com/pemfs-for-healing-diabetic-foot-ulcers) This indirect action can take longer (up to 60 days) to produce results than direct PEMF stimulation at the ulcer site. This means that stimulating neutrophils in one part of the body may activate the adenosine receptors circulating under the magnetic field sufficiently to benefit inflammation in other parts of the body. Direct stimulation of the ulcer would activate other mechanisms of healing action of PEMFs to result in faster healing, such as increased collagen production.

Nevertheless, even local treatment with a PEMF at sufficient intensities may help inflammation in the rest of the body indirectly. However, the adenosine stimulated by PEMFs has a very short half-life and would require frequent repeat treatments or treatments over extended periods.

Summary

Using PEMFs to reduce inflammation in the body, which is common to a vast majority of health conditions, is assisted by a "guardian angel," adenosine and the adenosine receptor. This new research, that shows an impact of PEMFs on this receptor, gives important guidance in choosing the magnetic field intensity necessary, in any areas of the body with inflammation, to produce the best results. We no longer have to resort to guessing about which magnetic field intensity to choose to best help the body to heal.

References

- Antonioli L, Blandizzi C, Pacher P, Haskó G. Immunity, inflammation and cancer: a leading role for adenosine. *Nature Reviews Cancer* 2013 (13): 842–857.
- Borea PA, Gessi S, Merighi S, Varani K. Adenosine as a multi-signaling guardian angel in human diseases: when, where and how does it exert its protective effects? *Trends Pharmacol Sci.* 2016 Jun;37(6):419-434.
- Cañedo-Dorantes L, Soenksen LR, García-Sánchez C, et al. Efficacy and safety evaluation of systemic extremely low frequency magnetic fields used in the healing of diabetic foot ulcers—phase II data. *Arch Med Res.* 2015 Aug;46(6):470-8.
- Chen JF, Eltzschig HK, Fredholm BB. Adenosine receptors as drug targets — what are the challenges? *Nat Rev Drug Discov.* 2013 April; 12(4): 265–286.
- de Kleijn S, Bouwens M, Verburg-van Kemenade BM, et al. Extremely low frequency electromagnetic field exposure does not modulate toll-like receptor signaling in human peripheral blood mononuclear cells. *Cytokine.* 2011 Apr;54(1):43-50.
- Massari L, Benazzo F, De Mattei M, et al. CRES Study Group. Effects of electrical physical stimuli on articular cartilage. *J Bone Joint Surg Am.* 2007 Oct;89 Suppl 3:152-61.
- Moorthy HK and Venugopal P. Measurement of renal dimensions in vivo: A critical appraisal. *Indian J Urol.* 2011 Apr-Jun; 27(2): 169–175.
- Ongaro A, Varani K, Masieri FF, et al. Electromagnetic fields (EMFs) and adenosine receptors modulate prostaglandin E(2) and cytokine

release in human osteoarthritic synovial fibroblasts. *J Cell Physiol.* 2012 Jun;227(6):2461-9.

- Palmer TM and Trevethick MA. Suppression of inflammatory and immune responses by the A2A adenosine receptor: an introduction. *British Journal of Pharmacology* (2008) 153 S27–S34.

- Varani K, Gessi S, Merighi S, et al. Effect of low frequency electromagnetic fields on A2A adenosine receptors in human neutrophils. *Br J Pharmacol.* 2002 May;136(1):57-66.

- Varani K, Vincenzi F, Ravani A, et al. Adenosine receptors as a biological pathway for the anti-inflammatory and beneficial effects of low frequency low energy pulsed electromagnetic fields. *Mediators Inflamm* (2017) 2017:2740963.

- Varani K, Vincenzi F, Targa M, et al. Effect of pulsed electromagnetic field exposure on adenosine receptors in rat brain. *Bioelectromagnetics.* 2012 May;33(4):279-87.

- Vianale G, Reale M, Amerio P, et al. Extremely low frequency electromagnetic field enhances human keratinocyte cell growth and decreases proinflammatory chemokine production. *Br J Dermatol.* 2008 Jun;158(6):1189-96.

- Vincenzi F, Padovan M, Targa M, et al. A(2A) adenosine receptors are differentially modulated by pharmacological treatments in rheumatoid arthritis patients and their stimulation ameliorates adjuvant-induced arthritis in rats. *PLoS One* (2011) 8(1):e54195.

- Vincenzi F, Ravani A, Pasquini S, et al. Pulsed electromagnetic field exposure reduces hypoxia and inflammation damage in neuron-like and microglial cells. *J Cell Physiol* (2017) 232(5):1200–8.

- Vincenzi F, Targa M, Corciulo C, et al. Pulsed electromagnetic fields increased the anti-inflammatory effect of A_2A and A_3 adenosine receptors in human T/C-28a2 chondrocytes and hFOB 1.19 osteoblasts. *PLoS One.* 2013 May 31;8(5):e65561.

Going 'Low and Slow'

In the going "low and slow" approach, low refers to intensity and slow refers to treatment time. Both need to be considered when using PEMF therapy. In a sense this process can also be referred to as a ladder, starting on the lowest rung and climbing the ladder from rung to rung until the desired level is reached. Getting to the top of the ladder is not always the goal for treatment but it is worth knowing what can be accomplished or tolerated. After one's limits are known, there will be a sense of how much work there needs to be done to reach the top of the ladder as fast as possible.

The Need for Going 'Low and Slow'

The need for going "low and slow" is to determine the body's sensitivity to, or readiness for, magnetic field stimulation. PEMF therapy is a form of "physical" therapy, as opposed to pharmacologic (drug) therapy, nutritional therapy, counseling, or procedures. The magnetic field passes through the body stimulating the production of charge in the tissues which then translates into a multitude of physiologic, biochemical, and immune responses. Every person's body is in a unique state or condition before beginning PEMF therapy. The unique state of every individual has to be accounted for in initiating a course of PEMF treatments.

Who Is Most in Need of Going 'Low and Slow'?

The people who are the most sensitive to PEMFs are in most need of going "low and slow." These include individuals who are sensitive to sound, computer terminals, electronics, EMFs, microwave ovens, smells, etc. People who are especially vulnerable often include those with fibromyalgia, chronic fatigue syndrome, neurologic syndromes, medication sensitivities, multiple allergies, poor tolerance for even low doses of medications, in a very weakened state, and very low blood pressure. People who have undergone long hospital stays, extensive radiation or chemotherapy, and/or who are prone to high anxiety states are also likely to be most vulnerable. If you suspect you are in one of these categories or expect to have sensitivity, then you should certainly follow a "low and slow" protocol, and maybe even a very slow protocol. Individuals who react even to the lowest levels of intensity and even minimal treatment time may not be candidates for PEMF therapy until the clinical situation causing their sensitivity has been adequately addressed.

Frequency-Based Versus Pulse-Based PEMFs

In my experience, individuals are more likely to have sensitivity reactions to frequency-based PEMFs than to pulse-based PEMFs, even if the PEMF systems are very low-intensity. Those who have reactions to frequency-based PEMFs are also most likely to be very reactive to environmental magnetic fields (EMFs) that I discussed in Chapter 2. When there is a lot of inflammation in the body, multiple frequencies presented to the body don't allow the body enough time between frequency sets to settle down and return to baseline. When individual pulses are presented to the body, especially at higher intensities (not necessarily the highest intensity), the body has less overall stimulation being thrown at it. Even here, with higher intensities, people will often find "sweet spots," where the intensity is still working to help the body but is not too high to be irritating.

Athletic Training or Rehabilitation Analogy

The use of PEMF therapy is somewhat like athletic training or physical rehabilitation. You don't get off the couch and run a marathon the next day without training for it. The more deconditioned you are the more training you will need before you are ready to run such a race. Training for playing professional football is considerably different than training for professional baseball. Training for specific tasks will be unique to the tasks as well as the person. During training, the fitness of the person will be tested by the activities performed. The level of fitness for the activity will determine how aggressive the training can be until finally the goal is achieved. After that it is a matter of maintenance.

Athletic training is a stop-start or stair-step process. You train, you test, you retrain, you retest, etc., until the goal is achieved. Since PEMFs stimulate so many different processes in the body, PEMF stimulation is like athletic training.

In both cases, you are pushing the body to its capacity to handle the stimulation. Obviously, some people are in much better condition or shape than others. As a result, their progress toward their goals will be faster.

Variations in PEMF System Intensity and Time Settings

Most PEMF systems have magnetic field intensity settings, ranging from minimum to maximum. Most also have timers or clocks that can be set for the desired treatment time. Often, however, treatment times need to exceed the limits of the PEMF system's timers or clocks. In that situation, the individual will determine the goal treatment time and may need to reset the program multiple times or use their own timer.

Optimal Goal for Intensity

The optimal goal for intensity is to be able to reach or use the maximum intensity, even if only temporarily. This is done to test one's limits for tolerability and the vitality of the tissue, organ, or the entire body. Once the maximal time and maximal intensity is tolerated, then any time or intensity may be able to be set to do the work in the body that is desired or needed. It is not a goal to always maximize the time and maximize the intensity for continuing treatment.

Not Everyone Needs to Go "Low and Slow"

For the average person, for those without significant disability, with maybe a few aches or pains, and no significant organ health problems, in average shape and with reasonable stamina, there will be very little time spent on "low and slow." They will fairly quickly advance to middle and higher levels of time and intensity. Those who are already in great shape, have lots of stamina, are regularly working out, even aerobically, with no significant health issues, would go high intensity and could treat for as long as they wanted or needed.

These could be patterns of increasing intensity and time:

- Medium intensity and normal pace
- High intensity and fast pace

PEMF System Time and Intensity Settings

You have to understand your PEMF system's time and intensity settings in order to most effectively benefit from your PEMF treatments. There are many possible variations:

- two intensity settings, one time setting for 20 minutes
- four intensity settings, one time setting repeating indefinitely in 30 minutes cycles
- 10 intensity settings, time set in 10-minute increments up to continuous
- one intensity setting, 10 programs with fixed 30-minute cycles
- 10 basic programs of fixed time cycles with PC capability to set time and intensity individually
- five intensity settings, in 5 or 10 minute cycles
- 10 intensity settings, time set in one hour increments up to 12 hours.

Once your system's time and intensity settings are understood, then you have to define your own "low and slow" protocol. Most of the time, very low- to medium-intensity systems can be advanced in time and intensity very rapidly.

Examples of "Low and Slow" Protocols

Here are examples of advancing intensity and treatment time faster than "low and slow." The first is a medium pace of advancement for a system with 10 intensity levels combined together for a total of 60 minutes of treatment time:

Medium pace			
step	intensity level	treatment time - mins	day
Step 1	1	5	1
Step 2	3	15	2
Step 3	5	30	3
Step 4	8	45	4
Step 5	10	60	5
Step 6	10	60	6

Medium pace			
step	intensity level	treatment time - mins	day
Step 7	10	60	7
Step 8	10	60	8
Step 9	10	60	9
Step 10	10	60	10
Step 11	maintain		11
Step 12	maintain		12

The second is a faster pace of advancement for a similar PEMF system:

Fast pace			
step	intensity level	treatment time - mins	day
Step 1	1	15	1
Step 2	5	30	2
Step 3	10	60	3
Step 4	maintain		4
Step 5	maintain		5

Normal and Slow Protocols for a PEMF system with 10 intensity levels

Normal protocol			
step	intensity level	treatment time - mins	day
Step 1	1	5	1
Step 2	2	10	2
Step 3	3	10	3
Step 4	4	15	4
Step 5	5	15	5
Step 6	6	30	6

Normal protocol			
step	**intensity level**	**treatment time - mins**	**day**
Step 7	7	30	7
Step 8	8	45	8
Step 9	9	45	9
Step 10	10	60	10
Step 11	maintain		11
Step 12	maintain		12
Step 13	maintain		13
Step 14	maintain		14
Step 15	maintain		15
Step 16	maintain		16
Step 17	maintain		17
etc	maintain		etc

Slow protocol			
step	**intensity level**	**treatment time - mins**	**day**
Step 1	1	5	1
Step 2	1	5	
Step 3	1	5	
Step 4	2	10	2
Step 5	2	10	
Step 6	2	10	
Step 7	3	10	3
Step 8	3	10	4
Step 9	3	10	5
Step 10	4	15	6
Step 11	4	15	7
Step 12	4	15	8
Step 13	5	15	9
Step 14	5	15	10
Step 15	5	15	11

Slow protocol			
step	intensity level	treatment time - mins	day
Step 16	6	30	12
Step 17	6	30	13
Step 18	6	30	14
Step 19	7	30	15
Step 20	7	30	16
Step 21	7	30	17
Step 22	8	45	18
Step 23	8	45	19
Step 24	8	45	20
Step 25	9	45	21
Step 26	9	45	22
Step 27	9	45	23
Step 28	10	60	24
Step 29	10	60	25
Step 30	10	60	26
Step 31	maintain		27
Step 32	maintain		28
Step 33	maintain		29
Step 34	maintain		30
Step 35	maintain		31
Step 36	maintain		32
Step 37	maintain		33
etc	maintain		etc

"Magnetic Sandwich" Therapy

PEMF treatment results for larger treatment areas are often better when two PEMF applicators are used simultaneously on either side of a body area. Magnetic fields always drop off significantly and naturally as the magnetic field travels away from an applicator through space or through a body. The body is like space to a magnetic field. So, the magnetic field intensity on the other side of the body or a body part will always be lower than the part near the applicator.

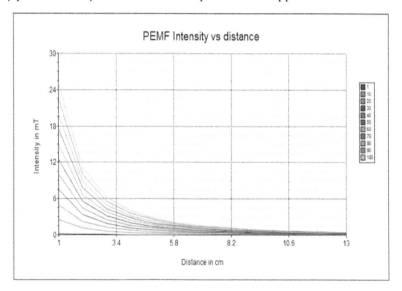

graphically represented this is what rapidly declining intensities look like
the color codes for the starting intensities in mT are in the legend to the right on the graph

Figure 1. From *Pawluk W. Clinical dosimetry of extremely low-frequency pulsed electromagnetic fields. Chapter 17. In Dosimetry in Bioelectromagnetics, CRC Press, publication Jan 2017, Markov M, Editor.*

One of the ways to measure this loss of intensity is using the inverse square law. This graph (**Figure 1.**) shows that a magnetic field of 100 mT (1000 gauss) at the surface of the applicator, within 1 cm (0.39 in) away, will have dropped down in intensity to around 25 mT (250 gauss), or only one quarter of its original intensity. This is a very rapid drop in magnetic field intensity, and applies to all magnetic fields.

Since one of the most common uses of PEMFs is to reduce inflammation, and the optimal magnetic field intensity to help with inflammation by affecting the adenosine receptor is about 15 gauss, the inverse square law has to be considered (see Appendix A). So, to achieve this optimal inflammation reducing intensity in the tissue that has the inflammation, the initial intensity of the magnetic field needs to be considered. For example, if the inflammation is at:

- 1 inch into the body, about 200 gauss will be necessary.
- 2 inches into the body 540 guss will be needed.
- 4 inches into the body 1820 gauss will be needed.
- 6 inches into the body about 3840 gauss will be needed.

These calculations apply to only one applicator. However, there are different calculations when combining two applicators opposite a target body tissue or organ.

What if two applicators can be combined opposite each other, each one losing intensity with distance? This solution is called a PEMF "magnetic sandwich." Each applicator provides a predictable magnetic field applied opposite another applicator, whether of equal or different intensity. This approach allows more uniform and higher-intensity magnetic fields to penetrate deep throughout the body, to help heal deeper tissues and organs. In scientific terms, it acts approximately like a "Helmholtz coil" setup.

This classic PEMF setup provides two coils of equal intensities, with the same circumference, placed at a specific distance apart from each other. (**Figure 2.**) The magnetic field of each coil, coil 1 and coil 2, has a maximum intensity very near the coil. This intensity drops off per the inverse square law as the magnetic field moves away from the applicator. But each magnetic field from each coil combines with the magnetic fields of both. In **Figure 2.** below, coil 1 on the left has a field line that begins to drop off until it essentially meets the declining field line of the coil to the right of it, coil 2. The overall fields of the two coils (overall line) combine to being a bit less than double (ie, the number 1 on the side of the chart) of each one separately (each one peaking at about 0.6). Where the two fields meet in the middle, that is, where the coil 1 line meets the coil 2 line, halfway between the two coils, the magnetic field is about half of the intensity from each one. So, practically speaking, the magnetic field in the middle between the two coils does not get to be less than about half of the field strength of each coil. See the Field Strength legend to the right of the chart.

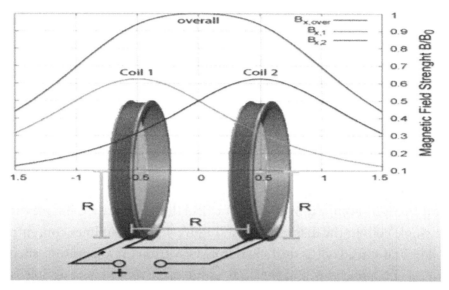

Figure 2. From *https://medcraveonline.com/IJBSBE/creating-the-new-generation-coils-to-generate-a-uniform-magnetic-field-using-for-medical-applications-simulation-and-analysis. html*

The diagram below (**Figure 3.**) shows the relative field intensities more clearly based on the center of the circular magnetic coil and the distance from that center.

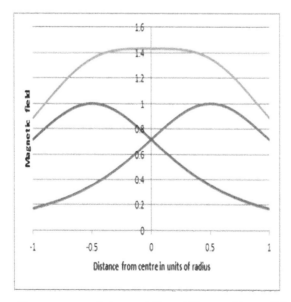

Figure 3. From https://homepages.abdn.ac.uk/j.s.reid/pages/Maxwell/Legacy/MaxCoil.html

Of the three curves in this graphic the two lower ones, right and left are from two side-by side, equal sized and equal strength coils. The numbers in the center line represent the relative magnetic field intensity. The upper curve is the total combined field from the two coils, about double (~1.4) the point of crossing of the individual coil field strengths at the center line (~0.7). This center area is the region of a relatively uniform magnetic field, between the two coils. This is why the "magnetic sandwich" produces the best potential magnetic field in the center between two oppositely placed applicators, for the treatment of tissues deeper in the body, for example, lungs, heart, kidneys, bowel, spine, etc.

If these vertical Helmholtz-type magnetic coils are placed on their sides (horizontally), and a body (or body part) is placed in between, the body will receive a relatively even, stronger magnetic field that it would at the same distance from a single coil. In the diagram below, **Figure 4.**, the field lines concentrate in the middle and spread out as the field moves away from the applicators, encircling the two sets of applicators and the body at the same time. This example is two-dimensional. The magnetic fields generated are actually three-dimensional, somewhat pictured as a doughnut with a hole in the center, with the doughnut itself being the magnetic fields.

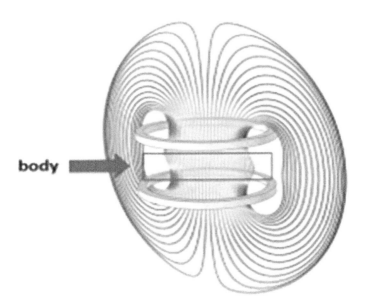

Figure 4. Adapted from https://www.comsol.com/forum/thread/134841/beautiful-streamlines-for-magnetic-field-lines-of-helmholtz-coils

To be accurate, this is not going to be technically an exact Helmholtz coil set-up. The principal still applies and will vary with the magnetic field intensity, the circumferences of the magnetic coils, the distance between the two coils and the thickness of the body or body part in between the coils. Nevertheless, the goal of this "magnetic sandwich" is to create a more uniform, wider and higher intensity magnetic field in which the body is treated, with the expectation of producing better health results more efficiently with less treatment time.

The concept of the "magnetic sandwich" only applies when two applicators are placed opposite each other. The farther apart the applicators are the weaker the magnetic field will be between them. So, to achieve the best results, relative to the inflammation-reducing example of needing 15 gauss at the area of inflammation, higher-intensity applicators will be needed when the distances between them are farther apart.

There are many variations to this type of "magnetic sandwich." There are PEMF systems that will allow various combinations of coils:

- two whole-body pads, with one or more coils inside each,
- one whole-body pad combined with a smaller pad,
- two smaller pads, of equal or varying sizes.

Some PEMF systems allow a whole-body pad that can be run at the same time as a local or regional pad, or a combination of these.

To treat smaller areas of the body with the highest intensity "magnetic sandwich," two stronger smaller applicators would work better, for example, treating across a knee, shoulder, or hip. Whole-body therapy can be provided with a significant benefit with a strong single whole-body applicator combined with a higher-intensity local applicator based opposite the whole-body pad.

The "magnetic sandwich" concept would not apply when applicators are placed in different parts of the body away from each other.

Resources

Other Books by Dr. Pawluk

Power Tools for Health: How pulsed magnetic fields (PEMFs) help you
This book teaches about basic concepts on the topic of magnetic fields, how PEMFs affect various body functions, how research has shown that PEMFs help with at least 50 different health conditions, how to select a PEMF system, how to use a PEMF system, and precautions and contraindications.

Magnetic Therapy in Eastern Europe: a review of 30 years of research (with co-author Jiri Jerabek)
  While magnetic field therapy did not originate in Eastern Europe, there was a significant development in the technology and the beginnings of research in magnetic field therapies in Eastern European countries. This book is a highly summarized review of the science and studies at the time, largely unknown in the English-speaking world, originally written in Eastern European languages and translated into English. This research is a big breakthrough in our understanding of what magnetic field therapy is, how it works, and how effective it is.

Websites

DrPawluk.com—extensive information about PEMF therapies and the various conditions they can help.

PEMFTrainingAcademy.com—established to develop objective information to train professionals in PEMF therapy.

EMF-portal.org—massive, university-based bibliographic database on extremely low-frequency (ELF) PEMFs, EMFs (including environmental and occupational exposures) and high-frequency magnetic therapy.

Device-Specific Websites

- FlexPulse.com
- BioBalancePEMF.com
- TeslaFit.com
- PEMF120.com
- MediThera-usa.com

Dr. Pawluk's Published Articles and Chapters

- Pawluk W. Coronavirus, Immunity and Use of Pulsed Electromagnetic Fields (PEMF's). J Med - Clin Res & Rev. 2020; 4(5): 1-8.
- Pawluk W. Use of a PEMF to treat complex TBI with Brain Gauge and Rivermead outcome measures. *The Journal of Science and Medicine*, 2020-03-10.
- Pawluk W. Clinical Use of Pulsed Electromagnetic Fields (PEMFs), In *Pulsed Electromagnetic Fields for Clinical Applications*, 2020-03-09.
- Pawluk W. The role of pulsed magnetic fields in the management of concussion and traumatic brain injury. *J. Science and Medicine*, 2019 (1): 1-12.2019-11-04
- Pawluk W. Clinical Dosimetry of Extremely Low-Frequency Pulsed Electromagnetic Fields. In *Dosimetry in Bioelectromagnetics*, 2017-05.
- Pawluk W. Magnetic Fields for Pain Control. In *Electromagnetic Fields in Biology and Medicine*. 2015-03-02.
- Pawluk W. Magnets, Meridians, and Energy Medicine: An Interview with William Pawluk, M.D., M.Sc. *Alternative and Complementary Therapies*, 2002-04.

About the Author

William Pawluk, MD, MSc, is a previously American board-certified family physician with additional training in acupuncture, homeopathy, hypnosis, energy medicine, and bodywork. He has had academic faculty appointments at a number of universities, including Johns Hopkins, and was the Clinical Director of the University of Maryland's Complementary and Alternative Medicine Program. He co-hosted a weekly health radio show at www.wcbm.com for ten years. In addition, he is an international expert in the medical use of electromagnetic fields with over thirty years of experience. He appeared on *The Dr. Oz Show* regarding use of magnetic therapy devices for helping pain. As part of his work with this technology, he previously wrote *Power Tools for Health*, a comprehensive book examining the scientific rationale for the use of PEMF therapies and a review of 50 health conditions for which PEMFs have been studied and shown to have significant benefits. In addition, he has written book chapters and articles, and has done numerous TV, radio, podcast, and magazine interviews on magnetic field therapies, and conducted research on the use of various kinds of electromagnetic systems on wound healing and other applications. He routinely teaches practitioners about the appropriate use of magnetic therapies. He was formerly Vice President of the North American Academy for Magnetic Therapy. To be able to continue to educate both the public and practitioners and help make this valuable technology available to consumers, he has established an authoritative website www.DrPawluk.com, reviewing the science of pulsed electromagnetic field (PEMF) therapy and various PEMF therapy options. He currently practices functional and holistic medicine in Baltimore, Maryland.

Made in the USA
Las Vegas, NV
26 November 2022

60340102R00236